D0812590

PANDEMIC POLITICS: THE DEADLY TOLL OF PARTISANSHIP IN THE AGE OF COVID

Pandemic Politics: The Deadly Toll of Partisanship in the Age of COVID

Shana Kushner Gadarian

Sara Wallace Goodman

Thomas B. Pepinsky

PRINCETON UNIVERSITY PRESS

PRINCETON AND OXFORD

Copyright © 2022 by Princeton University Press

Princeton University Press is committed to the protection of copyright and the intellectual property our authors entrust to us. Copyright promotes the progress and integrity of knowledge. Thank you for supporting free speech and the global exchange of ideas by purchasing an authorized edition of this book. If you wish to reproduce or distribute any part of it in any form, please obtain permission.

Requests for permission to reproduce material from this work should be sent to permissions@press.princeton.edu

Published by Princeton University Press
41 William Street, Princeton, New Jersey 08540
99 Banbury Road, Oxford OX2 6JX

press.princeton.edu

All Rights Reserved

Library of Congress Cataloging-in-Publication Data

Names: Gadarian, Shana Kushner, 1979- author. | Goodman, Sara Wallace,
    1979- author. | Pepinsky, Thomas B., 1979- author.
Title: Pandemic politics : the deadly toll of polarization in the age of
    COVID / Shana Kushner Gadarian, Sara Wallace Goodman, Thomas B.
    Pepinsky.
Description: Princeton : Princeton University Press, [2022] | Includes
    bibliographical references and index.
Identifiers: LCCN 2022006918 (print) | LCCN 2022006919 (ebook) |
    ISBN 9780691218991 (hardback) | ISBN 9780691219004 (ebook)
Subjects: LCSH: Trump, Donald, 1946- | COVID-19 Pandemic, 2020—Political
    aspects—United States. | COVID-19 (Disease)—Government policy—United
    States. | Medical policy—United States. | Right and left (Political science)—
    United States. | United States—Politics and government—2017-2021. |
    BISAC: POLITICAL SCIENCE / Political Ideologies / Conservatism &
    Liberalism | MEDICAL / Public Health
Classification: LCC RA644.C67 G334 2022 (print) | LCC RA644.C67 (ebook) |
    DDC 362.1962/414—dc23/eng/20220302
LC record available at https://lccn.loc.gov/2022006918
LC ebook record available at https://lccn.loc.gov/2022006919

British Library Cataloging-in-Publication Data is available

Editorial: Bridget Flannery-McCoy, Alena Chekanov
Jacket Design: Kevin Quach
Production: Erin Suydam
Publicity: James Schneider, Kate Farquhar-Thomson

Jacket Credit: © Davi Russo / Adobe Stock

Printed on acid-free paper. ∞

Printed in the United States of America

10 9 8 7 6 5 4 3 2 1

CONTENTS

LIST OF FIGURES

ACKNOWLEDGMENTS

We thank the National Science Foundation, the Russell Sage Foundation, the Cornell Center for the Social Sciences, the Campbell Institute of Public Affairs, and the Program for Conflict and Collaboration at Syracuse University for their generous financial support. These funders had no role in collecting, analyzing, or interpretating any of the data that we present here. YouGov collected the survey data that we use in this book; we thank Ashley Grosse and the rest of the YouGov team for their support all along the way. Special thanks as well to Emma Dreher, Ahmed El Sammak, and Kevin Zong for outstanding research assistance.

We were fortunate to work with Bridget Flannery-McCoy and Alena Chekanov to bring this project to completion. They and the rest of the Princeton University Press team made the editorial process easy and smooth, and Bridget helped us tell the story of this politicized pandemic clearly and fully. We thank them for their support and encouragement, especially welcome during the midst of a pandemic that upended everything about how we live and how we work.

We thank our many friends and colleagues, in real life and on Twitter, for helpful feedback and suggestions along the way. Thank you to colleagues at American University, Dartmouth College, the University of Denver, Harvard University, the University of Konstanz, the London School of Economics, McGill University, the University of North Carolina–Chapel Hill, Princeton University, Syracuse University, and the University of Wisconsin for hosting us at virtual talks where we received extremely useful feedback. Thank you to the schools, camps, and caregivers who safely cared for our children so we could continue to teach and research. The authors thank each other for their hard work, creativity, and persistence and for providing a productive outlet for a diverse menu of emotions. Last, we thank our families for their patience, support, love, and good cheer while the three of us found a way to think about the pandemic even more than most regular people. We dedicate this book to them: *to Mike, Jonah, Ethan, Ella, Adam, Micah, Silvia, Julie, Eli, and Anisa.*

Introduction

The floor of the Bank of Oklahoma Center in Tulsa was awash in red, white, and blue. Eager supporters of President Donald Trump were holding signs, wearing "Make America Great Again" hats, and sporting T-shirts with expressions ranging from "Guns, God, and Trump" to "Make Liberals Cry Again." The attendees were young and old but mostly white. Parents brought their children. There were memorabilia for purchase. Everyone inside the arena had their cell phones at the ready, eager to capture moments of the man of the hour.

Inside, it felt like a typical Trump rally. Outside, however, the atmosphere was tense. It was less than a month since George Floyd had been murdered by Minneapolis police office Derek Chauvin, and protesters had mobilized outside the venue carrying signs that read "Dump the Trump," "No Justice. No Peace," and "Defund the Police." Law enforcement was keeping a tight perimeter. Police brandished shields and clubs, and members of the Oklahoma Highway Patrol and National Guard were armed and ready. On the street—in big yellow capital letters—was written "BLACK LIVES MATTER."

But it was not just the presence of protestors that made the rally notable. What was truly exceptional was the timing. It was June 20,

2020, and Trump was having his first in-person campaign rally in four months—in the middle of a global pandemic.

In a typical election year, it would be unheard of for a president to take a four-month break from the campaign trail. This is particularly true for a candidate such as Trump who thrives on crowd applause. But this wasn't a typical year. The United States was in the middle of a global pandemic. The novel coronavirus SARS-CoV-2—commonly known as COVID-19—grew from an infection of zoonotic origin in Wuhan, China, in late 2019 into a public health emergency of global proportions. COVID-19 spreads through respiratory droplets produced when a person breathes, coughs, sings, sneezes, or speaks, and transmission is more likely when people are in close contact with one another, particularly when airflow is poor such as in indoor facilities. COVID-19 infections vary dramatically from person to person. Some carriers are asymptomatic; some experience fever, loss of smell and taste, and shortness of breath; and some end up hospitalized on respirators. And for millions, COVID-19 has proved fatal. The first death from COVID-19 in the United States was recorded on February 29, 2020. By the time of the June 20 rally in Tulsa, that number had reached 115,000 Americans. And by December 2021, over 800,000 Americans had died of COVID-19–related illnesses.

But you wouldn't know the country was in the throes of a public health emergency by looking at pictures from June 20. Almost everyone in the arena was unmasked, and there was no social distancing. Public health officials and experts had warned the campaign against holding an indoor rally, as COVID cases continued to climb in Oklahoma. But here were more than six thousand Trump supporters, coming out to see their president.[1] It wasn't a full house—the arena was only a third full—but Trump was back on the road as if the pandemic was over. During his remarks, he even quipped that unlike him, his Democratic opponent, former vice president Joe Biden, "remains silent in his basement." Biden was like millions of Americans: still at home, still socially distancing, still working online, and still navigating the real uncertainty of life during a pandemic.

Trump's Tulsa rally was a spectacle designed to project strength and "business as usual," confidently flouting public health recommendations and the commonsense precautions adopted by hundreds of millions of Americans during the pandemic. Biden eventually resumed campaigning but only in socially distanced parking lot events, while Trump kept up his in-person rallies, oftentimes held indoors. Republicans even tried to hold a traditional in-person national convention in Charlotte, North Carolina, but were forced to scale back to a hybrid format when the state government refused to allow the event to proceed at full capacity and without face masks.[2]

Tulsa and over a dozen similar campaign events held after would come to be described as "superspreader" events. Eight Trump campaign staffers tested positive for COVID after the rally,[3] and Tulsa health officials noted the rally "likely contributed" to a surge in new COVID cases.[4] One study estimated the collateral effect of these Trump superspreader events: nearly 30,000 confirmed COVID-19 cases, likely leading to more than 700 deaths.[5] Trump himself even became a vector. According to White House chief of staff Mark Meadows, Trump tested positive for COVID-19 on September 26, 2020. He then kept up an active campaign schedule for almost a week, knowingly exposing more than 500 people—from fundraisers to staff to Gold Star families to Democratic candidate Biden at the presidential debate in Cleveland, Ohio—before being hospitalized at Walter Reed National Medical Center on October 2.[6] Trump received cutting-edge experimental treatment and walked out of the hospital three days later. Upon returning to the White House, he was photographed immediately removing his mask with a still-active case of COVID-19 in the presence of White House staff. He tweeted "Don't be afraid of Covid . . . Don't let it dominate your life . . . I feel better than I did 20 years ago!" The same could not be said for the more than 210,000 Americans who had died by that point.

Politicizing a Pandemic

It is difficult to describe the devastation that the COVID-19 pandemic has wrought in the United States. Rich and poor, red states and blue states, Black and white, coastal and inland, metropolitan and rural—no corner of America was unaffected. The first known deaths occurred in mid-February in Santa Clara County, California.[7] In March 2020 alone, more Americans died from COVID-19 than the number killed in the September 11 terrorist attacks. By the end of April, the death toll surpassed the number of U.S. military personnel who died during the Vietnam War. By December 2020, at around three thousand deaths per day, each day was a 9/11. By June 2021 when just over half of Americans had received at least their first dose of a COVID-19 vaccine, the total number of deaths had passed six hundred thousand. By December 2021, this grim figure passed eight hundred thousand. Even with a vaccine widely available, the United States was still seeing thousands of deaths per week during the last months of 2021—a figure that far exceeds the death toll from the seasonal flu.[8]

The catastrophic death toll of the COVID-19 pandemic in the United States was not inevitable. The novel coronavirus strain—SARS-CoV-2, which came to be called COVID-19 (*CO* for corona, *VI* for virus, *D* for disease, and 19 for the year in which it was first identified)—proved novel in more ways than one. Biologically, it was a deadlier strain of the generic coronavirus. It was also novel in the scope and rate of spread. From the first identified case in Wuhan in December 2019, it spread globally in just weeks. Although deadlier diseases such as SARS and Ebola had seen outbreaks in the previous decades, the scale of the COVID-19 pandemic was unequal to any health crisis in recent memory.

And COVID-19 was particularly novel as a public health emergency. Health is not an inherently polarizing issue—everyone wants to be healthy and for their families to be safe. Diseases such as Alzheimer's, opioid addiction, and cancer do not differentiate between Americans based on their sport allegiances, musical tastes, or partisan preferences.[9] When polio was paralyzing and killing children in the United States, Americans across the political spectrum sent three million dimes to the White House and helped fund a polio vaccine.[10] And during a public health crisis such as a pandemic, we might expect our differences to fall away as people seek out information about what is happening and how to be safe.[11] In the case of COVID-19, that did not happen.

Moreover, as the scale of the crisis became clear, we might have expected that people would pull together to support swift government action to overcome it. Economic crises such as the Great Depression (1929–1933) and the Great Recession (2007–2009) created massive public demand for policies that expanded the scope and size of the federal government to protect citizens from the worst of the financial fallout. Terrorist attacks and military crises have historically increased presidential approval as feelings of solidarity and patriotism grow and criticism from opponents fall away.[12] Nowhere was this rally-round-the-flag effect more apparent than after the 9/11 attacks, when "United We Stand" banners hung in American homes and George W. Bush's approval ratings climbed to over 90 percent.[13] This coming together, in the case of COVID-19, did not happen either.

The pandemic in the United States was always going to be bad. We can think of the United States as a medical patient with a set of preexisting conditions that make them susceptible to illness. One preexisting condition was a decaying health care system in which insurance company interests played an outsized role in costs and coverage. A second preexisting condition was deep social, economic, and racial divisions that, combined with unequal access to health care, perpetuated structural inequality. The third preexisting condition was President Trump, obsessed with projecting strength to ensure his own reelection, gutting bureaucracies tasked with coordinating emergency responses, refusing to take responsibility for managing the crisis, and nurturing a cult of personality that revolved around his unchallenged authority.

But nothing proved more consequential for deepening the COVID-19 crisis than the fatal comorbidity of partisan polarization. Polarization refers to a tendency of parties, movements, and individuals to locate themselves on the extremes of a political spectrum rather than in the center. It is the "simultaneous presence of opposing or conflicting principles, tendencies, or points of view."[14] Democracy is inherently conflictual and competitive, but polarization distances people from one another, reducing the potential for consensus and, in its extreme form, civility. As political scientists Jennifer McCoy and Murat Somer write, "polarizing politics always carries the risk of taking on a life of its own, eviscerating crosscutting ties and nonpartisan channels for compromise, and becoming pernicious."[15]

In short, polarization divides the "we" of "we the people" into an "us" versus "them." Individuals flee the center, where cross-group dialogue and compromise take place, and move to the extremes. And in the United States, this centrifugal force is powered by partisanship. Two parties—Democrats and Republicans—divide the American electorate.

In the United States today, partisanship is not merely the candidate you choose or the policies you support. Partisanship in America is a social identity. It is a suite of opinions, experiences, and characteristics that define not just who you vote for[16] but also, increasingly, *who you are.* Importantly, partisanship is a social identity because it is not just about how you feel individually but also how you present yourself and relate to others, both those who hold the same partisan identity as you (your copartisans) and those who do not (your partisan opponents).

Of course, individuals hold many social identities, including gender, religion, class, education, and personality. But in the United States today, many of these identities are becoming aligned with partisanship.[17] Historically, for example, observant Christians in the United States were core constituencies of both the Republican and Democratic parties. Today, white evangelical Christians overwhelmingly vote for Republicans.[18] Rural Americans have historically voted for both Republicans and Democrats, but today rural whites increasingly align with the Republican Party.[19] For these reasons, political scientist Lilliana Mason describes partisanship as a "mega-identity, with all the psychological and behavioral magnifications that implies."[20]

When partisanship is a social identity, it connects the idea of *who* is a Democrat or Republican to *what Democrats or Republicans do* and *who they listen to.* For instance, if Americans approached partisanship programmatically—that is, by examining the issues they cared about and seeing which party best espouses them— voters would abandon their partisan identity when parties changed their positions. But rather than change or update their partisanship when parties change positions, strong partisans (that is, those who strongly identify with one party) change their positions to match the party with which they identify.[21] There is no better evidence for this proposition than the norm-shattering experience of the 2016 presidential election. The Republican Party, long viewed as the party of American global capitalism, found itself led by a politician who railed against global trade and in favor of protectionism. Once the party changed, so did the preferences of many of its supporters. In other words, Americans remained loyal to their partisan identity rather than to their policy beliefs. This is what political scientist Julia Azari notes is the toxic combination of "weak parties and strong partisanship," the willingness of party members to follow a president and party even as they move away from core principles.[22]

American politics has not always been characterized by extreme partisan polarization. The country's winner-take-all electoral system produces a two-party system in which both Republicans and Democrats must appeal to multiple social groups to form a viable electoral coalition. But whereas once there were ideological differences within parties (e.g., conservative Democrats, liberal Republicans), ideology now so closely aligns with partisanship that liberals vote for Democrats and conservatives vote for Republicans. Even most independents lean toward one party or another and behave in ways that resemble partisans.[23]

Citizens are good at taking party cues because Americans have sorted into partisan social groups that bring their social identities in line with their partisan affiliations.[24] Take again the example of rural white Americans. The process by which rural whites have become a bedrock Republican constituency has two implications. First, rural whites may no longer know anyone who is also a rural white but who is not a Republican. In previous eras, Americans' social worlds included both Democrats and Republicans even if they were all of the same economic or occupational background. These cross-cutting social ties were once a key factor in undermining partisan divisions in American society but are now less common and more tenuous.[25] Whereas common social and economic bonds once over-rode partisan divisions, today Americans on the Left and the Right just do not interact as much as they used to.

The second implication of partisan sorting is more ominous. If partisanship is a "mega-identity" that increasingly aligns with other social identities, then it follows that one can mobilize partisans without appealing to partisanship itself. A campaign that is relatively certain that rural whites share its partisan orientations is just as effective in mobilizing their votes by appealing to their rural or white identity as by appealing to their views on agricultural policy. This also incentivizes politicians to use messages targeted at specific group identities rather than messages that appeal across groups.

Therefore, in the same way that we often hear about red states and blue states, we can think of "red" and "blue" Americans. These aren't just words that describe one's politics; instead, they capture a way of life. For instance, during a colorful interview between Michael Anton, a former Trump national security official, and National Public Radio host Steve Inskeep, Anton identified himself as a "red person" who had formerly been a "blue person."[26] A blue person might listen to National Public Radio, drive a Subaru, recycle, watch independent films, support pro-choice politics, and live in a blue state. A red person might drive a truck, watch Fox News, attend an evangelical Christian church, and support Blue Lives Matter. And, as it turns out, red and blue Americans respond differently to a pandemic.

Deep partisan polarization created two pandemic realities in America: one where the pandemic was taken seriously and one where the pandemic was an inconvenience. For many Americans the pandemic meant washing hands, wearing masks, avoiding contact with loved ones, canceling travel, and waiting for a safe vaccine or a proven treatment. For others the pandemic was overblown, mostly a problem for the old and infirm similar to the seasonal flu and certainly not a virus that would require major changes to how

Americans lived. Many among this group were skeptical of science and vulnerable to misinformation about the virus and vaccines. The consequences have been tragic, as those who ignore public health guidance have become particularly vulnerable to falling victim to the coronavirus themselves, thus prolonging the pandemic.

When it comes to a communicable virus that requires collective action, partisan polarization undermines a government's ability to respond effectively. At the highest levels of government, polarization made the federal response slower and less effective. Polarization determined which states would receive federal aid, on what terms states would mitigate viral spread, and which children would attend school in person or online. It determined which experts to listen to and who citizens should trust. It determined who wore masks and who did not. It fostered an environment of low trust in government and in each other. In total, partisan polarization produced a public response to the pandemic in which individuals assessed risks, formulated attitudes, and participated in certain health-related behaviors (or not) because of their party identification.

But this was not inevitable. Yes, America faced difficult structural and social preconditions that would make any pandemic hard. Yes, Americans were sharply divided by partisanship at the outset of the crisis. But polarization is not an inevitable barrier to collective action or to a coordinated, effective response to a pandemic. Partisan and other forms of polarization are common around the world,[27] and deeply divided countries such as the United Kingdom, South Korea, and Taiwan did not make partisanship the lens through which to see or experience the COVID-19 pandemic. Partisan divisions may be deeper and wider in the United States than in any other advanced democracy,[28] but this did not make their manifestation in response to COVID-19—over issues ranging from perceptions of the government's handling of the crisis to mask wearing and contact tracing—inevitable.

The crucial factor that differentiates the United States from other high-income democracies is that the Trump administration chose to make the pandemic political. In the early days of COVID-19, there was a cacophony of conflicting messages, both within and between the scientific community and politicians, as politicians were figuring out what to do and as scientists continued to learn what the virus was and how it evolved. When people are concerned about health crises, they usually trust medical experts more than political leaders and want to hear from them.[29] These early days were the window of opportunity during which political leaders faced a choice: they could put experts out front and center and assemble a united, bipartisan strategy to combat the virus, or they could choose to exploit partisanship, activating political divisions to further their individual and partisan goals. The Trump administration chose partisanship.

What does it mean to "choose partisanship?" America's national leaders chose to preserve a strong economy in an election year, chose an image of strength over the potentially worrisome look of mobilizing resources early, and chose not to encourage deference to trusted public health leaders. Instead, the president and conservative media publicly and repeatedly disagreed with public health experts about how serious the coronavirus pandemic was and what types of policies could effectively manage it.[30] The active undermining of experts began with the president, seeped into agencies over which he had significant influence such as the Centers for Disease Control and Prevention, was amplified by conservative media outlets, and trickled down to state governors and mayors. And most of all, it influenced the behavior of the millions of Americans who looked to him for leadership.

Having multiple conflicting messages—and an executive who undercuts his own health bureaucracy—meant that Americans had to decide about how to evaluate the threat from the coronavirus and subsequently how to react. Given these conflicting cues, Americans listened to the leaders of their parties. This led to sharp partisan differences in the ways that ordinary Americans responded to the crisis.

This is our argument. The core explanation for America's disastrous response to COVID-19 is partisanship. The Trump administration and its partisan allies chose to politicize the pandemic by associating it with Trump's own fate in office. That decision cast the subsequent response to the COVID-19 pandemic as primarily about partisan politics rather than public health. This partisan response was all-encompassing, touching everything that the pandemic touched, from health behavior to policy views to worries about the election that occurred during the pandemic's peak. And as these differences persisted, they metastasized. Partisanship undermined Americans' social solidarity—their willingness to adopt behaviors to protect others and sometimes themselves—and became the core framework through which Americans interpreted and elected officials reacted to the pandemic. Those differences in opinions and the differences in the behaviors that follows have cost hundreds of thousands of American lives. And after two years of pandemic politics the policy landscape is forever changed, as formerly bipartisan issues—such as measles and polio vaccine requirements for schoolchildren and trust in experts—are now politicized like never before.

Surveying a Pandemic

Why did California and Nevada issue stay-at-home orders but neighboring Utah and Wyoming did not? Why was the president of the United States telling Americans that COVID "will go away. Just stay calm. It will go away" while hospitals were at capacity and nurses and essential workers protested outside for protective gear such as face masks? Should we be wiping down our mail with disinfectant? Can I see my neighbor if we're outside and socially distant? Where can I buy toilet paper? Should I wear a mask outside? Are we flattening the curve? How much longer are we supposed to work from home while also supervising our kids in online school? Do you think we're going to have to cancel our summer vacation? Is the government doing all it can to protect me, my family, and my community?

These are questions that we, like all Americans, started to ask in March 2020. As large segments of American economic and social life moved online and at home, we also saw our lives overturned by the force of the pandemic. As political scientists, we were specifically attuned to observing the politics of this shift. And as specialists in political processes and behavior—both in the United States and around the globe—we were paying attention to political information and how our fellow Americans were reacting to it. Despite the suggestion that it "will go away," the early stories of mounting caseloads, overrun hospitals, quarantined citizens, and lockdowns coming out of China and Italy were impossible to ignore.

Recognizing the inevitability of COVID-19 reaching the United States, we decided to pool our skills to study American attitudes and behaviors. Each of us is an expert in a different field of politics: emotions and external threat from terrorism to health scares, mostly in the United States (Gadarian); citizenship and democratic threat, including immigration and electoral interference, mostly in Europe (Goodman); and economic crises and democratic backsliding, mostly in Asia (Pepinsky). Our areas of interest and our existential worries started to blend into the same conversation. We wanted to know who in America shared our worries. We wanted to know if Americans would rally together to fight this collective challenge, or if—as we fearfully suspected from years of research—politics would dominate the U.S. response. And we realized that we could provide a view of the emerging crisis that did not come from the echo chamber of social media or the cacophony of cable news.

Ramping up a large research project to survey Americans on their behaviors and attitudes in response to an emerging health crisis is no small task. Social scientists at federally funded universities are unlike researchers at think tanks and polling firms in that our research plans need to be approved by in-house ethics review committees. In addition, university researchers need to independently obtain funding and coordinate with a contracted survey company to draft up a list of questions. This survey then needed to go into the field, that is, out to our survey respondents. We did all of this in the first two weeks of March 2020. We even wrote down our theoretical expectations about what we thought we might find—specifically, that we would see partisan differences in COVID-19 attitudes and behaviors—and shared them in a public repository. In social science, this is referred to as "preregistering" our research and analysis and is used to increase credibility and reduce hindsight bias. With approval from our ethics boards and emergency funding from the National Science Foundation in a Rapid Response Research Grant, our first survey of Americans launched on March 20 as we ourselves were transitioning to working from home and our kids began learning remotely.

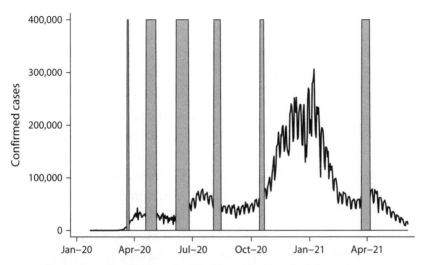

Source: https://covid.cdc.gov/covid–data–tracker/#trends_dailytrendscases

FIGURE I.1. Survey waves

In all, we surveyed ordinary Americans six times, from March 2020 (as states started to lock down, with schools moving to virtual formats and mass cancellation of events) to March/April 2021 (after the inauguration of President Joe Biden and alongside a mass rollout of COVID vaccines). Each wave gives us a different snapshot of America as the pandemic waxed and waned (see figure I.1). We were also able to tap into other events capturing the American public over the year. We could ask questions about, for example, racial justice following the murder of George Floyd (wave 3), the challenges of reopening schools (wave 4), the stakes of the upcoming presidential election (wave 5), and attitudes about vaccines (wave 6). An astute reader might look at this figure and question why we did not have a survey in the field during the peak of the pandemic. For us, the most critical time period was capturing attitudes before the election (wave 5) and after inauguration (wave 6) to see if a partisan change in power produced shifts in policy support or government trust.

At a basic level, our surveys are similar to the standard public opinion surveys released as part of the election cycle. They are designed to be nationally representative, meaning that respondents are chosen randomly but in ways that ensure they reflect, more or less, all adult Americans. This is important: because our respondents are a random but representative sample of all Americans, we can use our surveys to infer what the American population at large was thinking throughout the pandemic. The idea that a survey sample can be representative of a larger population is the bedrock of public opinion research, and we follow this logic as well.

That said, our surveys differ from the standard election poll in two notable ways. First, they are much larger than standard samples: we started with three thousand survey respondents in March 2020, which is about three times as many respondents as we find in most polls. This gives us a great deal of what statisticians call "statistical power," the ability to identify differences among groups of Americans with a high degree of precision. Smaller surveys can give us an overview of all Americans but might not be powerful enough to detect how subgroups of Americans differ—for example, how attitudes might differ by income, race, or religion. To explore the complexity of Americans' political responses to COVID-19, we need to collect data on more Americans.

Second, unlike standard election polls, our surveys follow the same individuals over time. This is known as a panel survey design. Public opinion research firms normally draw a sample of, say, 1,000 Americans to conduct a poll, and then when they want to conduct another poll, they draw a new sample of 1,000 Americans. Our strategy was to recontact the same people we polled in the first round every time we conducted a new survey round. In this book, we call each of the rounds of surveys a survey *wave*, and our respondents whom we interview multiple times are our *panel* of respondents. Following the same individuals in a panel survey is more costly and time-consuming than drawing a fresh sample for each wave, as the survey firm has to recontact the same individuals and incentivize participation. However, this strategy gives us unparalleled insights into such things as the rigidity or flexibility of beliefs as well as the effect of contextual (e.g., local COVID caseload) or circumstantial (e.g., becoming unemployed) factors over time. In the last survey wave in March/April 2021 (supported by a grant from the Russell

Sage Foundation), we added what is called an "oversample" whereby we interviewed an additional set of nonwhite respondents outside of our panel, including 450 Black respondents, 450 Asian American respondents, and 450 Hispanic respondents. These additional respondents allow us to more reliably understand how minority communities fared during the pandemic and what their experiences were with vaccines.

Our Roadmap

In tracing the evolution of health behaviors, attitudes, worries, and policy preferences over the course of the pandemic, we illustrate the early and persistent role of partisanship in shaping individual responses to COVID-19. Despite rising caseloads, uncontrolled spread, and unprecedented loss of life, even taking into account localized factors in an attempt to move away from the national context, partisanship defined both elite and mass responses to the pandemic early on. Once set, the partisan course of the pandemic never deviated.

We develop this argument over ten chapters. Our goal is to produce a definitive account of the politics of the COVID-19 pandemic in the United States, from how it became partisan to the consequences of that choice and from individual worries and policy attitudes to health-related behaviors such as wearing a mask and getting vaccinated. A comprehensive account necessarily begins before the pandemic reached American shores. Chapter 1 sets the stage by describing in detail what we have labeled "preexisting conditions," which we foreshadowed in this introduction. They include a decaying and politicized health care environment, economic and racial inequality, Trump himself, and, above all, partisan polarization. We think of these conditions as time zero, what epidemiologists would describe as the time before an outbreak threshold when a pathogen starts reproducing at high rates.[31] While these factors would make the U.S. outbreak bad, the choice to politicize the pandemic—attaching partisan identity to behaviors and attitudes—made it uniquely worse. Each of these factors on their own would challenge a collective or effective pandemic response; their interaction proved deadly.

Chapter 2 details the onset of the pandemic from January until April 2020. While covering only a short period of time in the long arc of the COVID-19 pandemic, we argue that elite cues, media amplification, and partisan choices in these early critical days were sufficient to permanently affect the trajectory and severity of the pandemic. The series of choices that follow—from early reopenings in the summer of 2020 to Trump rejecting the image of mask wearing even after he became sick with COVID and including differential endorsements and rates of vaccination in red versus blue states—would replicate these early elite patterns. In detailing how the COVID-19 pandemic began to rip through America's communities, we also see how the interaction of preexisting conditions made the American pandemic uniquely worse. Here we draw a number of comparisons to other countries, from the United Kingdom to Brazil, to illustrate how preexisting conditions such as populist leaders and polarization would make for a bad pandemic, but none make partisan politicization inevitable.

Chapters 3 through 10 move from elites and micropolitics to the focus of our analysis: individuals. The partisan pandemic was all-encompassing—it affected social, economic, and political attitudes. But it begins with health. In Chapter 3, we ask about basic health behaviors. Who washed their hands more often? Who wore masks? Who stopped traveling? Partisanship was consistently the strongest predictor of these health behaviors; specifically, Democrats exhibited more prohealth behaviors than Republicans. Chapter 4 moves to Americans' worries about the pandemic and the role that emotions play in health behavior and blame attribution. In focusing on these emotional motivations, we see Democrats expressing anger, disgust, and anxiety and more often seeking out information, while Republicans consistently report feeling hopeful.

Chapters 5 through 7 move from individual behavior and emotions to policy attitudes. Chapter 5 begins with health policy: Should the government enforce lockdown measures? Should the government monitor people's movements? Chapter 6 shifts focus to the economy: What effect did COVID-19 and the economic shutdown have on our respondents? How did experiences such as unemployment affect attitudes about economic policy and government priorities? What should the government do about the economic distress of millions of Americans? Chapter 7 considers immigration policy: Who supports the closure of international borders? Who supports the quarantining of Americans? In each of these policy domains, attitudes strongly divide by partisanship along almost every dimension.

Chapters 8 and 9 situate the pandemic within the context of broader social issues. The pandemic coincided with two of this century's most significant threats to the United States as a liberal democracy: the exposure of rife racial inequality and police brutality in the wake of the murder of George Floyd, and the contested 2020 presidential election. Chapter 8 examines the intersection of the pandemic and race, exposing and raising awareness of the deep inequality in illness and death experienced by Black and other minoritized American communities. This chapter also explores violence against Asian American communities who were unfairly scapegoated as vectors of infection, an injustice that immigrant communities and their descendants often experience during pandemics.[32]

Just as equality of citizens is a core tenet of democracy, so are free and fair elections. Chapter 9 looks at the direct assaults on the integrity and independence of the U.S. electoral system. From unfounded concerns about illegal voters to the reliability of vote by mail, American democracy entered the pandemic on precarious footing, but these claims and conspiracies made it worse. By the time Trump-supporting insurrectionists stormed the U.S. Capitol on January 6, deep wounds had already been inflicted.

Chapter 10 closes out the empirical chapters by turning to the politics of vaccination. Policy experts—and millions of eager Americans—optimistically hoped that the arrival of vaccines would usher in the end of the pandemic. Yet, conservative media figures, antivaccination activists, misinformation campaigns, and enduring holdouts had other plans. In looking at vaccine hesitancy, availability, and incentives, we again see how partisanship shaped vaccine uptake. Failing to reach herd immunity by President Biden's July 4, 2021, goal created fertile community conditions for the new delta variant to develop and take root across America. Here we saw the most needless but foreseen consequence of a partisan pandemic: large death tolls in Trump-supporting communities despite a widely available vaccine that was found to be highly effective in preventing death.[33]

In our concluding chapter, we ask a fundamental question: Could it have been different? Our argument throughout is that a partisan pandemic was not inevitable, but was there any point along the way where the country could have changed course? We argue that with different leadership less focused on an electoral logic along with a more robust public health infrastructure, the outcome could have been different and better. Had the pandemic started in a geographic area more critical to Trump's reelection campaign, the response from the White House would have likely been more constructive. What do we learn from this pandemic that may help the country navigate the next threat, be it a health scare, a terrorist attack, or climate change? We chart out lessons for policy makers about the importance of having the perspectives of social scientists in helping to shape reactions to health crises. Masks, vaccines, and rapid tests cannot end the pandemic if a substantial portion of the public will not use them. Social scientists can work with public health policy makers to understand how identities such as partisanship can create powerful barriers to uptake.

The COVID-19 death toll is one aspect of the pandemic that we as a nation have yet to fully reckon with. An art installation on the National Mall in Washington, D.C., in September 2021 displayed almost seven hundred thousand white flags, each representing one American lost to the pandemic. As we finish writing this book (in December 2021) that number has surpassed eight hundred thousand, and the pandemic is still our daily reality. The surge of the new omicron variant means that discussion about off-ramps from mask wearing and resuming normalcy have been put delayed once again. The pandemic is not over.

Another part of the pandemic that we have not reconciled is our truly divided country. Partisanship was not merely a political identity; it was a social identity that saved some and killed others. This is why the U.S. pandemic was so unlike the pandemic in other democracies. As our book shows, the partisan divide was set in stone early on and has endured. Across so many attitudes and behaviors, partisanship remains strong and consistent. Partisanship even made the pandemic worse because it politicized every possible solution to COVID-19, from what we wear to how and whether we vote in the next election. And absolutely no solution to a communicable virus will work if it is only adopted by some. The forces that make our political identities strong are the very same that weaken intergroup trust when community needs it the most. With partisan identities more powerful than ever, postpandemic democracy looks more precarious than ever.

The pandemic is still with us. It is represented in the loved ones missing from family dinner tables, the jobs that were never recovered, the symptoms of the so-called COVID long-haulers, the learning setbacks facing an entire generation of children—we could go on. It is also in the guilt and the anger; it is in the mistrust between so-called red people and blue people. We as Americans must understand this pandemic so as to reconcile the past and attempt to move forward together. But it is not something we leave behind. Like the virus, pandemic politics has become endemic too.

1

America's Preexisting Conditions

Before patient zero—a thirty-five-year-old man in Snohomish County, Washington, who had recently traveled to Wuhan, China—fell ill with COVID-19 in mid-January 2020 and long before the words "coronavirus" and "COVID" entered the collective lexicon, the United States was already poised for a difficult pandemic. Every country in the world faced the challenges of managing an unprecedented public health emergency, but almost no advanced democracy responded as inefficiently and ineffectively as did the United States. Why? The rest of the book will talk about the politics of the pandemic and how political choices were made that wreaked incalculable consequences for Americans. In this chapter, we lay the groundwork for understanding the politics of the pandemic by focusing on the context in which those choices were made.

This chapter overviews a series of institutional and political vulnerabilities that precede the onset of the pandemic. We describe these as *preexisting conditions*, structures and politics that were already weakening the policy-making environment on January 1, 2020. These preexisting conditions are deep partisan polarization; Donald Trump himself, relying on a charismatic personality and populist politics to make decisions that would preserve his popularity in an election year; (3) the crumbling and outdated U.S. health care system; and (4) systemic racial and economic inequality. These preexisting conditions primed the United States for a bad pandemic, one particularly vulnerable to partisan politicization. On their own, each of these preexisting conditions would make mitigating a pandemic hard. Together, their interaction made the American COVID pandemic uniquely awful.

Preexisting Condition #1: Partisan Polarization

It is hard to overstate the influence of partisan polarization on U.S. politics, much less the COVID-19 pandemic. Polarization was the most endemic and ultimately consequential preexisting condition for how the United States responded to the pandemic. Without polarization, an erratic president buoyed by charismatic political authority would be subject to greater discipline from within his own party, and bipartisan efforts to hold him accountable for his actions would have been easier to sustain. Polarization, on the other hand, actually shields politicians from facing the consequences of their choices.

As we explained in the introductory chapter, polarization creates a political environment in which the partisan center is abandoned in favor of more extreme partisan positions and the parties move further apart without the benefit of cross-cutting positions. In the U.S. context, partisan polarization at the level of party elites means that leaders are focused more on attacking their opponents and signaling their partisan loyalty than on making good policy or looking for bipartisan solutions to common problems. This extends to the wider population as well, as Americans have become increasingly polarized socially. Most worryingly, partisan polarization in the United States does not just reflect growing divides on policy matters but also captures the *moralization* of differences as "good" versus "evil." Scholars describe this emotional valence as "affective polarization" whereby disagreement becomes distrust. Put succinctly, "Democrats and Republicans both say that the other party's members are hypocritical, selfish, and closed-minded, and they are unwilling to socialize across party lines, or even to partner with opponents in a variety of other activities."[1]

How did partisan polarization become such a dominating feature of everyday political and social life? As a general observation, most Americans pay little attention to politics most of the time.[2] When they have little information on an important topic, such as the economy, foreign policy, or a novel health crisis, they draw on their social identities for cues on how to respond,[3] process information,[4] and interpret events.[5] This means that people's sense of *who they are*, based the social groups with which they identify, shapes *what they think*.

Many kinds of social groups—from one's gender to economic class to favorite sports team—convey a sense of belonging and identity in a social world. But in the United States today, partisanship is one of the strongest of these identities.[6] It is a source of meaning and pride and a shortcut for identifying who is similar to you and who is unlike you.[7] Partisan identity is a heuristic that simplifies what would otherwise be complex and multilayered distinctions between people who share their policy outlooks on specific issues and those who do not.

Thus, partisanship as a social identity does not merely guide individuals on political choices such as who to vote for[8] and what policy positions to adopt[9] but also, increasingly, on choices such as who to like and treat with respect and dignity and who to dislike and treat with hostility.[10] One of the most consistent findings in the social sciences is that people prefer their own social groups (ingroups) to members of groups they are not part of (outgroups) and will actively discriminate against outsiders, particularly when it comes to allocating resources.[11] People will even avoid interacting with members of an outgroup on a day-to-day basis.[12] As a sign of just how powerful the political effects of such outgroup antipathy can be, scholars of political behavior have found that disliking supporters of the opposing party motivates voting choices more strongly than liking members of your own party: Democrats and Republicans are more motivated to vote based on their dislike for their partisan opponents than on their own party's positions.[13] Partisans view supporters of the other party as morally suspect. Opponents become enemies; disagreement becomes antagonism. Partisans view the political leaders of the opposing party in the same way.

As Americans increasingly follow partisan cues to cultivate social networks of people similar to them, this process of "partisan sorting" creates partisan "siloes" in activities, hobbies, and news sources.[14] Even economic decisions, such as what kind of car to purchase, can become correlated with partisanship.[15] And this sorting has increased over time,[16] accelerated by a media environment that provides partisan news to partisan viewers. Viewers of MSNBC and Fox News are simply going to receive different information and perspectives on any given issue. For instance, Fox News devoted only a fraction of its new coverage to Hurricane Maria, which swept across Puerto Rico in 2017, relative to MSNBC and CNN.[17]

These differences in informational supply are sustained by the psychological tendencies of social identity. Strong partisans seek out information that reaffirms their previous views[18] and discount information that counters those views,[19] because in the language of social psychology they derive self-esteem from their "ingroup identity." Put another way, we can understand partisan behavior in psychological terms as a form of self-expression. As Ezra Klein describes in *Why We're Polarized*, "When we participate in politics to solve a problem, we're participating transactionally. But when we participate in politics to express who we are, that's a signal that politics has become an identity."[20]

As a preexisting condition to the pandemic, partisan polarization meant that Americans were predisposed to accept information from political leaders of their most favored political party even if that information was inaccurate and reject information from political leaders of their partisan opponents even if that information was accurate, designed to keep them safe, and based on sound medical advice.

In the U.S. political system, the political leader who commands the most attention is the president; presidents' position of power means that they are in the media spotlight, and unlike Congress and other political bodies, the president speaks with a single voice.[21] The public generally takes cues on what issues to be concerned about from the leaders of their own party[22] and will use the president's position to guide their own policy preferences.[23] This means that if a Republican president announces a policy position about some issue area in which a Republican voter is uncertain or uninformed, Republicans may conclude that it must be a position that they too support. A Democrat in the same position, by contrast, may conclude that it is a position they oppose.

One implication of this way of thinking about politics is that people are more likely to accept messages from the political leaders and the president of their own party but can use policy positions from the other party to adjust their views. In addition, because most Americans do not pay close attention to politics and are not strongly ideological, public attitudes are flexible enough to take a variety of positions to reflect those of party leadership. To observe how this works, take the example of attitudes toward the Vietnam War, which started under Democratic president Lyndon Johnson and continued under a Republican president after Richard Nixon's election in 1972. Support for the war was high at the beginning as elites of both parties and the mass media broadcast prowar messages, but over time as the hawkish position was more firmly espoused by Republican leaders such as Nixon and Democratic party support softened, liberals in the public grew to oppose the war while conservatives remained supportive, particularly those most attentive to the issue.[24]

President Trump's election is a stark illustration of the strength of partisan polarization in contemporary U.S. politics. Unlike the Vietnam War era, there is significantly less overlap in the parties' positions on issues such as the economy, trade, and foreign policy.[25] At the elite level, despite the early hope that there would be some common ground between congressional Democrats and Republicans on issues such as infrastructure and prescription drug costs, there was little bipartisanship in Congress in the Trump years. Trump's policy agenda—such as the Muslim immigration ban and the economically nationalistic "Buy American" program—was a significant departure from existing Republican Party platforms, yet most establishment Republicans rallied behind the president and moved in lockstep with Trump's priorities. For instance, only a handful of Republicans opposed the Muslim immigration ban, most notably including Senators John McCain and Lindsey Graham.[26] Even future vice president Mike Pence denounced a ban against Muslims as "offensive and unconstitutional" when Trump first floated the idea on the campaign trail.[27] Cowed by the strength of Trump's brand within the Republican Party, though, former Republican adversaries such as Ted Cruz, Chris Christie, and Lindsey Graham became some of the president's loudest cheerleaders.

This extreme polarization was mirrored in the public as the decline of bipartisanship produced a stronger alignment of partisanship with ideology and other social identities. In the wake of the 2016 election, the United States witnessed a surge of activism in the form of volunteer networks advocating for liberal policies under the banner of the "Indivisible" movement, a women's march, and progressive groups running candidates down-ballot across the country, in all a resistance movement composed of a coalition of different groups that were all intent on opposing Trump policies.[28] And there was mobilization on the political Right too, from neo-Nazis and Proud Boys in Charlottesville to what morphed into a QAnon miasma of Trump election truthers, COVID denialists, and conspiracy-minded fabulists who touted that Washington elites ran a child sex-trafficking ring.[29]

Of course, partisanship and policy views are not set in stone. People's views do change in response to major, disruptive life experiences.[30] Emotions, particularly anxiety and empathy[31] but also sheer self-interest,[32] can override partisan cues. But partisanship is sticky. Once it becomes the prism through which politics is refracted, it also guides the way that people search for and accept information.

On the eve of the pandemic, this polarization had reached heights unrivaled in modern American history.[33] We might even describe the winter of 2020 as its zenith. The House of Representatives held presidential impeachment hearings that were prompted by a whistler-blower complaint about quid pro quo in a phone call between Trump and Ukrainian president Volodymyr Zelensky. No matter how critical members of Congress may have been of the president in private, every congressional Republican lined up behind Trump, casting their lot with him for the course of the 2020 electoral cycle. No Republican member of the House voted to send the impeachment articles to the Senate. The Senate vote to remove the president failed by a vote of 47 to 53, with no Republican senators voting to remove Trump.

Popular opinion echoed this elite polarization as partisans lined up for and against the president. According to a poll by Monmouth University, 92 percent of Democrats and 52 percent of independents supported the impeachment, compared to only 13 percent of Republicans.[34] Approval of Trump's presidency showed a similar pattern: over time, it was the most polarized by party than any other president since the advent of scientific polling.[35] In a January 2020 Gallup poll run during Trump's first impeachment, there was an 87 percentage point gap between Republicans' approval of Trump (94%) and Democrats' approval rating (7%). As these stark figures illustrate, Americans were deeply divided, riven by partisanship and increasingly polarized into two distinct camps defined by their partisan identity. Even independents—a third of the American public—were caught in partisan divides. While there is a set of independents who do not see themselves as close to either party, most typically lean (and vote) in either a Democratic or Republican direction, acting more like partisans than truly independent voters.[36] Polarization really describes a plurality of Americans on any given issue.[37]

There is a tendency for Americans to believe that every election is the most important in their lifetime. But in the context of a divisive president who had just survived an impeachment proceeding and had transgressed nearly every governing norm in American politics, the 2020 election was already expected to be the most important election in half a century. Americans plainly understood it as such. With the presidential election on the horizon for November, by early January 2020 those on the Left and on the Right had every incentive to view any new political issue through a partisan lens.

Preexisting Condition #2: President Trump

Polarization on its own makes effective policy making difficult. But a president with weak commitments to democratic norms who is disinterested in the work of governance makes it harder still. President Trump's governing style was erratic and divisive, from his brash, uncensored speaking manner and his caps-locked Twitter screeds to his repeated ad hominem attacks on Democrats and Republicans alike. These personal affections may be distasteful, but they are not the reason we characterize Trump as a pandemic preexisting condition. Other Republican presidents may have pursued similar policies as Trump and may even have been as polarizing. We are not arguing that having a Republican president condemned America to an ineffective response because of any specific ideas or policy commitments of the Republican Party. Rather we are arguing that features of Trump himself proved damning in crisis: his specific leadership style, based on charismatic authority and patronage, and his pursuit of political priorities that projected an image of economic and political strength rather than problem solving and good governance.

Trump's vanity was both the source of his braggadocious leadership style and the tool by which he identified trustworthy advisers, who tended to be longtime friends, family members, or business associates. As an extension of his outsized personality and projected images of success, Trump collected a large base of supporters to convey what Max Weber describes as "charismatic authority." This is a type of political authority that emerges when an individual is viewed as having the power to rule because of his unique personal qualities, reflecting a belief that the leader is a "savior, a prophet, or a hero."[38] Charismatic leaders do not need to actually *have* exceptional qualities to style themselves as such or to be viewed by segments of the mass public in this way. In the words of Jennifer Merolla and Elizabeth Zechmeister, "What is alone important is how the individual is actually regarded by those subject to charismatic authority, by his 'followers' or 'disciples.'"[39] In times of crisis, however defined, individuals even value "strong leadership more highly than partisan affiliation, making some politicians seem more charismatic than they otherwise would." In his 2016 speech accepting the Republican Party nomination for president, Trump outlined an America in the midst of chaos and violence. He argued his case for presidency by saying that he was singularly fit to repair the damage, stating "I alone can fix it." This personalization of politics presaged how he would govern during the later public health crisis—through a fixation on his own electoral prospects.[40]

But decades of research by scholars of politics around the world have shown that charismatic leaders do not merely sidestep or outshine political parties. Rather, they transform parties, subverting party organizations and internal hierarchies and tying career advancement within the party to personal relationships.[41] Charismatic authority also reduces the costs of party organization "because they involve not much more than an unstructured mass of people rallying around a leader."[42] Charismatic authority is powerful because it is highly personalistic, but since it is concentrated in one individual, it is also weakly institutionalized and cannot, for instance, be transferred with the same strength to individuals who are not Donald J. Trump. This means that the longevity of Trumpism is hard to sustain without Trump as the leader of the Republican Party.

As an extension of this charismatic authority and as a means to consolidate and protect his power while in office, Trump cultivated a menagerie of trusted advisers based on loyalty rather than performance, expertise, or skill. He embraced patronage and favoritism to donors, family members, and business associates at a level that was unprecedented in modern American history. From Louis DeJoy (Republican donor) as postmaster general to Ben Carson (a neurosurgeon) as secretary of housing and urban development, key executive branch appointments were held by partisan loyalists who had no substantive expertise or governing experience. Trump's closest and most trusted advisers were his own family members. His administration conceived of public policy and federal programs in clientelist terms, to be awarded to supporters and withheld from opponents rather than to be administered using neutral and objective criteria.[43] In practice, this meant that very senior positions—positions that would be critical in pandemic policy design and emergency response—were held by individuals who were loyal to the president but lacked critical experience or were uninterested in coordinating across bureaucracies, working with states, identifying appropriate contractors to obtain vital supplies, and the myriad other tasks a government faces in an emergency.

Alongside his disregard of expertise, Trump hollowed out the federal bureaucracy. Several important positions in the federal government were held by acting directors, reflecting Trump's disdain for the Senate approval process as well as his belief that acting directors would be easier for him to control. Key positions in the federal bureaucracy—those most necessary for an effective public health response—were either vacant or filled by temporary appointees. A study by the Brookings Institute counted an astonishing number of vacant positions across key cabinet-level departments: 44 percent vacancies in Senate-confirmed positions in the Department of Education, 17 percent in Health and Human Services, and 65 percent in Homeland Security.[44] In July 2019, the Centers for Disease Control and Prevention's epidemiologist embedded in China's disease control agency left the position. Instead of appointing a replacement, the Trump administration eliminated the role,[45] leaving no American in China to monitor the public health situation when the pandemic broke out in January 2020.

In the context of extreme partisan polarization in the United States, however, Trump was never penalized by his supporters for the excesses of his leadership style or his failures of governance. He was simply a divisive figure, adored by his supporters and detested by his opponents. Never in the course of his administration did he reach 50 percent job approval in Gallup's polling data, and his disapproval ratings were almost consistently higher than his approval ratings, a phenomenon never before seen in the modern political era, as shown in figure 1.1.

There was little relationship between the state of the economy, executive decisions, and political events, on the one hand, and mass support for Trump, on the other. This is evidence of an administration that was not rewarded for effective governance or punished

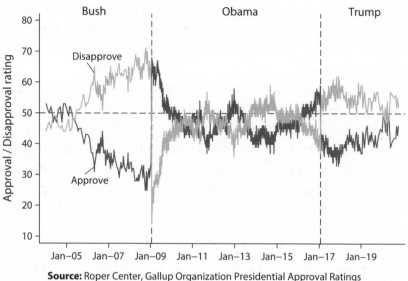

Source: Roper Center, Gallup Organization Presidential Approval Ratings

FIGURE 1.1. Presidential approval ratings, 2004–2020

for ineffective governance but one that was highly focused on the man himself.

By contrast, previous presidents were deeply affected by controversial and unpopular decisions. George W. Bush, after receiving a buoy of support following 9/11, suffered massive popularity losses in the fallout of the Iraq War and the mishandling of Hurricane Katrina. Barack Obama's popularity swung widely over the two terms of his presidency, as early support due to the financial crisis gave way to more divisions over the size and scope of the federal government. In a preview to the polarization around COVID-19, issues around health and health care such as the Affordable Care Act became not only partisan but also more closely connected to racial attitudes and beliefs about the beneficiaries of a more expansive health care system.[46]

But Trump never needed a majority of Americans to give him positive approval ratings. In the American political system, one wins reelection not by obtaining a majority of the popular vote but instead by capturing key states. As Andrea Schneiker has argued, Trump's particular brand of charismatic appeal—not simply as a populist but

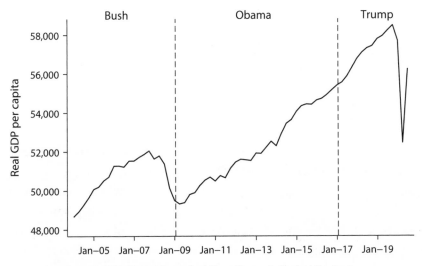

Source: FRED, United States Real Gross Domestic Product Per Capita

FIGURE 1.2. Economic performance, 2004–2020

as a "superhero" with unique authority and knowledge that establishment politicians and other establishment elites lack—can explain both his particular choice of policies and the appeal that they have among his supporters.[47] Specifically, for Trump this meant a singular focus on economic growth.

Trump inherited a strong economy from his predecessor and, following nearly a decade of steady growth under President Obama (see figure 1.2), quickly attributed America's successes as his own. Trump saw economic performance as integral in his bid for reelection. In January 2020 on the coattails of an impeachment, he was at Davos telling the World Economic Forum about the U.S. economic boom. His almost singular obsession with economic indicators would lead to tweets pronouncing "Did you hear the latest con job? President Obama is now trying to take credit for the Economic Boom taking place under the Trump Administration" (February 17, 2020), in response to a mid-February jobs report, and, two days later, "Highest Stock Market In History, By Far!" (February 19, 2020). While we know now what was happening behind the scenes (which we detail closely in chapter 2), this projection of economic success and singular focus on maintaining a positive narrative in the wake of an impeachment hearing was critical to understanding how decisions would be made during crisis.

Preexisting Condition #3: A Broken Health Care System

President Trump did a lot of damage to the architecture of American government. But the bureaucratic landscape he inherited was hardly suited to managing a global pandemic, especially when it comes to the U.S. health care system. Every American probably has or has heard a story of someone calculating the costs of visiting a doctor or calling an ambulance before making a decision about whether something is medically necessary, or planning a surgery based on financial rather than medical timelines (i.e., to meet annual deductibles). Such anecdotes—unthinkable in most advanced industrial economies—are sadly common in the United States.

Health care costs in the United States are far higher than in every other advanced economy, and at the same time, coverage is woefully inconsistent, outdated, and incomplete. To show just how American health care outcomes compare to those of other high-income economies, in figure 1.3 we compare the United States with other wealthy countries in Western Europe, North America, and East Asia along four dimensions: infant mortality rates, maternal mortality rates, life expectancy, and a composite index of health care policy quality.[48] This gives a holistic picture of health care across advanced industrialized countries.

The United States is easily visible in each of these four plots because of how unusual and off-the-line it is. By the numbers, the United States is wealthier than all but a handful of countries in the world. But in the top row of figure 1.3, we see that the United States nevertheless has higher infant and maternal mortality rates than any other country to which we have compared it. And the bottom row shows that the United States has the lowest life expectancy of any of these countries and near to the lowest health care policy ranking.

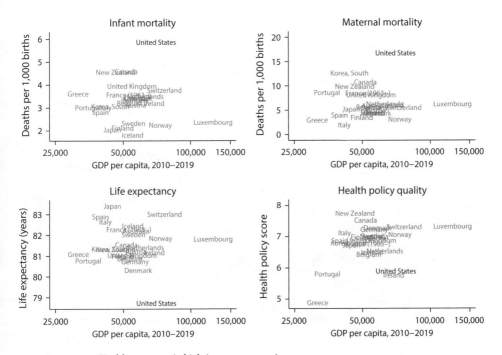

FIGURE 1.3. Health outcomes in high-income economies

We are not proposing that high infant mortality rates make a country vulnerable to COVID-19. Rather, our point is that all of these health indicators reflect the comparatively poor quality of the U.S. health care system. Given how wealthy the United States is as a country, its health care outcomes are abysmal.

We can go further to underline America's outlier status. In figure 1.4, we compare countries in terms of their health expenditures. Once again the United States stands out—and not in a good way. The United States spends far more in absolute terms than any other advanced economy on health care, and far more relative to the size of its economy as well. Strikingly, these high costs are borne equally by the public sector and the private sector: the United States ranks near the top of all countries in terms of how much the both the government spends and the private sector spends on health care.

So, what makes health care outcomes so bad in the United States? And if health care outcomes are so bad, why does American health

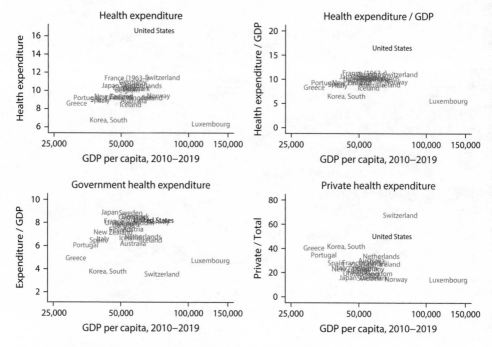

FIGURE 1.4. Health care expenditures in high-income economies

care cost so much? There are a number of factors at play, but at root is the absence of a robust public health insurance scheme that covers all Americans and de-marketizes health care delivery. The market for health care is not like markets for other goods and services, as economist and Nobel Prize laureate Kenneth Arrow noticed decades ago.[49] Health care markets feature unparalleled levels of uncertainty about the value of the "goods" being consumed, a bewildering array of licensing requirements for providers, and, most importantly, extreme inelasticity of demand: people who need emergency care are in no position to comparison shop, haggle, or refuse care that is more expensive than they can afford.

In all advanced economies, the solution to the imperfections of health care markets is health insurance combined with a health care system that features a strong role for government in managing costs. In the United Kingdom, for example, most doctors are employees of the National Health Service, which controls costs as a matter of government policy. Private insurance is still available, but the National Health Service offers a baseline coverage for everyone as a social right. In Germany, both employers and employees pay into nonprofit health care funds, which cover the remaining population. The United States is utterly different, maintaining a health care system that relies on market mechanisms more than does any other high-income country. Americans pay for health care in many different ways: through employer-subsidized insurance or a health maintenance organization, by purchasing health insurance individually, by paying for health care out of pocket, through Medicare or Medicaid, or through the Veterans Administration. And for a long time, many Americans did not have health insurance at all (a gap that the Affordable Care Act was designed to fill).

Higher costs do not produce better health outcomes. Rather, they produce greater inequality in outcomes. For those with means, American health care is world-class. For those without, that world-class American health care is generally unavailable. It is not hard to see how adding a highly infectious virus to the mix would create even further confusion and stresses on the system, when so many Americans are worrying about the costs of both obtaining a diagnosis and getting the treatment they need.

America's federal structure—with key national health care policies administered by the states—only compounds the challenges of quality health care delivery. Some states have long histories of chronic underfunding in health care as well as low taxes coupled with low trust in government.[50] For instance, access to care, quality of care, and overall health outcomes differ drastically from state to state, with states such as Hawaii and Massachusetts at the top and Arkansas and Mississippi at the bottom.[51] News outlets can run click-bait articles about the "best and worst states" to be in when you have a heart attack from these differences (and for the record, you're better off heading to a hospital in New Jersey than in Oklahoma).[52] This highlights how health outcomes depend not just on federal government priorities but also on how they are implemented across the states.[53]

This has particular consequences for racial inequality in health care outcomes.[54] When there was a tuberculosis outbreak in the predominantly Black rural community of Marion, Alabama, in 2016, high incidence rates were attributed not just to "generations of limited health care access" but also to "distrust of public health officials."[55] In fact, the outbreak started two years earlier, but patients had been reluctant to disclose their contacts to public health officials ("The phrase that every single case uses is, 'I don't want nobody knowing my business'"). Many pointed to the legacy of the Tuskegee experiment, when Black men were denied penicillin as part of a study of untreated syphilis in the 1930s in Macon County, Alabama, as a cause for such distrust of public health officials.

The weaknesses of the American health care system in response to pandemics were already laid bare as recently as the global Ebola virus outbreak.[56] In September 2014, a Liberian citizen visiting the United States tested positive for Ebola in Dallas, Texas. He passed away in October. There were in total only eleven cases of Ebola in the United States and only two cases where the virus was contracted *in* the United States, both nurses who worked with the victims. The only other death was a doctor who contracted Ebola while in Africa.

The Obama administration's response to this Ebola outbreak displayed all of the hallmarks of America's fragmented health policy landscape: the challenges of using federal authority to conduct contact tracing and coordinate state responses, the lack of policy tools to establish common standards for testing and treatment across the country, the independent role played by hospitals themselves in making key decisions about treatment and protection, and a decentralized financial model leading to questions about who would pay for it all. In one case, it was reported that the cost of treating two patients at the University of Nebraska Medical Center exceeded $1 million, and it was unclear who would be footing the bill.[57] One of the nurses who fell ill with Ebola subsequently filed a lawsuit for negligence against her hospital's parent company, claiming nurses did not receive proper training or equipment.[58] The Ebola outbreak was also characterized by partisan division, as Republicans were much more critical of the US disaster preparedness than Democrats. For instance, Republican lawmakers were critical that Tom Frieden, director of the Centers for Disease Control and Prevention

(CDC), allowed an exposed nurse to board a commercial flight and supported a travel ban for incoming flights from Ebola-affected regions.[59]

After its much-criticized response to the Ebola outbreak, the Obama administration created a pandemic response team and a play-book for avoiding some of these very problems of coordination and federal management given the inevitability of a future outbreak. The Trump administration would discard both (as we will see in chapter 2), revealing how these preconditions of President Trump's leadership style and the U.S. health care system would interact in fatal ways.

Preexisting Condition #4: Inequality

Underneath it all—under the polarization, unique leadership style, a gutted bureaucracy, and bad health care policies—rests a fundamen-tally unequal society. We mentioned above how American health care institutions produce racial inequality in health outcomes, but this is only one facet of American inequality. The United States is among the world's wealthiest democracies, and also one of the world's most highly unequal societies.

Figure 1.5 presents two different ways to measure income inequality. On the y-axis in the left-hand figure is the Gini coefficient, which is a measure of how unequal a country is. The Gini coefficient ranges from zero (a scenario in which every person in the coun-try has the same income) to one (a scenario in which one person has all of the income in a country and everyone else has nothing). The y-axis in the right-hand figure, by contrast, is the ratio of the amount of disposable income held by those at the 90th percentile of income and those at the 10th percentile of income. The message is the same however you measure inequality: the United States is the most unequal advanced economy in the world.

Inequality itself is not inherently a problem for responding to a pandemic; governments that care about their citizens will do their best to provide resources and treat communities in need. But the interaction of inequality with unaffordable and incomplete health

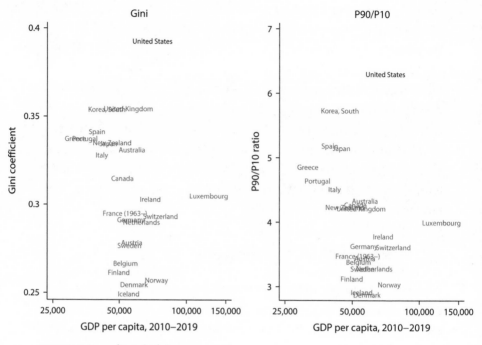

FIGURE 1.5. Inequality in high-income countries

care institutions (not to mention the fact that most quality health care for the working-age population is tied to employment) produces an entirely segmented health care experience. Underfunded hospitals are inevitably those that are overburdened. Individuals who can afford emergency care, experimental treatment, costly prescriptions—and those who can afford to eat healthy and exercise to reduce comorbidities—will invariably have better health outcomes than those who cannot.

The danger of American inequality becomes acute when we observe how economic inequalities overlap with racial inequalities. Racial inequality has deep roots in American politics,[60] anchored in nearly every dimension of American political, social, and economic life. Black Americans and Latinos are more likely to experience unemployment than Asian or white workers.[61] Median household income for Black Americans trails every other ethnic group.[62] Black Americans are less likely to be homeowners.[63] Black men are incarcerated at far higher rates than Latinos, who far exceed rates of white men.[64] Specifically, while Black Americans comprise about 12 percent of the adult U.S. population, they constitute 33 percent of the U.S. prison population.[65] Black men are also 2.5 times more likely to be killed by police than white men.[66] Minoritized communities experience homelessness at higher rates than whites.[67] School districts with a majority of student of color receive billions less in K–12 education funding than do predominantly white school districts.[68] Relatedly, there is a widely documented racial achievement gap, from grades to standardized tests to graduation rates. Black citizens are less likely to vote than whites, and both are more likely to vote than Hispanics and Asian Americans.[69] And Black Americans systematically experience worse health care outcomes, from maternal health to inadequate access to doctors to what one study calls a weathering effect, in which "chronic exposure to social and economic disadvantage leads to accelerated decline in physical health outcomes."[70] In short, there is no area of American life untouched by racial inequality.

These racial disparities in health are older than the United States itself. And yet health policy making has become more racialized since the Obama administration. Specifically, as Michael Tesler has argued, because the Affordable Care Act was championed and passed by a Black president, Americans came to associate health care with race.[71] As a result, Americans' attitudes about race and discrimination are now better at predicting their attitudes toward health policy than has ever been the case before. Race-based opposition to Obama's presidency not only fueled opposition to health care reform but also drove public opinion about the economy and several other issues.[72]

It is here that we see the link between anti-Obama attitudes and Trump's electoral base in 2016. Trump voters were overwhelmingly white, and his rhetoric and campaign style consistently played on racialized tropes in American society in an appeal to that voter base. Trump's campaign slogan—"Make America Great Again"— was described as a racist dog whistle, speaking directly to "those who have felt a loss of status as other groups have become more empowered,"[73] that is, white Americans in postindustrial cities struggling to regain social prestige and political power. In one study, Trump voters indicated a strong belief that Blacks are "less deserving than 'average Americans.'"[74] Add to this a growing split between urban/suburban middle-class voters and rural and working-class voters—the former aligning with the Democrats and the latter with Trump's Republican Party—and it is plain that the polarization that we addressed above is associated with a whole host of racial, class, and geographic divisions.

We see in the case of inequality how these preexisting conditions interact. The partisan politics of American health care exacerbates racial disparities in health access and health outcomes. Over the past four decades, states with more generous social and economic policy had higher life expectancy than states with more conservative social policy.[75] This has direct implications for racial disparities in health outcomes, as states led by Republican governors and legislatures were less likely to have expanded Medicaid eligibility through the cost sharing of the Affordable Care Act, and the nonexpansion states were more likely to have large populations of Black residents.[76] And as we will see, these states were also slower to shut down the economy at the earliest part of the pandemic (if at all), earlier to reopen, and less likely to have mask mandates; these policies were all linked with more cases among residents.[77]

The deep problems of poverty, inequality, and a weak welfare state are easier for politicians to overlook when the overall economy is running well. But even steady economic growth hides deep vulnerabilities. The median household family incomes for Black Americans is 37 percent lower than that for white non-Hispanic Americans. The difference for Latinos of any race is roughly 22 percent; for Native Americans the difference is 26 percent.[78] This means that although poverty and economic insecurity themselves present major risks to pandemic response, we will not be able to fully grasp those risks without careful attention to the racialized dimensions of poverty and inequality in the United States.

None of these observations are new. Anyone paying attention to American politics in January 2020 would have reported that Americans were highly politically polarized; that health care inequality was a pressing challenge; that race, class, status, and geography were essential for understanding American democracy; and that the president of the United States was fundamentally unserious about any of these problems. What few could have predicted, though, was just how dangerous these preexisting conditions would be in the context of a pandemic, and how fundamentally they would shape the Trump administration's response to the COVID-19 pandemic.

These preconditions also serve as a useful instrument for how we think about the United States in comparative perspective. The United States is certainly unique, and the confluence of these factors is atypical but not without precedent or comparison. There are other countries that struggle with deep polarization (the United Kingdom), federalism (Germany, Canada), and deep racial and economic inequality (Brazil). These cases are instructive benchmarks as we observe the pandemic timeline unfold in the United States. While we certainly learn important policy lessons and pandemic management possibilities from all states, those that lack America's preconditions may be able to leverage social and government trust to encourage citizen behavior (e.g., Denmark and Sweden) and implement policy in a way the United States would never be able to achieve, much like comparisons to nondemocratic contexts. It is to this timeline and these comparisons that we now turn.

2

Politicizing the Pandemic

In March 2020, Massachusetts hospitals were soliciting donations. But this was unlike their typical ask. They didn't need money. They needed safety goggles, masks, and other personal protective equipment (PPE) for frontline workers. In the emergency rooms, nurses and medical staff were reusing single-use masks. Outside the hospitals, nurses were holding up signs imploring passersby for donations. Personal appeals were made to construction companies and research labs, with one nurse worrying "I'm praying, I'm hoping that we don't end up like Italy, but what if we do?"[1] The local news was showing pictures of workers in garbage bags instead of gowns and fashioning masks out of bandanas.

Even if hospitals had received millions of dollars to support purchases of PPE, they would have had no way to spend it. The sudden surge in demand for surgical masks and N95 respirators disrupted the global supply chain and exceeded existing capacity to manufacture them, creating acute shortages worldwide. Ninety percent of surgical masks sold in the United States are made overseas,[2] and China was making around half of the world's masks. But even American-owned companies that manufactured masks in China were not exporting them, for these companies too faced acute shortages. Peter Navarro, an adviser to President Donald Trump on manufacturing and trade, described this step as Beijing opting to "nationalize effectively 3M, our company."[3]

Back in Massachusetts, hospital executives, along with state and local governments, were scrambling to get supplies. The state's Republican governor, Charlie Baker, managed to place an order for 3 million N95 respirator masks, only to see them seized at the port in New York by the Federal Emergency Management Agency (FEMA).[4] Similar reports were coming from across the United States—from ventilators in Colorado to thermometers in Florida to testing supplies in Washington—with one official in Massachusetts asking "Are they stockpiling this stuff? Are they distributing it? We don't know."[5] The next time Governor Baker attempted to supply his state with masks, he relied on the New England Patriots football team, using the team's private airplane to bring 1.2 million N95 masks to Boston.[6]

How did it come to be that states were in bidding wars against one another and fighting with the federal government to obtain desperately needed health supplies? The answer is not surprising, but it is unsettling. As a former assistant secretary to the Department of Homeland Security observed, "For decades, we have worked disasters the same way. The locals execute, the states coordinate and the feds support. . . . The federal government under Donald Trump has decided it is going to essentially go to war, create a parallel response apparatus, and it's winning. That's the problem."[7]

We know from chapter 1 that the United States faced preexisting conditions that would make the pandemic difficult in any case. Partisan polarization, Trump's leadership style, a crumbling health care infrastructure, and endemic economic and racial inequality would make a public health emergency such as COVID-19 challenging. But these preexisting conditions did not mean that a calamitous response was inevitable. At the outset of the pandemic there was a window of opportunity, a moment during which effective messaging by health experts and bipartisan endorsement of an active government response could have unified the country. Americans might have united in response to the COVID-19 pandemic, as they have in many previous external crises.[8] On January 29, 2020, the worst-case scenario (detailed in a memo by Navarro to the president) put American deaths at half a million.[9] Looking back at that prediction from December 2021, with the United States having passed eight hundred thousand deaths, we now have a sad appreciation of the gravity of the crisis that was unfolding. This chapter looks critically at those early days when American politicians and media elites politicized the pandemic.

The pandemic's earliest days were characterized by neither uniform expert-led messaging nor an effort to rally the public around a common message of shared sacrifice for the common good. Rather, the Trump administration downplayed the threat of the pandemic, adopting a divisive crisis management strategy that put polarizing figures such as the president out front. The emergency management strategy playbook was thrown out in exchange for patronage and deliberate inaction. The administration did not just abandon its responsibility to protect the most vulnerable Americans—the sick and infirm and those living in assisted living facilities and prisons—but also abandoned all Americans while portraying the pandemic as no less than a political conspiracy against the Trump administration. These choices led millions of Americans to understand the pandemic in partisan terms, that is, to align with what was good for their "team" rather than for the country. It was not inevitable that the COVID-19 pandemic would become a partisan issue, but the Trump administration's choices made it so.

This chapter presents a timeline of the first critical months of 2020. The pandemic has endured for years, but we need only look at these early months to establish our central argument: early decisions to politicize the pandemic solidified a pattern of attitudes and behaviors that would characterize the entire pandemic, from mask wearing and vaccines to attitudes about economic recovery and school reopening. Essentially, by April 2020 we already knew everything we needed to know to understand the politics of the COVID-19 pandemic. The pandemic ballooned from a health crisis into a social crisis as the partisan approach to COVID-19—forged in the pandemic's earliest days—became its central feature.

We start this chapter by examining how policy choices were made in the context of America's preexisting political conditions, specifically polarization and Trump's presidential style, to show how politics exacerbated—and in turn was exacerbated by—these preexisting conditions. Building on the foundations of chapter 1, we show how the Trump administration's choices created a uniquely American COVID-19 pandemic. And to illustrate just how distinct the American experience with COVID-19 was, we consider how the U.S. political response differed from the politics of COVID-19 in other countries. Many countries were similarly handicapped in confronting the pandemic, with populist leaders or uneven access to health care, but none politicized the pandemic as much—or as successfully—as Trump.

A Small Window of Opportunity

The first confirmed case of COVID-19 in the United States was diagnosed on January 21, 2020, but it was not on the radar of most Americans or news organizations. COVID-19 was something happening in China or in Italy—it was not yet an American problem. The United States had its own issues to confront, including impeachment hearings and presidential primaries. With the Dow Jones at an all-time high and strong jobs numbers, President Trump focused his reelection campaign on the economy, conveying a message of strength to overshadow the impeachment proceedings. To the extent that Americans were paying attention to China at all, it was in light of Trump's much-touted "historic" trade deal. On January 17 Trump retweeted conservative Fox host Laura Ingraham, who said "Years from now, when we look back at this day, nobody's going to remember Nancy [Pelosi]'s cheap theatrics, they will remember though how President Trump brought the Chinese to the bargaining table and delivered achievements few ever thought were possible."

For its part, the Democratic Party was selecting its presidential candidate for the November 2020 general elections, having winnowed a field of twenty-nine candidates down to six: Joe Biden, Pete Buttigieg, Amy Klobuchar, Bernie Sanders, Tom Steyer, and

Elizabeth Warren. At a January 14 debate in Des Moines, Iowa, not a single candidate mentioned a health crisis in China. Any mentions of China were in the context of putting pressure on North Korea to cease nuclear weapons buildup (Biden) and the profiting of multinational corporations and loss of jobs domestically caused by Trump's trade deal (Sanders).

But although the American public was not looking to China in January 2020, infectious disease and medical experts were. In December 2019, officials were already concerned that the World Health Organization (WHO) and the Centers for Disease Control and Prevention (CDC) had been slow to address the virus.[10] Behind the scenes, health officials and members of the Trump administration were receiving startling information about the unfolding pandemic and attempted to convey the seriousness of the crisis to the president. Health experts were raising the alarm on the critical need to procure surgical masks for frontline workers.[11] The CDC began to develop a diagnostic test for COVID-19, and on January 20, one day before the first confirmed case in the United States, travelers from Wuhan, China, started receiving health screening at three U.S. airports.[12] This was three days before Trump reported having received his first warning: "On Jan. 23, I was told that there could be a virus coming in, but it was of no real import. In other words, it wasn't, oh, we have got to do something, we have got to do something. It was a brief conversation."[13]

The intelligence community was rallying; Robert O'Brien, Trump's fourth and final national security adviser, warned the president on January 28 that "this will be the biggest national security threat you face in your presidency. . . . This is going to be the roughest thing you face."[14] That same day, a senior medical adviser at the Department of Veterans Affairs wrote in an email to a group of public health experts, "Any way you cut it, this is going to be bad."[15] By this time, a Chinese scientist had already confirmed that the novel coronavirus could be transmitted from human to human, and the WHO had issued a global health emergency. Navarro sent a stark memo to Trump on January 29 warning of trillions in economic losses.[16] Trump was warned about COVID-19 more than a dozen times in his President's Daily Brief during January and February.[17]

The United States was not alone, of course. Every country in the world would need to face down the pandemic, each with its own set of preexisting preconditions. And there was a range of preparations taking place. Some countries—particularly those in Asia—had recent experience with pandemics such as SARS, Middle East respiratory syndrome (MERS), bird flu, and swine flu. For instance, South Korea authorities, having learned lessons from handling MERS,[18] were prepared with a test for COVID before the first domestic case was diagnosed. Their government also performed comprehensive testing and contact tracing with a MERS protocol already in place. And they had an infrastructure for central government purchasing of PPE already in place. Their curve would peak by the end of February, before the United States had even put mass testing in place.[19]

Other high-income democracies that did not have recent experiences with pandemics faced sizable coordination challenges. Germany, however, despite the sizable challenges of a federal system, entered the pandemic with its detailed National Pandemic Plan,[20] released on January 16, involving early mobilization and coordination between local health authorities and the Robert Koch Institute (Germany's public health agency). Elective surgeries were pushed back, hospitals shared data with a federal website to map out their supply chain needs, and extra intensive care facilities were built just in case.[21] One of the first diagnostic tests for COVID-19 was also developed in Germany before its first case of COVID was diagnosed on January 27. And because the German health care system is decentralized and consumer-oriented, coupled with a robust sector of private laboratories, testing could scale up quickly across the country.[22]

The United Kingdom was considerably less prepared than Germany and, perhaps, a closer comparison to the United States at the time. The United Kingdom had its first confirmed cases by the end of January just as Brexit, its deeply polarizing exit from the European Union, was being finalized. And like the United States, the government of Boris Johnson was slow to respond (as *The Times* described February, it was "22 days of dither and delay").[23] Numerous clusters emerged as a result, overwhelming contact tracing measures and necessitating a legally enforced national lockdown starting

March 23. Yet this was not the most negligent case. Sweden, which chose a controversial no-lockdown model, relied on social trust and voluntary compliance to pro–social health behaviors rather than control measures. One study found that "UK mortality would have approximately doubled had Swedish policy been adopted, while Swedish mortality would have more than halved" if Sweden had adopted British strategies.[24]

In looking at the United States in comparison during these earliest days, we see that there are a lot of models to choose from. Countries with similar preconditions faced similar obstacles of coordination and mobilization. Here, we see an early window of opportunity. Experts saw the pandemic as inevitable; awareness was being raised globally, and Americans were still poorly informed about this evolving situation. COVID-19 was not yet politicized in America. As a novel public health threat, it represented a blank slate about which people did not have prior convictions one way or the other. The president's choices in this moment were critical. Multiple experts and his own advisers were urging him to act. By mid-January news organizations were covering the Wuhan lockdown and the emerging global outbreaks, but the American public heard relatively little from the president. On January 22 he tweeted, "One of the many great things about our just signed giant Trade Deal with China is that it will bring both the USA & China closer together in so many other ways." On January 24 he echoed this admiration: "China has been working very hard to contain the Coronavirus. The United States greatly appreciates their efforts and transparency. It will all work out well."

This is the first time the American public heard from the president about the coronavirus at all: *it will all work out well.* The message to Americans was reassuring, not designed to inflame partisan passions among either Republicans or Democrats. And in fact, the first national politician to tie COVID-19 to American politics was none other than Joe Biden. On January 27, then-candidate Biden wrote in an op-ed in *USA Today* that "the possibility of a pandemic is a challenge Donald Trump is unqualified to handle as president."[25] But candidate Biden's prescient warning was little noticed at the time. Instead of ad hominem attacks against Biden, Trump's usual response to political opponents, Trump simply tweeted "We are in very close communication with China concerning the virus. Very few cases reported in USA, but strongly on watch." The rest of his tweets that day focused on the impeachment ("The Witch Hunt continues!") and the China trade deal.

When we reflect on late January 2020, we see the first inklings of the political implications of COVID-19. Yet the pandemic had not yet been politicized in the United States. There is a subtle but important difference between *politics* and *politicization*. It is entirely normal to expect that Americans' views about the pandemic would follow their political orientations. Constitutional conservatives, for example, may reasonably ask whether the federal government possesses the authority to pass vaccine mandates for federal employees. Progressives should wonder about the implications of America's unequal health care system during a national public health emergency. That's just normal politics. To some extent, we expect Republicans and Democrats to disagree about how to respond to the COVID-19 pandemic because they generally disagree about the size and scope of government. But we also expect them to agree about the basic nature of the pandemic and the urgent need to manage it responsibly.

When we say that the pandemic was politicized, we mean specifically that a subset of American political and media elites—led by Trump—cast the COVID-19 pandemic as essentially *about* politics. When a presidential candidate such as Biden pens an op-ed that criticizes the sitting president's policy preparedness for a pandemic as inadequate, he is focusing on how voters should evaluate a politician's performance in a time of crisis. When a president alleges that the pandemic is a conspiracy by the deep state and the establishment media to harm his reelection chances—the Democrats' "new hoax" following the first impeachment—he is politicizing the pandemic. The public discourse is no longer about the scale of the threat, the appropriate policy response, or their public health implications. It is about whether you support a president who calls the pandemic a hoax and blames the Democrats for not supporting him.

We make our position plain here: it is Trump who politicized the pandemic. We do not disagree that once he launched his Twitter tirades about how unfair the COVID-19 pandemic was to him, Democrats responded in kind. Once the pandemic was politicized, it was hard for any Democrat or Republican to opt out of the partisan bickering. But only one party held the White House, and only one person sat in the Oval Office. Perhaps if Democrats had occupied the White House in early 2020, a Democratic president would have politicized the pandemic just as Trump did. But in point of fact, it was Trump who as commander in chief made the fateful decision to portray the COVID-19 pandemic as a partisan political issue. And following his characteristic tactic of personalizing all matters related to politics and policy, he chose to cast the debate in terms of identity: to support Trump was to share his views about the pandemic. Trump turned the pandemic into a litmus test of loyalty.

Messages of reassurance and portrayals of confidence and strength were deliberate, rhetorical choices by Trump. In a series of interviews with *Washington Post* reporter Bob Woodward, Trump admitted to purposefully underplaying how dangerous the corona-virus was to the public during this time. "I wanted to always play it down," he said. "I still like playing it down. Because I don't want to create a panic."[26] In the same interview, he also admitted to Wood-ward that "it's also more deadly than your—you know, your—even your strenuous flus" but publicly would attest "This is a flu. This is like a flu."[27]

As Trump was downplaying the threat in public, what was he doing in terms of policy? Trump had been briefed repeatedly by experts about the threat that COVID-19 posed but deliberately did not act on that information until January 27. On that date he assembled a coronavirus task force led by Alex Azar, secretary of housing and human services. But like many of Trump's administrative appointments, task force members were largely appointed for loyalty, not expertise; the twelve-member group included only two medical health professionals: CDC director Robert Redfield, a controversial virologist who inspired little confidence,[28] and Dr. Anthony Fauci, a deeply respected immunologist who was little known outside of medical circles. On January 31, the president also signed a proclamation banning all travel between the United States and China due to the risk of infection, boasting on February 2 that "we pretty much shut it down coming in from China." Trump would return to the "China ban" often, crediting himself with a forceful early response.

But February was also full of policy missteps. As health officials were begging Trump to obtain more masks and PPE, on February 7, the same day the WHO warned of a "limited stock of PPE,"[29] Secretary of State Mike Pompeo announced that the United States was donating over seventeen tons of medical supplies to China.[30] A day later, answering questions at the World Economic Forum, Trump stated he was aware of the first case in the United States and that he was not worried about a pandemic: "We have it totally under control. It's one person coming in from China, and we have it under control. It's—going to be just fine." Matt Pottinger, deputy national security adviser and former *Wall Street Journal* reporter in China, guided by experiences in South Korea and Japan, recommended that masks be delivered to the White House in mid-February, but senior administration officials directed staffers not to wear them.[31]

Instead of acting on these warnings coming from members of his own administration, Trump kept a normal schedule. He went golfing and on a trip to India, all while the task force was running worst-case scenarios that made it clear that quarantine, isolation, and mitigation efforts needed to be put in place immediately.[32] On February 24 Trump tweeted, "The Coronavirus is very much under control in the USA. We are in contact with everyone and all relevant countries. CDC & World Health have been working hard and very smart. Stock Market starting to look very good to me!" This was the first time he had tweeted about the coronavirus since February 7—surprising for such a prolific tweeter. On February 26 Trump reported that there were only fifteen cases of COVID-19 in the country and that "within a couple of days [it is] going to be down to close to zero."[33] And Larry Kudlow, the president's National Economic Council director, told CNBC that "we have contained this. I won't say airtight, but it's pretty close to airtight."[34]

The inconvenient truth about image management and projections of strength is that you can only control the narrative for so long before the news and weight of global events will outpace you. As early as February 5, Senator Chris Murphy (D-CT) tweeted, "Just left the Administration briefing on Coronavirus. Bottom line: they aren't taking this seriously enough. Notably, no request for ANY emergency funding, which is a big mistake. Local health systems need supplies, training, screening staff etc. And they need it now." As outbreaks emerged around the world, Trump's silence and gaslighting conveyed a message of indifference and unseriousness.

To make matters worse, the virus was spreading without detection across the United States because there was no comprehensive program to test, trace, and isolate. The WHO issued protocols for countries to manufacture tests for "diagnostic detection of 2019-nCOV" on January 17, building off the German model,[35] but the United States chose to develop its own test. On February 5 the CDC began shipping its test to public health labs across the country, but within days these tests were reported to be unusable, and this would remain the case for almost a month.[36] An investigation by Health and Human Services would later document how this catastrophic error was a product of myriad dysfunctions and system failures, including lack of leadership and coordination at the federal level.[37] In one instance, a CDC employee admitted that it was not "politically possible" to copy the WHO test under Trump: "Imagine the backlash we would have had if the CDC had said, 'Hey, yeah, let's use a German test.'"[38]

As state health agencies waited for the CDC to fix its faulty diagnostic tests, hospitals were not permitted to use the WHO-distributed test,[39] and clinical and commercial labs were prohibited from developing and using their own. Trump declared on February 26 that "we're testing everybody that we need to test"; in reality, only three states had any testing capacity at all.[40] It was on this same day that the CDC confirmed the first U.S. case of COVID-19 through community exposure, that is, in a patient without recent travel history or known exposure to a positive patient.[41] By the time the Food and Drug Administration authorized the CDC test in late February and in the absence of market competitors, the limited availability of tests meant that they had to be rationed. Michael Shearer and other *New York Times* staff writers would refer to February as "the lost month" that made containment impossible.[42] As we emphasized in chapter 1, a gutted federal bureaucracy and a wobbly and unequal health care system would have handicapped the ability of the United States to respond to the pandemic, but the Trump administration's deliberate inaction crippled the public health authorities from the pandemic's earliest days.

Meanwhile, the travel ban that Trump had signed back in January to stop travelers from China coming to the United States was no ban at all, merely a set of restrictions. Travelers with American passports were still admitted, as were tourists returning from China and residents of Hong Kong and Macao, who were not subject to restriction. An estimated 430,000 people came to the United States from China in the period after the ban was put into place on more than 1,300 direct flights from China arriving at seventeen U.S. cities with uneven CDC screening protocols.[43] Yet, Trump repeatedly circled back to his "China travel ban" as a great achievement, boasting in a February 28 tweet that "I was busy calling early BORDER & FLIGHT closings, putting us way ahead in our battle with Coronavirus. Dems called it VERY wrong!"

By late February—with only a handful of diagnosed cases in the United States but with the general lack of testing making it impossible to know how widespread the pandemic was—the window of opportunity was closing. Democrats were pushing for more transparency and preparedness behind the scenes, but there were few COVID-related tweets by members of Congress in the entire month of February. For instance, between February 19 and February 25 only 3 percent of tweets were about COVID-19, but by the following week this number would jump to 15 percent.[44] Meanwhile, Trump was publicly claiming that "it's going to disappear. One day—it's like a miracle—it will disappear."[45] Republicans were also blaming Democrats for politicizing the pandemic, with Trump characterizing their criticism of his administration's handling of the pandemic as a "new hoax." The right-wing media followed in lockstep with his public message. Rush Limbaugh stated on his radio program that "it looks like the coronavirus is being weaponized as yet another element to bring down Donald Trump. Now, I want to tell you the truth about the coronavirus. . . . Yeah, I'm dead right on this. The coronavirus is the common cold, folks."[46] A Fox News anchor claimed that the virus was another attempt to impeach Trump.[47]

This emerging focus on the president's political fortunes rather than pandemic preparedness is what turned policy disagreements into partisan politicization. Instead of confronting criticism about the lack of preparedness by announcing new plans for how to manage the pandemic or even reassuring (falsely) that preparations were sufficient so that Americans should feel safe, Limbaugh was instructing his listeners to think about Trump first and the nation's health second—if at all. This subtle change in emphasis had devastating consequences by tying the news about the pandemic to opinions about the president. Rather than responding to ongoing news about the spread of the coronavirus with greater demands for government action or personal sacrifice, those who supported Trump had been primed to discount the news itself.

The American people were hearing from Trump and were also hearing from the media, but they were not hearing from health experts in February. This is different from other high-income countries that found that communication was a key factor in establishing early compliance and—to recall a saying of the time—to "flatten the curve." For instance, Taiwan prioritized frequent and transparent communication with the goal of reaching as many residents as possible. To do so, Taiwan flooded information outlets with high-quality material, from YouTube and memes to broadcast media. Taiwan's digital minister Audrey Tang helped to develop a map with real-time updates about mask supplies in pharmacies.[48] A unified government response focused on high-quality information helped to align Taiwanese citizens with government priorities.

In the end, Trump only began to take the pandemic seriously when it was clear that it would have dire effects on the U.S. economy that would be impossible to hide. CDC spokesperson Dr. Nancy Messonnier was the first person from within the government to make a public statement that conveyed the seriousness of COVID-19 to the American public. Her February 26 warning included recommendations for telework, closing schools, and cancellation of mass gatherings, and she concluded that "I understand this whole situation may seem overwhelming and that disruption to everyday life may be severe. But these are things that people need to start thinking about now."[49]

Messonnier's warning fully undercut Trump's carefully cultivated image of strength. Her statement spooked investors, producing a 1,000-point dive in the Dow Jones Industrial Average. Messonnier was removed from her position the very next day, and Trump expressed privately his desire to fire her altogether.[50] This clarion call ended the myth that "all would be fine," but it was still an image that Trump attempted to maintain. He started tweeting about the novel coronavirus every day, congratulating the CDC and his task force appointees for "doing such a fine job" while bragging about low numbers.

As the reality of the virus began to set in, the gap between official commentary and everyday experience grew wider and wider. Trump was projecting confidence, while CVS and Walgreens were warning Americans about hand sanitizer shortages.[51] Privately, on February 29 Navarro received a dire warning from virologist and Trump adviser Steven Hatfill, who said, "In truth we do not have a clue how many are infected in the USA. We are expecting the first wave to spread in the U.S. within the next 7 days."[52]

David Frum, in an essay for *The Atlantic* titled "This Is Trump's Fault," wrote about this critical juncture, and it is worth quoting here at length:

> By February 28, it was too late to exclude the coronavirus from the United States. It was too late to test and trace. . . . It was too late to refill the stockpiles. . . . It was too late to produce sufficient ventilators in sufficient time. But on February 28, it was still not too late to arrange an orderly distribution of medical supplies to the states, not too late to coordinate with U.S. allies, not too late to close the Florida beaches before spring break, not too late to bring passengers home from cruise lines, not too late to ensure that state unemployment-insurance offices were staffed and ready, not too late for local governments to get funds to food banks, not too

late to begin social distancing fast and early. Stay-at-home orders could have been put into effect on March 1, not in late March and early April."[53]

On March 1 the United States reported its second death from COVID-19, and New York reported its first positive case. The first high school in the Seattle area closed after a student and parent tested positive. It was not too late for a forceful response, but the window on a unified nonpartisan response was practically closed. Acknowledging the reality of the situation would undercut Trump's image of confidence, contradicting his insistence that the pandemic was either a minor inconvenience or a partisan conspiracy. In placing image management above proactive public health measures, Trump not only activated partisan loyalty but also aligned political sides with a false dichotomy between following the science versus following their partisan leaders.

We call this a false dichotomy because there is no inherent trade-off between following science and partisan loyalty. For instance, Democrats and Republicans were both as likely to get a flu vaccine before the pandemic.[54] Fully aware of his polarizing nature as president and on the coattails of such a charged impeachment proceeding, Trump could have put epidemiologists on his coronavirus task force, mobilized FEMA and its procedures for disaster response, directed emergency funds to the states, and put scientists out front and supported their messages. Even an embattled president could have unified the country by endorsing the evolving science, activating existing protocols, invoking policy mechanisms to ramp up domestic production of PPE, and speaking to the American people with direct honesty. This is what a nonpoliticized response would have looked like. And it is entirely possible for even polarizing heads of state to lead a nonpoliticized response, as illustrated by countries such as the United Kingdom, South Korea, and Taiwan that are bitterly divided over politics.

Trump chose differently. With every day that he remained silent, he lost the ability to establish a narrative that could supersede the thoroughgoing partisan differences characterizing American politics. And with every day spent gaslighting Americans, telling them not to believe their own eyes and instead focus on his own successful leadership, the pandemic became worse. By early March, the disjuncture between Trump's narrative and the pandemic reality put us through Alice's proverbial looking glass. By the first week of March, the window of opportunity for a unified response was closed. The pandemic was already partisan.

Deflection and Denial

The first survey of Americans' views of COVID-19 of which we are aware is a Reuters/Ipsos poll released on March 6, 2020, when Trump was still publicly downplaying the seriousness of the coronavirus.[55] Already by this date there were stark differences in how Republicans and Democrats thought about COVID-19. Democrats were twice as likely as Republicans to believe that COVID-19 was an "imminent threat to the United States." After a month of downplaying and conservative news coverage that minimized the seriousness of COVID-19, it is not difficult to explain this divergence. As Jennifer McCoy, an expert on polarization and its consequences for democracy, observes, "Our hyper-polarization is so strong that we don't even assess a potential health crisis in the same way. And so it impedes our ability to address it." Indeed, hyperpolarization divided Americans, affecting how they think of themselves, their partisan allies, their political opponents, and the news that they encounter. The consequence was a polarized partisan media environment, one that made COVID-19 not just about public health also but a referendum on the Trump administration.

Partisan polarization, like other preexisting conditions, would make it hard to manage a pandemic. But preexisting conditions did not mean that deep partisan differences over health behavior and attitudes were inevitable. As we show in the following chapters, there were Democrats willing to support strong border controls (an immigration position typically held by Republicans) and Republicans willing to support strong measures for COVID economic relief (a welfare position typically held by Democrats). And there is nothing inherently partisan about protective measures; for example, one can imagine a scenario where Republicans strongly endorse mask mandates if it means getting the country back to business. Yet such measures, like many other health behaviors, became partisan issues.[56] Even as attitudes toward COVID-19 itself settled into partisan camps during the first wave, there was cooperation across partisan lines to flatten the curve in both Democratic- and Republican-led states.[57] Individuals respond to elite cues and behaviors, and elites—foremost among them Trump and the mass media—chose partisanship. In the absence of nonpartisan leadership, partisan messaging created partisan conflict over what was a fundamentally nonpartisan public health emergency.

We can draw on other countries' experiences to see how divided places managed the pandemic's politics differently. Recall that the United Kingdom is similarly polarized as the United States, most recently along the political issue of Brexit, finalized on February 1, 2020.[58] Brexit could have been an easy issue for dividing public opinion during the pandemic in the United Kingdom, where obtaining PPE, closing borders, and prioritizing economic openness could all have become political issues. But in a March 30 YouGov poll of British adults, a majority across the political spectrum agreed that the coronavirus outbreak had brought the United Kingdom together.[59] By late April Prime Minister Boris Johnson, having recently recovered from coronavirus, would emphasize that "if we can show the same spirit of unity and determination as we've all shown in the past six weeks then I have absolutely no doubt that we will beat it."[60] While classically upbeat and optimistic, this messaging also recognized the British public's impatience with lockdowns and shared suffering. This type of optimistic but honest messaging and unity could have occurred in the United States. Moreover, this solidarity persisted: in June 2020 the British public overwhelmingly agreed with the statement (89%) that "people have a civic duty to self-isolate for 14 days if they have been in contact with somebody who had been diagnosed with coronavirus."[61]

In the first week of March 2020, Trump continued to project optimism without honesty. On March 2, the eve of Super Tuesday, he held a rally in Charlotte, North Carolina. When asked about the health implications of a large gathering, Trump asserted, "I think it's very safe." On March 3 he toured National Institutes of Health and spoke about Phase I trials for a potential vaccine, and Azar confirmed sixty cases in the United States and forty-eight repatriated cases. And the very next day Trump stated that "a lot of people will have this and it's very mild." He also said in an interview on Fox News that he thought the death rate reported by the WHO was "really a false number."

March 6 was a busy day. Trump signed into law the COVID-19 Preparedness and Response Supplemental Appropriations Act, which dedicated billions to pandemic response. Trump also toured the CDC in Atlanta while also taking time to criticize Democratic governor of Washington Jay Inslee, who was urging the president take the virus more seriously.[62] Meanwhile, ten states reported their first case that day.

By this time Trump's messaging became erratic, simultaneously blaming Democrats, denying the severity of the pandemic, and boasting falsely about his administration's accomplishments. While at the CDC he asserted, "Anybody that wants a test can get a test." This was simply not the case. In reality, just under two thousand tests were performed on March 6.[63] Meanwhile, COVID was spreading without detection, Americans were emptying supermarket shelves, and sellers were price gouging for hard-to-get items such as hand sanitizer.[64] Many Americans had the impression that the COVID-19 pandemic was concentrated in the epicenters of Washington State and New York City, and on March 8 Surgeon General Jerome Adams said he believed that COVID-19 was contained in certain areas of the country.[65] On March 9, Trump compared COVID-19 to the seasonal flu on Twitter: "So last year 37,000 Americans died from the common Flu. It averages between 27,000 and 70,000 per year. Nothing is shut down, life & the economy go on. At this moment there are 546 confirmed cases of CoronaVirus, with 22 deaths. Think about that!"

That same day, the coronavirus task force addressed the nation on television. Trump began by declaring that the coronavirus was "very much under control" and spoke about tax relief and the hotel and cruise industries, flanked by Vice President Mike Pence and the surgeon general. Dr. Deborah Birx spoke about how to keep workplaces, schools, and restaurants safe, saying "communities are at the center of this" in reference to a set of guidelines available online. Other task force members focused on nursing homes, telehealth options, and the oil market. The message was that the pandemic was under control and that the administration had its hands on the wheel.

But in reality, Americans started to realize the magnitude of the pandemic even if they did not yet appreciate how long the effects would last. Organizations were beginning to cancel events without direction from the federal government, a step that Fauci called "prudent." Meanwhile, Ohio State University suspended in-person instruction, and California was banning large events. Northern Italy was already in quarantine, Ireland canceled all of its St. Patrick's Day parades, and Israel was requiring anyone who entered the country—citizens and nonnationals alike—to self-quarantine for fourteen days. The city of Madrid, Spain, announced that it was closing all schools, nurseries, and universities.

March 10, 2020, might have been the last day that Trump felt in control of the narrative. Publicly he uttered perhaps his most ignominious words to reporters at the U.S. Capitol: "We're prepared, and we're doing a great job with it. And it will go away. Just stay calm. It will go away." To be fair, he may have believed this. Fauci, Birx, the surgeon general, and others all seemed to be on the same page: this was a virus that predominately affected the elderly, triage should be focused on instances of community spread, and young adults without underlying health conditions should take precautionary measures such as washing their hands. Behind closed doors, Republican senators were urging Trump to make Fauci "the face of the federal government's response" because "he has credibility" and "speaks with authority."[66]

The next day, the National Basketball Association suspend the remainder of its 2020 season after Utah Jazz player Rudy Goberts tested positive. This augured a cascade of cancellations across American public life: sports, music, arts, and ultimately schools.

Basketball is a multibillion-dollar industry with global reach. That the National Basketball Association felt that the virus was serious enough to cancel the entire remaining season, in the absence of federal guidelines, brought the reality of COVID-19 home for Americans. The government was saying and doing one thing, but Americans were living and observing something else.

That evening, the president made remarks about COVID-19 from the Oval Office for the first time. Trump began his address with "From the beginning of time, nations and people have faced unforeseen challenges, including large-scale and very dangerous health threats" and spoke about "early, intense action," referencing his travel ban from China. He also compared the U.S. successes with conditions in Europe and extended the travel ban to include twenty-five European countries (the United Kingdom and Ireland were added later). He spoke about maintaining good hygiene but reassured businesses and investors, who had just seen the Dow drop 1,400 points only two days after a loss of 2,000 points: "This is not a financial crisis, this is just a temporary moment of time." Trump concluded his address by declaring that "the virus will not have a chance against us. . . . We have the best economy, the most advanced health care, and the most talented doctors, scientists and researchers anywhere in the world. We are all in this together. We must put politics aside, stop the partisanship, and unify together as one nation and one family."

This was the nonpartisan, unifying message that would allow an effective national response to the pandemic. But the very next day, Trump tweeted to millions of followers that "Sleepy Joe Biden was in charge of the H1N1 Swine Flu epidemic which killed thousands of people. The response was one of the worst on record. Our response is one of the best, with fast action of border closings & a 78% Approval Rating, the highest on record. His was lowest!" Even as Trump was posturing as a "wartime president" by finally taking the pandemic seriously, he—like the conservative media—continued to liken it to "seasonal flu."[67]

But of course, COVID-19 was not like the seasonal flu, and evidence from other countries easily foretold what would happen next.

Some countries, such as South Korea and China, were already past their peak. Caseloads in South Korea had been on the decline since February 29 largely due to comprehensive testing and screening as well as an intensive set of mitigation policies, from monitoring positive individuals who do not require inpatient care to providing food, toiletries, and psychological support to make quarantine easier.[68] By mid-March, China was also ending lockdown of most of Hubei Province (with a population of fifty-six million), while its capital city Wuhan stayed in lockdown another two weeks. Lockdowns in China were severe: the only people on the streets were police and emergency personnel. But in an authoritarian single-party regime, Chinese officials are not accountable to an elected legislature or to citizens and are unconstrained in their ability to monitor and surveil their citizens. Italy, by contrast, had locked down Lombardy and fourteen other provinces, affecting sixteen million residents.[69] But Italy is a democracy, so it combined a series of inducements and controls to keep caseloads low after lockdown. Germany, while not locked down yet, was already testing at scale—including asymptomatic people, which we now understand is key to managing the coronavirus's spread.

By early March, COVID was probably spreading uncontrollably in every state. Yet almost no one was being tested; whereas the United States was testing hundreds of Americans a day, other countries with much smaller populations were testing thousands. On the local news Americans were seeing hospitals inundated with patients. Workplaces were shuttering on the heels of governors' orders. Preschools were closing. The everyday experience of most Americans stood in sharp contrast to the Trump administration's messaging.

By mid-March, it was already too late to stop the partisan politics of COVID-19 in the United States. In a March survey from the Pew Research Center, 79 percent of respondents who primarily watched Fox News as their main source of political news said that the news media had "greatly" or "slightly" exaggerated the risk from coronavirus. This compares to 54 percent who watched CNN and 35 percent who watched MSNBC.[70] Trump's early strategy of denying the pandemic's severity and then blaming Democrats had become the dominant political narrative.

On March 15, a *New York Times* opinion essay by columnist David Leonhardt soberly indicted the president's early response to COVID-19: "He could have taken action. He didn't."[71] And in the absence of presidential leadership and action, states, communities, companies, and cultural organizations took matters into their own hands to—as Yascha Mounk of *The Atlantic* worded it in his March 10 column—"cancel everything."[72] On March 16, six counties in the San Francisco Bay Area announced a "shelter in place" order. California issued the first statewide stay-at-home order on March 19. By late March, nearly every aspect of American life had been affected by COVID-19: schools were closed across the country, all but the most essential businesses were shuttered, casinos were closed in Las Vegas, and air travel had ground to a halt. Democratic presidential nominee Joe Biden released his first advertisement targeting the president's handling of the COVID-19 pandemic. Biden's point was plain: "Trump knew. He failed."

If Trump had ever wanted Americans to take the pandemic seriously, he undermined that goal both by resorting to partisanship blame and simultaneously undercutting nonpartisan efforts to manage the crisis with tweets such as "WE CANNOT LET THE CURE BE WORSE THAN THE PROBLEM ITSELF" and, in what was heard by supporters as a deliberately ambiguous statement regarding the CDC face mask recommendation on April 3, "It's going to be, really, a voluntary thing. You can do it. You don't have to do it. I'm choosing not to do it, but some people may want to do it, and that's OK. It may be good. Probably will."[73] All the while, Trump and his press briefings would keep an eye on when the economy would reopen again: first it was in fifteen days, then reopening by Easter. By April 17 he was tweeting "LIBERATE MICHIGAN!" to encourage the armed Michigan protestors who took to Lansing to oppose COVID stay-at-home orders issued by Democratic governor Gretchen Whitmer.

Attaching a partisan valence to public health efforts counts as one of Trump's more dangerous decisions, one that traded American lives for short-lived face-saving in an election year. This was a risky game, one that some Republican state governors were unwilling to play at the outset of the pandemic. For instance, Governor Mike DeWine of Ohio—an avowed conservative Republican—departed early from Trump, becoming a notable "follower of science" by frequently deferring to director of the Ohio Department of Health Amy Acton.[74] DeWine canceled the 2020 Democratic presidential primary a day before the scheduled election on March 17, only to a have a judge overrule his decision. Acton then closed the polling centers due to a health emergency. Trump loyalists tried to curb DeWine and Acton's authority, especially after DeWine's cautious extension of Ohio's stay-at-home "Stay Safe Order" until May 29, long after Trump's goal of reopening after Easter. In May, state House Republicans put forward a bill to limit the Ohio Department of Health's powers by requiring that health closure extensions be approved by a joint legislative committee. Protestors also started to show up at Acton's home, and by summer she had left her position.

But Ohio's DeWine and Massachusetts governor Charlie Baker were exceptions among state-level Republican officials. Most Republican governors followed in lockstep Trump's tone and leadership. Eight governors—all Republican—decided against issuing statewide stay-at-home orders altogether. One explanation for this policy choice was that there was no nationwide order from the CDC, which Trump was always reluctant to issue. But Republican governors also associated public health measures with individual liberty. Governor Kristi Noem of South Dakota stated plainly that "the people themselves are primarily responsible for their safety" and upheld the U.S. Constitution as a mechanism "prevent[ing] us from taking draconian measures much like the Chinese government has done."[75]

Framing the pandemic as a choice between government mandates and personal freedom would become a consistent theme in subsequent months. This distinction was perhaps best summarized by South Carolina governor Henry McMaster: "We are not ordering people to stay at home, but from the very beginning we've been telling people to stay home."[76] Opposing pandemic measures became synonymous with opposing government authority and preserving personal liberty. This type of "rugged individualism"[77] played right to the core of Trump's antiestablishment, antielite voter base, who viewed those who followed pro–social health behaviors and stay-at-home orders as "sheep."

These themes—downplaying the seriousness of the pandemic and linking it with individual rights and personal choice—were the predominate elite cues from Republican leadership. In a polarized political landscape, Democrats would predictably organize around another set of messages (although opposing Trump is itself sufficient to motivate many Democrats). An essay in the journal *Science* studied Twitter messages as cues sent to the public by members of the U.S. House and Senate during the onset of the pandemic.[78] The essay's authors found that Democrats not only talked about the pandemic more but also that their tweets more frequently emphasized health content and consequences for the American worker. By contrast, Republican tweets—when focusing on the pandemic—mentioned China and American businesses. These nonoverlapping messages produced what the authors label as an "elusive consensus." Republican and Democratic elites were speaking about the pandemic in fundamentally different ways as they communicated fundamentally different concerns to their constituents. While privately they were working together to pass emergency legislation—Trump signed the Coronavirus Aid, Relief, and Economic Security Act (CARES) into law on March 27 after a contentious but ultimately productive bipartisan effort—the public messaging by political parties was quite different. As parties and political elites settled on a partisan message, the mass public followed.

These divisive messages from political leaders were amplified through the partisan media environment, and media elites also generated their own messaging that strengthened their ideological side. Put baldly, CNN and MSNBC spoke about the pandemic differently than Fox News and—in extremist manifestations—Newsmax and One America News Network (OANN). And while we could typically ignore the far-right propaganda and disinformation of a channel such as OANN or Breitbart, Trump gave these outlets unprecedented legitimacy by issuing them press passes to be part of the White House press corps. He even retweeted these extreme-right outlets while simultaneously denigrating mainstream media, thus legitimizing them to a wider audience of followers: "I watch and listen to the Fake News, CNN, MSDNC, ABC, NBC, CBS, some of FOX (desperately & foolishly pleading to be politically correct), the @nytimes, & the @washingtonpost, and all I see is hatred of me at any cost" (March 22).

How was the conservative media discussing COVID? We know that at the outset, conservative media alleged that the COVID-19 pandemic was not as bad as the numbers made it seem to be and openly stated that information about the pandemic was being manipulated in order to harm Trump's reelection chances. They even forwarded a narrative that the emerging pandemic was the Democrats' fault. Breitbart, for example, pushed the line that Democrats had ignored the pandemic in their drive to impeach Trump.[79] Aside from this commentary, conservative media also forwarded dangerous misinformation. Fox News zealously promoted hydroxychloroquine, an unproven and potentially dangerous COVID-19 "treatment," nearly three hundred times between March 23 and April 6.[80] On March 21, Trump began to echo this dangerous claim on Twitter: "HYDROXY-CHLOROQUINE & AZITHROMYCIN, taken together, have a real chance to be one of the biggest game changers in the history of medicine." An OANN host even encouraged Americans to get coronavirus to build immunity.[81] And while mainstream news sources attempted nonpartisan coverage—and frequently called out their Fox News counterpart for dangerous disinformation—they nevertheless aired Trump's coronavirus press briefings each day without attempting to fact-check his claims.

Media outlets are the primary source of information about current events for most Americans. Research on COVID-19 and the media has found that the news Americans watch had a direct effect on their attitudes and behavior. Fox News viewers were more likely to travel,[82] less likely to socially distance,[83] and less likely to purchase hand sanitizer and masks.[84] Shockingly, these same conservative media outlets were a primary "intelligence" source for Trump himself. In one example, Trump reported in an interview on Fox that he got information on ventilator needs by watching Sean Hannity.[85] Trump even lifted footage of Hannity positively discussing Trump's handling of the pandemic and presented it during the televised April 13 coronavirus task force briefing.

This narrative only brings us to early April. Yet through elite messaging, party rallying, and the mass media, the pandemic was already politicized. From early denial and deflection to a combative offensive, the message from the Trump administration was all partisan.

Federalism and the States: COVID-19 Politics beyond Washington

The story of the pandemic so far has largely been one of Trump's pathologies, making decisions in a polarized political environment to safeguard his electoral prospects. But one of the key takeaways to early inaction is that much of the COVID-19 response was relegated to the states. The last piece of the early pandemic story is understanding what happened between the federal government and the states. In it, we see some of America's unique pathologies, namely how federalism and the states' uncoordinated health care systems stymied early efforts to contain the pandemic.

In America's federal system, state governments play a central role in managing public health crises, but the federal government acts as an essential coordinator, with federal emergency declarations allowing it to channel resources to states in need. This is not dissimilar to the pressures facing Germany, in which because of its federal constitutional structure, *Länder* (state) minister-presidents have a lot of authority. Chancellor Angela Merkel was reluctant to lead from up front, which would inevitably produce a much-criticized belated response, with one expert writing that "there's 'Keep-calm-and-carry-on' and then there's burying one's head in the sand."[86]

But the U.S. response was not simply belated; it was also uncoordinated, chaotic, and inconsistent, a response that dangerously pitted states against the federal government—and states against each other—in bidding wars for PPE. When the president disavowed himself of responsibility ("No I don't take any responsibility at all")—but, oddly enough, not authority ("When somebody is the president of the United States, the authority is total")—the emergency response would necessarily be centered in the states. Yet the sober truth is that the federal government could not have fully responded to the pandemic even if it wanted to. In a survey of federal workers during the pandemic, only one-third of respondents indicated that their agency was of adequate size and quality to fulfill the mission of the agency.[87] This is the consequence of both the long-term decay of federal bureaucracies and Trump's disinterest in governing and personnel management.

The federal government's own inaction explains why resources were scarce to begin with. In January and early February, the United States was still exporting PPE to China. And as global supply chains ground to a halt, the coronavirus task force did not make the national stockpile a priority, and the president did not invoke the Defense Production Act. This law allows the president to redirect domestic producers to make critical goods in support of the nation in times of emergency. Trump was both late to use it (having criticized it as antibusiness and likening it to nationalization)[88] and moderate in its use when he did. On March 18 he invoked the Defense Production Act but stopped short of implementing it to force production on certain goods, such as ventilator parts and PPE. Instead of ordering domestic companies to produce, say, more face masks and promising them bulk purchase orders from the U.S. government, any supply that was produced was subject to bidding wars on the open market. Distilleries would begin to produce hand sanitizer and clothing manufacturers would start to make masks, but they did this to meet market demand, not because they were responding to the Trump administration's orders.

As the states could not rely on the federal government and its depleted national stockpile for assistance, they instead had to fend for themselves. Without federal government coordination, states competed against one another—and even against the federal government—to secure masks and other essential goods. With all states trying to acquire ventilators to treat critically ill COVID-19 patients, bidding wars started driving prices up.[89] Some states formed alliances, such as California, Oregon and Washington's Western States Pact, to cut down on bidding wars and improve allocation. And in several instances, notably California, the federal government would only assist in supplying the state with (in this case) cotton swabs if Governor Gavin Newsom asked Trump personally and thanked him publicly.[90] Maryland governor Larry Hogan, a Republican, put his state's COVID-19 testing supplies under the watch of the Maryland National Guard,[91] fearful that the federal government might confiscate it, as reports had circulated of such actions by FEMA in other states.

Rather than using existing infrastructure to support the pandemic response, the Trump administration relied on business contacts outside of government for solutions. The administration tasked senior White House adviser and Trump son-in-law Jared Kushner to head a coronavirus supply chain task force to supply states with ventilators and PPE. Kushner's strategy relied on private industry connections and personal relationships instead of the infrastructure at FEMA, and the task force itself was composed of inexperienced volunteers.[92] By all accounts—including a prominent whistleblower complaint—this federal procurement operation was a disaster. In the aftermath, Kushner sough to deflect blame. "The notion of the federal stockpile was it's supposed to be *our* stockpile," he said during one press briefing. "It's not supposed to be states' stockpiles that they then use."[93] This is quite obviously false, a display of not only shocking incompetence but also callous indifference to the welfare of hundreds of millions of Americans.

It is not clear exactly why the federal government proved so unable or unwilling to coordinate the state-level responses and why it attempted to strategically shift responsibility and authority to the states. There are at least three potential explanations, none of which are mutually exclusive. First, it may have been entirely accidental and a consequence of administrative incompetence, with ill-prepared advisers such as Kushner playing key roles in the White House's coronavirus task force. Second, it may have been ideological, consistent with the Republican Party's conservative beliefs in limited government. In reference to demands for PPE, a *Vanity Fair* exposé reported Kushner remarking that the "free market will solve this" and "that is not the role of government."[94] This explanation simultaneously (and conveniently) also exculpates Trump from obligation and responsibility.

A third possibility is that the Trump administration's unwillingness to coordinate the states was political, and that the Trump administration deliberately refused to coordinate an early national response and help the states in greatest need as a way to punish Democratic-led states, states that would not help his reelection campaign. In the same *Vanity Fair* article, a meeting attendee remarked that "in hindsight it's not crazy to think it was some purposeful belief that it was okay if [Andrew] Cuomo had a tough go of it because [New York] was a blue state."[95]

Regardless of motivation, no one was held accountable for the administration's catastrophic failures. So, with the vacuum of federal leadership, states were left to fend for themselves, and much of their decisions would be shaped by partisanship, yielding an uneven patchwork of state-level responses. Republican governors as well as governors from states with more Trump supporters were either resistant to adopting or slower to adopt stay-at-home policies such as social distancing.[96] There were some notable exceptions: DeWine, Baker, Hogan, and Vermont governor Phil Scott—all Republicans— were early adopters of social distancing guidelines in their states. But by and large, the story in the states replicated the story at the federal level: Republican Party governors and Republican-dominated states aligned with the Trump administration's politics.

Meanwhile, Democratic-led states not only implemented stay-at-home orders early—states such as California, Illinois, and New Jersey were among the first but also among the hardest hit—but were also among the last in lifting shutdown orders. A study by the CDC shows that states with stay-at-home orders were able to reduce population movement and thus reduce community spread of COVID-19.[97] And as the scientific community's understanding of the virus evolved to identify the necessity of face masks (the CDC recommended on April 3 that all Americans wear them), that too would be framed as a policy suggestion to be implemented with state discretion. Trump remarked at an April 23 press briefing that he had "no problem with face masks, if the governors want to do that."

Meanwhile, most Americans were not protesting. Small businesses were shuttered along with businesses and schools. Most Americans were at home. By the end of 2020, the American economy had lost nine million jobs, with losses concentrated in leisure and hospitality sectors as well as bars and restaurants and other low-paying industries. This is over three times as many jobs lost in the United States as in the European Union (a community of twenty-seven member states and a combined population of nearly five hundred million people). While the European Union states largely maintain robust health care and employment retention schemes,[98] the United States instead relied on stimulus checks and compensation. In the United States, almost forty million Americans filed for unemployment by May 2020,[99] and only a third of Americans ended up back in their old job after six months.[100] Without a comprehensive social safety net such as robust unemployment protections, many Americans found themselves behind on bills, unable to buy food, and evicted if their work hours were cut or their place of employment shut down.

Moreover, many of these job losses were in areas that could not move to remote work. And jobs classified as essential—from nurses to grocery store shelf-stocking—were disproportionately held by Black Americans.[101] Not only could essential workers not work from home, taking precautionary measures to protect themselves and their families, but they also couldn't supervise at-home learning. The early days of the pandemic created a sharp difference in experiences based on income, occupation, and race. Endemic inequality meant that some Americans could withstand the shock of a job loss or a pay cut with little trouble. Those with means not only have access to better health care services but are also more likely to be able to work from home—and thus enjoy more job security—and avoid contact with others, all essential practices for containing community spread of the virus. Meanwhile, many American workers faced a difficult trade-off between caring for themselves and their families and keeping their jobs and paychecks. In a stark illustration, as the *New York Times* was covering stories of Manhattanites retreating the city for their second homes upstate (a "a family compound meant for entertaining—not work")[102] and hiring tutors to run "pandemic pods" when schools went online,[103] you could also find examples of children without laptops or internet who had to sit in a parking lot outside of a McDonalds or a closed public library in order to "attend" class online or submit work.

By the end of April 2020, America had passed a grim milestone: one million confirmed cases of COVID-19. Americans' experiences in the pandemic at this time were very much a product of where they lived, which in turn was shaped by partisanship of those in charge. Meanwhile, the president was making increasingly worrying statements that undercut prohealth messaging, including about injecting disinfectant and "hit[ting] the body with a tremendous, whether it's ultraviolet or just very powerful light" (April 23); "that testing is, frankly, overrated" (May 14);[104] and that he was taking a preventative treatment not authorized by the Food and Drug Administration ("I'm taking it—hydroxychloroquine"). The president was also making decisions that abandoned federal responsibility. For instance, to encourage mask use and overcome supply chain issues, the United States Post Office and the Department of Health and Human Services drafted plans to send 650 million reusable face masks, or 5 masks per household, to every person in the country, but this plan was canceled by the White House to avoid "concern or panic."[105] These steps did not simply deny the pandemic; they made it worse. By the end of May, the number of COVID-related deaths in the United States had passed 100,000.

The Pandemic Settles In

As the virus spread beyond Washington and New York, it became a truly American catastrophe. Journalist Ed Yong wrote in a bold essay in *The Atlantic* in August 2020 that COVID-19 "defeated America" in that it "humbled and humiliated the planet's most powerful nation." The sad fact is that despite the many initial unknowns about the virus itself—how it spread, who is most vulnerable, how to treat it, and how best to avoid it—the trajectory of events in the United States had been predictable since the early days of spring. By the end of April, we knew everything we needed to know about how Americans would respond.

To restate one of our central arguments, the COVID-19 pandemic was always going to be bad because of America's unique preexisting conditions, but it was not inevitable that COVID would rip apart America. It could have been different. The United States entered the COVID-19 pandemic with a strong economy but a polarized political system, an image-focused president, a hollowed-out federal bureaucracy, and a health care system beset by inequality in access and quality of care. Yet there was a window of opportunity in February and early March when Trump could have put trusted health officials out front, reinforced their messages, unified Democratic and Republican leadership through bipartisan messaging, and put politics aside to flatten the curve. But when given the opportunity to take costly actions to protect American lives, the Trump administration too often decided to project an image of strong leadership and good news. When the pandemic proved too serious to ignore, Trump turned defensive, lashing out at his political opponents, deflecting blame, and relegating responsibility to the states without supporting them at the federal level.

Throughout this chapter, we have compared the United States to other high-income countries: the United Kingdom, Germany, South Korea, and Taiwan. The American experience with COVID-19 as a fundamentally political issue stands in sharp contrast to each of these countries, even though many of them are sharply polarized (the United Kingdom, South Korea, and Taiwan) or are a federal state (Germany) that requires coordination among many jurisdictions. Pandemic management under Trump was no less than disastrous, but the United States was not the only country to suffer so mightily from the COVID-19 pandemic.

In the end, the country whose experience perhaps most closely matches that of the United States, especially in those critical early months, is Brazil. Like the United States, Brazil is a federal state with a presidential system of government. Brazil is also a highly unequal society, with vast differences in state capacity and material welfare across the states that are a partial legacy of chattel slavery. And Brazil is led by a conservative populist with authoritarian ambitions, Jair Bolsonaro. Unlike Trump, Bolsonaro has a military background and leads only a very small party within the Brazilian government. But as president, his style, braggadocio, and right-wing populist positions are eerily reminiscent of Trump.

Bolsonaro politicized the pandemic, with dire consequences. Brazil's first documented case was February 26. On March 6 Bolsonaro got on television and said, "The moment is for unity."[106] By March 24, Bolsonaro was already stating that "our lives have to go on. Jobs must be kept. . . . We must, yes, get back to normal."[107] Repeating a favorite Trump line, Bolsonaro would also state on television that "it's just a little flu" and "people are going to die, I'm sorry. . . . But we can't stop a car factory because there are traffic accidents."[108] In addition to denying the severity of the virus, Bolsonaro prioritized keeping the economy open at any cost. He fired his minister of health in mid-April over disagreements on social distancing guidelines. Bolsonaro also issued an executive order to strip states of the authority to restrict people's movement during the pandemic,[109] which was quickly revoked by Brazil's Supreme Federal Court. His son, Senator Flavio Bolsonaro, would tweet a government video with the hashtag #obrasilnãopodeparar ("Brazil can't stop").

As Brazil's cities were left to implement patchwork solutions, Jair Bolsonaro lashed out at local officials who implemented restrictive lockdowns. Moreover, Brazil's Ministry of Health, despite the lack of scientific evidence, supplied the administration of Manaus—a city in the Amazon region suffering from severe outbreaks and a lack of oxygen at the time—with ivermectin and chloroquine as treatments.[110] The editors of *The Lancet*, a British medical journal, declared at the time that "perhaps the biggest threat to Brazil's COVID-19 response is its president, Jair Bolsonaro."[111] And like Trump, Bolsonaro eventually tested positive for COVID-19. But surpassing even Trump's desire to protect an image of strength, Bolsonaro reported that he would not take a COVID-19 vaccine.[112]

Based on early social distancing and quarantine practices, a mid-2020 study estimated that in the state of São Paolo, if suppression and transmissibility stayed the same, the best estimate was of

9,551 deaths by the end of the pandemic.[113] These early policies were in spite of Bolsonaro. The early practices did not hold, and by mid-November 2021 this figure was at 153,000. By January 2021, right before vaccinations became available, Brazil would suffer the second-largest number of losses in the world, behind the United States. Vaccination would also be a slow endeavor, because unlike in other Latin American countries such as Chile and Colombia, Bolsonaro did not negotiate a vaccine contract in 2020. And unlike Trump, Bolsonaro did not direct Brazilian pharmaceutical companies to develop their own vaccines.

For Trump, like Bolsonaro, unifying efforts to claim that "we're all in this together" were the exception rather than the rule. And they were short-lived, immediately undercut, or framed as a voluntary personal choice. In the end, COVID-19 is a community disease requiring community-level responses. And as the pandemic dragged on and the U.S. election got closer, appeals to unity would become scarce. Instead of hard questions and honest answers, Americans heard their president in daily press briefings talk up his administration's "great successes" and achievements. Right when Americans needed to trust public officials and learn about how to protect themselves from a global pandemic, Americans heard their political and media elites talk about the pandemic in essentially partisan terms.

No country is perfect. The United Kingdom made a mess of its early pandemic response, and one of its prime minister's trusted political strategists created national headlines by violating the national lockdown repeatedly. But we view these political errors as fundamentally different from the deceptiveness and mendaciousness of the Trump administration. In the end, it was duplicity and violation of trust that finally cracked public support for Boris Johnson's COVID measures when on December 2021 he was exposed as having held multiple illegal gatherings at Downing Street a year earlier, violating COVID lockdown rules while the rest of the country was spending Christmas apart from their families.

Without social solidarity and political trust, it is hard to demand sacrifices of a country's citizens. Countries such as France, Italy, the

Netherlands, and the United Kingdom have repeatedly been forced to return to lockdown conditions, and this is enabled by a sense that each government is not deliberately fanning the flames of partisan disagreement as part of their COVID-19 response. Government trust is also necessary if you want citizens to download contact tracing apps such as Germany's Corona-Warn-App, which has been downloaded by more than fifteen million Germans. But in the United States trust was low, and a return to lockdown was never viable. Even during the winter of 2020–2021, the worst wave of all, shops and restaurants were open even though millions of schoolchildren were still learning from home.

Instead of building trust and solidarity, America's political elites chose partisanship. And no country was as politically polarized as the United States. A Pew study in the spring of 2021 looked at comparative attitudes on retrospective COVID-19 restrictions across eleven democracies.[114] The top-line finding is that the ideological Right was more likely to think there should have been fewer restrictions on public activity, but in the United States the gap between the Right (fewer restrictions at 52%) and left (at 7%) was enormous. The next closest gap was half that size (Australia, with a 21-point difference). The Netherlands and South Korea had among the smallest gaps, both at 11-point differences. Simply put, no other high-income democracy was as politicized and polarized as the United States.

Once set in motion, partisan politics proves sticky. Not even strong countermessaging attempts by Republican Party stalwarts such as former vice president Dick Cheney and former California governor Arnold Schwarzenegger could move Republican attitudes on mask wearing; skepticism had already been set by Trump's public behavior and cavalier attitude to the CDC recommendation. Trump's opposition was deliberate; he and his advisers saw it as an opportunity to exploit as a "cultural wedge issue."[115] Sadly, the implications were felt only months later. States with Republican governors that enjoyed a lower incidence of COVID-19 at the beginning of the pandemic could afford to downplay the threat. They may have even genuinely believed that coastal states were exaggerating or that claims were overblown. But while these states had low COVID-19 caseloads in the first wave, they experienced higher caseloads for the rest of the pandemic.[116]

Partisan politics has suffused the COVID-19 pandemic in the United States. We have shown how the pandemic was mishandled in Washington and how its implications trickled out into the states. But we have yet to see how ordinary Americans have responded: whose behaviors have changed and what Americans thought and felt about the pandemic as it has unfolded over time. It is to these behaviors and attitudes from March 2020 and the subsequent year that we now turn.

3

To Mask or Not to Mask

THE BEHAVIORAL RESPONSE TO COVID

Wash your hands. Stay home. Wear a mask. Use hand sanitizer. Those were the lessons that millions of Americans were learning quickly in March 2020. "Social distancing" entered the collective vocabulary. Health officials warned people not to touch their faces or shake hands and to avoid blowing out birthday candles. The *Today* show compiled a list of songs that people could sing for twenty seconds while washing their hands, including "Happy Birthday," Dolly Parton's "Jolene," and "Stayin' Alive'" by the Bee Gees.[1] Gloria Gaynor filmed herself singing "I Will Survive" while washing her hands, and Neil Diamond reworked "Sweet Caroline" to include the lyrics "hands washing hands."[2] People reacted to these directives by clearing supermarket shelves of soap and hand sanitizer along with toilet paper, creating nationwide shortages.

It is hard to overstate the magnitude and swiftness of the changes to American life in the first months of the pandemic. Businesses, movies, and sports arenas all closed, neighbors and friends now harbored potentially deadly germs, and events such as weddings and funerals were suddenly dangerous vectors of disease. Millions started working from home, often homeschooling children at the same time, while millions of others lost their jobs. Within weeks, a little-known company called Zoom became the go-to replacement for in-person meetings, classes, and happy hours. Americans were wiping down their mail, packages, and groceries. Live television shows were suddenly broadcasting out of people's living rooms instead of studios, with small children, normally in school, running through the background of the news and comedy sketches. Bars, restaurants, concerts, travel, March Madness, Disney World—it all closed down.

Health agencies from the World Health Organization to the Centers for Disease Control and Prevention (CDC) to local health departments all recommended staying home, not mixing households for social events, staying out of public transit, and, later, wearing masks when in public. States required quarantines for those who had flu-like symptoms, and new worrisome symptoms seemed to crop up daily: loss of taste and smell, nausea, or "COVID toes."[3] Not everyone stayed home even as mitigation measures were still in place. Celebrities such as Kim Kardashian threw lavish parties,[4] and politicians such as Gavin Newsom broke rules such as no indoor dining that they had implemented themselves.[5] Celebrities aside, what determined whether everyday Americans followed the health recommendations or whether they ignored them, continuing on with life as normal?

The pandemic's preconditions shaped who was able to adopt the health guidance fully at first. Social determinants of health such as income, age, housing, and access to insurance all made following directives easier for those with more resources. The advantage for those with more resources was compounded, since people with higher incomes also tend to have fewer underlying health conditions and work in less public-facing jobs.[6] Economic precarity meant that many low-income workers in high-risk jobs such as meatpacking, transportation, and retail could neither stay home to ride out the pandemic nor afford time off if they became ill. An employment-based health care system meant that many people who found themselves unemployed were also suddenly uninsured and might not seek medical care even if they felt sick. People of color are more likely than white Americans to live in denser neighborhoods and in multigenerational housing, making social distancing more difficult.[7]

These structural issues matter in determining people's capacity to follow best practices, but they do not tell the whole story. This was a fraught time for ordinary Americans who wondered about how the virus spread, how deadly it was, how long the pandemic would last, whether they could get a test, and so forth. They looked toward their political leaders at the time and saw vast differences in how the parties discussed the pandemic and whether people should even be concerned. In late February President Donald Trump assured the public that there were very few cases in the United States, and in early March 2020 he was still on the campaign trail in Pennsylvania, Tennessee, and Florida holding fundraisers and doing town halls with no social distancing or masks apparent, a visual sign of how belated and reluctant the Trump administration's response to the pandemic was.[8] Democrats in Congress discussed the coronavirus earlier on and more often than their Republican counterparts and focused on the threats to public health and American workers.[9]

Partisanship became a fundamental determinant of Americans' health behaviors and beliefs in response to COVID-19. In a context of reluctant leadership and high uncertainty, these diverging signals from political leaders shaped Americans' choices about which health recommendations to follow. Democrats would follow Democratic leadership to express more concern and be stricter in following the rules, while Republicans would take Republican cues and be less worried and less likely to report following CDC recommendations.

Partisanship not only determined health behavior and beliefs in the early weeks of the pandemic but also continued to matter throughout the pandemic. By late April 2020 after a brief period of what looked like a collective effort to shelter at home—reducing the stress on health services by flattening the curve—a combination of anxiety, hardship, and fatigue motivated partisan efforts to reopen the U.S. economy, encouraged by Trump and Republican governors. With some concluding that the worst was already over even as caseloads grew, Republican-led states such as Alabama, Georgia, Idaho, and Tennessee began to reopen. From this point onward Democrats' and Republicans' health behaviors diverged, and this divergence became an enduring feature of the COVID-19 pandemic in the United States. The patterns in health behavior that we observed in March 2020, which were driven by partisanship rather than by risk, were set in that early period and continued over time, even as the virus moved with deadly force into more rural, conservative areas. Health behaviors responded not to the risks on the ground but instead to the messages that came from party leaders.

Health Behavior in March

By the end of March, the pandemic had driven the American economy to a near standstill. The first wave of our survey—March 20–23—coincided with this first spike in cases. It was fielded one day after stay-at-home orders in California (March 19), the first state to do so, and coincided with subsequent orders in Illinois, New Jersey, New York, and six other states. Dozens more would follow.[10] With our survey out so early in the pandemic, we were able to see how Americans were reacting to the crisis right as it happened.

No survey can cover everything, so we designed our survey with the objective of capturing how Americans were changing their health behaviors in both easy and difficult ways as well as how their demographic profiles (e.g., race, ethnicity, income, gender, partisanship) shaped those responses. Based on this, we chose eight health behaviors in wave 1 of our survey that ranged from easy and low-cost behaviors (more handwashing and purchasing hand sanitizer, for instance) to costly and involved (visiting the doctor and self-quarantining). Notably, on wave 1 we did not ask about mask wearing because the CDC was unequivocal that only people who worked in health care or were caring for infected people needed to wear masks, and the surgeon general was actively discouraging the public from buying masks because there was a shortage of personal protective equipment for health care workers.[11]

Some behaviors were publicly observable (e.g., leaving home), while others were private (e.g., handwashing). We would not necessarily expect partisan or other demographic differences to appear for

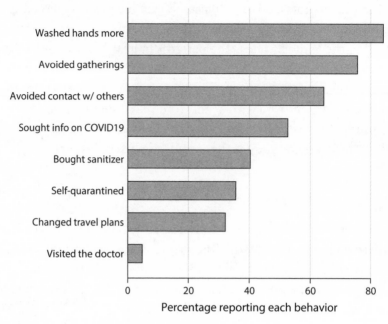

FIGURE 3.1. Health behaviors, March 20–23, 2020

a behavior such as handwashing, which costs little and is normally done by oneself. If behaviors were meant not just to protect people from coronavirus but also to signal something to others about how seriously they took the virus, then behaviors such as mask wearing and social distancing, which were public gestures, would be clearer signs that health behaviors had a political meaning as well.

Figure 3.1 shows the percentage of our three thousand survey respondents who reported each of these eight health behaviors. It is quite evident from the figure that Americans were aware of the pandemic and were responding to it. By mid-March, the vast majority of Americans were washing their hands more frequently than they had previously; many were also avoiding social gatherings and contact with others. Far fewer people reported that they were taking more stringent measures such as self-quarantining or changing travel plans, though in a Gallup poll around the same time 64 percent reported canceling or postponing travel, and 80 percent reported avoiding travel by airplane, bus, subway, or train.[12] In the same poll respondents were also asked about keeping kids home from school, which—because of statewide stay at home orders—quickly shot from 37 percent (March 13-15) to 84 percent a week later (March 23–29). Other national surveys showed the same general trends: most Americans were changing their social behaviors in response to the pandemic.

If these figures were the whole story, there would be reason for optimism. Avoiding social interactions was one of the most important things people could do to manage the spread of COVID-19, and most Americans were doing just that. While only four in ten Americans reported purchasing hand sanitizer, supply chain problems meant that it was hard for Americans to buy hand sanitizer even if they wanted to.[13] Most of our respondents did not report visiting a doctor, but this may have been a sign of precaution, whereby individuals were minimizing exposure where possible, and a reflection that few across America were yet severely ill.

These aggregate figures do not tell the whole story, though. Americans experienced the pandemic differently depending on where they lived, what they did for a living, and who they were. Frontline workers such as medical professionals, bus drivers, grocery store workers and other essential workers, people who could not work at home, and those living in congregate or multigenerational housing were more likely to be exposed to the virus. Economic conditions forced certain workers to leave their homes more frequently and use mass transit, increasing the chance for being infected by the virus. People with less access to health care and those living in poorer communities, rural communities, and communities of color were also more vulnerable to both getting the virus and dying from it. The elderly and those with compromised immune systems were also likely to become very ill once exposed, and as we saw, some of the hardest-hit communities in the earliest days of the pandemic were retirement, hospice, and nursing homes.

If people weighed their risk for disease most heavily in deciding to change their behavior, we might expect that there would be differences based on the individual characteristics of people that led them to be more at risk or more able to adopt recommended behaviors. Wealthier Americans might be better able to work from home and avoid social gathering, but low-income service workers in grocery stores or driving buses might be more likely to be exposed to COVID. To understand how Americans processed the earliest stages of the pandemic, we examine how Americans changed their health behaviors and how that varies by their economic, social, and political characteristics.

DID BEHAVIOR DIFFER BY INCOME?

We first looked at how the early behavioral response to COVID-19 differed by income (figure 3.2). Our expectation was that if the pandemic was experienced unequally, then those with the means to adapt to the pandemic would be more likely to do so than those with more limited means. And that is what we found: those who reported the highest levels of income were most likely to report nearly every behavior, with decreasing levels of compliance for people with lower household incomes. These results confirm that the aggregate numbers in figure 3.1 actually masked substantial heterogeneity among Americans.

These figures tell a story of opportunity; high-level income jobs migrated to remote telework. Architects, lawyers, and professors had jobs that could be mostly completed from home with minimal accommodations and the income to start ordering grocery and meal delivery, whereas lower-income Americans had fewer opportunities to isolate or stay at home. For many, their jobs became reclassified as "essential work" as warehouse packaging, mail, grocery store employees, and meat-processing workers became vital components to keep the economy going and help other Americans stay at home. It is not a coincidence that these worksites were the location of among the most rampant and early outbreaks. The early costs of the pandemic were disproportionally borne by the poor, a point to which we will return in chapter 6, where we consider the economic impacts of the COVID-19 pandemic in the United States.

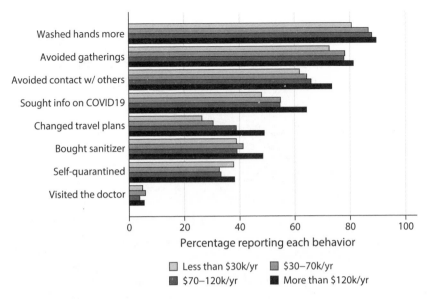

FIGURE 3.2. Health behaviors, by income

DID BEHAVIOR DIFFER BY LEVEL OF EDUCATION?

When we compared Americans at different education levels, we found a similar if somewhat more pronounced pattern (figure 3.3).

Clearly, education matters in explaining COVID-19 behaviors: those with higher education are more likely to report adopting nearly every behavior that we asked them. Although eight in ten Americans were avoiding gatherings, this was seven in ten among high school graduates and nearly nine in ten among those with postgraduate degrees. Differences in searching for information on COVID-19 also suggest that Americans of different education levels were experiencing the COVID-19 differently. In March 2020, information about the pandemic was prevalent but also rapidly changing and sometimes contradictory (i.e., were masks effective or should the public leave them for health care workers?), making navigating this tsunami of information difficult. People with more education looked for more information and were also more likely to translate that information into behavioral changes.

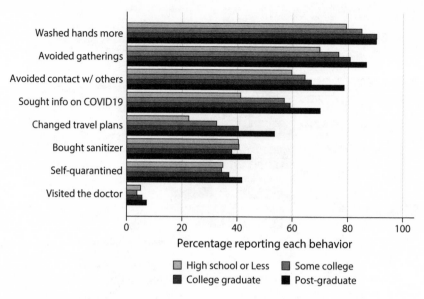

FIGURE 3.3. Health behaviors, by education

The patterns in COVID-19 health behaviors are so similar in figures 3.2 and 3.3 because income and education are so highly related in the United States.[14] This is particularly important, as it suggests that there are deeper socioeconomic differences—perhaps best understood as class—that distinguish Americans' COVID-19 responses. Again, we will have more opportunity to explore these issues in chapter 6, where we turn to the economic implications of the COVID-19 pandemic. For now, though, we can conclude that socioeconomic factors that differentiate Americans in so many other domains of American life also shaped their behaviors in response to the COVID-19 pandemic.

DID BEHAVIOR DIFFER BY GENDER?

We next looked at behavior by gender (figure 3.4). Our initial expectation was that men would be less compliant with health behaviors due to gendered expectations about vulnerability and that women would be more likely to take into consideration the interests of their entire family.[15] And indeed, across almost every response American

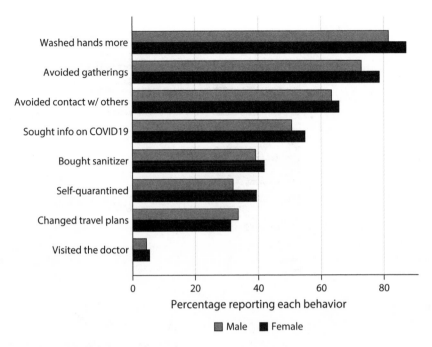

FIGURE 3.4. Health behaviors, by gender

women are slightly more likely than American men to report one of our COVID-19 health behaviors.

This pattern is noteworthy in just how consistent it is. These differences in gender are not the consequence of differences in income or employment by gender: in our sample the women are not more likely to be highly educated or to report higher incomes than the men.[16] And other studies find similar gendered patterns in COVID-19 compliance, where women take COVID more seriously than men by supporting restrictive policy measures and are overall more compliant with pro–social health behavior.[17] One study attributes this asymmetry to women being more likely to listen to medical experts and follow other countries' experiences.[18] In the same study, women also attribute their behaviors to feeling anxious and feeling responsibility for themselves and others. This evidence suggests that women feel more attuned to the implications of the pandemic for their families, and respond by exhibiting protective behaviors.[19]

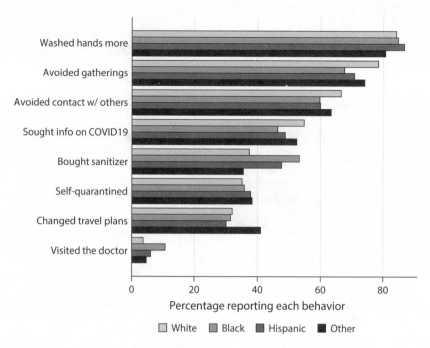

FIGURE 3.5. Health behavior, by race/ethnicity

DID BEHAVIOR DIFFER BY RACE AND ETHNICITY?

Next, we considered health behaviors by respondents' racial and ethnic identities. Respondents self-identified both their primary racial group and whether they identify as Hispanic or Latina/o. While America's racial and ethnic landscape is complex, we simplify these categories to facilitate comparisons in broad strokes. We divide respondents into four categories: White, Black, Hispanic, and Other. The category of "Other" is quite heterogeneous (it includes, for example, Asian Americans, Native Americans, multiracial people, and those who choose not to report their racial and ethnic identity). But even this simplified fourfold racial and ethnic classification helps to visualize differences across major groups effectively, as we see in figure 3.5.

Communities of color bore the earliest and deepest costs of the pandemic, with higher rates of hospitalization and death,[20] but we do not see major differences in individual behaviors, at least in the initial phase. The figures show that there was widespread prohealth behavior across racial groups. White Americans reported a greater propensity to seek information on COVID as well as avoid gatherings and contact with others, but Black and Hispanic Americans were more likely to purchase sanitizer and self-quarantine. Large majorities across racial groups were likely to wash their hands more. The lack of differences in behaviors across racial groups reinforces the idea that disproportionate effects of the coronavirus on minority individuals are largely the result of structural barriers to health (i.e., workplace safety, types of housing, inequality in health care access) rather than individual choices.

This view only skims the surface of the uneven experience of the pandemic on minority communities. Chapter 8 will look closely at different behaviors, attitudes, and experiences of COVID-19 among different ethnic and racial groups. Yet at the same time, research shows that as the pandemic progressed, African American men were least likely to know how COVID spread and less likely to be familiar with symptoms and left the house more.[21]

DID BEHAVIOR DIFFER BY EXPOSURE TO THE VIRUS?

Did the lived experience of COVID in one's community—burdening local health services and ripping through local nursing homes—motivate individuals to participate in more prohealth behavior? To answer this, we looked at differences in COVID-19 behavior by exposure to the COVID-19 virus itself. We used data from the COVID-19 Tracking Project,[22] which provided daily figures for the numbers of recorded COVID-19 diagnoses in each county in the United States as well as the number of recorded deaths from COVID-19 in that county. We matched these county-level data from March 23, 2020—the last day of our first survey—to our survey respondents' zip codes, which they reported as part of our survey. This gave us a very fine measure of the local COVID-19 experience at the time that our first survey wave was in the field. We considered this a conservative estimate, given how few people were being tested at the time.

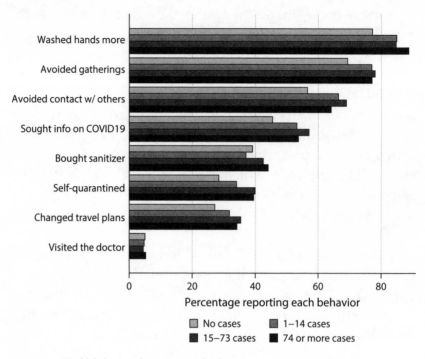

FIGURE 3.6. Health behaviors, by county caseloads

To compare experiences, we divide our survey respondents into four roughly equally sized groups: those living in counties with no reported cases at all, those living in counties with at least one but fewer than fifteen cases, those living in counties with between fifteen and seventy-three cases, and those living in counties with seventy-four or more cases. Figure 3.6 compares our survey respondents by county-level caseloads.

There was a marked difference in self-reported behavior between the highest case category and the no case category on items such as washing hands more, avoiding gatherings and contact with others, and seeking information on COVID-19. But for areas with diagnosed cases, we saw little difference because of scale. Recall that this snapshot was from mid-March, that is, before widespread testing or contact tracing was implemented anywhere in the United States. Information on local caseload was still limited, available as anecdotes on the local news, from social media reports of local hospital conditions, or on one of the nascent national dashboards aggregating county data, such as the COVID-19 tracker run by Johns Hopkins University.

All in all, our March survey told us a fairly consistent story that demographic and socioeconomic factors matter for understanding how Americans responded to the earliest days of the pandemic. These circumstances certainly shaped how an individual behaved in March 2020. Income, education, race and ethnicity, and local caseload all mattered. But how much of an individual's response was politically motivated? What role might have political factors played in shaping individual-level differences?

DID BEHAVIOR DIFFER BY PARTISANSHIP?

Finally, we looked at how Americans' behavioral responses to COVID-19 differ according to their political orientations. We can do this in a number of ways: looking at their partisan affiliations, their support for President Trump, or their position on an ideological scale of conservative versus liberal. Partisanship, ideology, and support for Trump were tightly aligned in the U.S. political system,[23] so it does not matter which measure of politics we use. Partisanship always matters, as we show in figure 3.7.

There were consistent political differences in Americans' early behavioral responses to COVID-19, with a roughly 10 percentage point difference on average between Democrats and Republicans. We see a nearly 20 percentage point difference between Republicans and Democrats in seeking information about COVID-19. In short, by March 23, Americans were already living in different worlds when it comes to COVID-19. These worlds were defined by politics.

Democrats and Republicans often disagree about health policy, that is, whether the federal government should run a health care system, how much to spend on health, and whether to expand programs like Medicaid and Medicare.[24] Yet, the health behaviors of individuals do not always vary. Republicans and Democrats report similar levels of good health and are equally likely to get a yearly flu shot most years and exercise at similar rates.[25] Like other areas

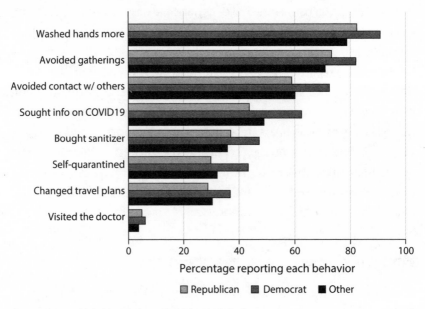

Washed hands more
Avoided gatherings
Avoided contact w/ others
Sought info on COVID19
Bought sanitizer
Self-quarantined
Changed travel plans
Visited the doctor

Percentage reporting each behavior

Republican   Democrat   Other

FIGURE 3.7. Health behaviors, by partisanship and ideology

of politics, though, the messages that come from political leaders can shape health preferences. During Barack Obama's presidency, Republicans were more worried about the Ebola outbreak and less likely to get an H1N1 vaccine,[26] reflecting low levels of trust in the president's handling of these crises. Even policies around nutrition and obesity, which are usually not structured by partisanship, can become driven by politics when connected to partisan figures.[27]

Even while majorities of Republicans reported washing hands more frequently and social distancing and certainly were not rejecting COVID-19 precautions altogether, the differences between parties are meaningful from both a political and public health perspective. From a political perspective, both Democrats and Republicans show early concern, but Democrats consistently report more (and more frequent) COVID-19 health behaviors. From a community perspective, an infectious virus can only be slowed with a majority of behavioral compliance or herd immunity, regardless of political beliefs. Therefore, in communities where Republicans predominate, health behaviors would be slower and less likely to halt the spread of COVID-19. Community spread cannot be stopped if four out of ten Republicans keep meeting with people outside their households. It also would mean that more convincing and pro-health messaging would need to take place in these communities, not less.

These differences persisted over time, as we will see below. Moreover, they grew. In the early days of the pandemic, a time of high uncertainty and low information, most Americans did adopt the costly behaviors needed to contain its spread, but the seeds of partisan disagreement over how to handle it were already sown.

IS IT REALLY ABOUT PARTISANSHIP?

As social scientists, one of the questions we must ask when looking at results like this is whether these behavioral differences are really about politics. After all, Americans' political affiliations and ideological orientations are as much a product of their social and economic circumstances as they are something inherent to their identities. Perhaps Democrats consume different kinds of news that gave them a different perspective on the seriousness of the pandemic, or perhaps Democrats tended to work in jobs that allow them to socially distance more effectively. If so, knowing that Democrats and Republicans are different does not tell us that they are different because of their political orientations or partisan affiliations.

We also know that there were sharp geographical differences in how COVID-19 spread through the United States. Those areas hit first by the pandemic included blue states such as Washington and New York, not red states such as Alabama and Idaho. Moreover, the crisis unfolded first in urban areas that are especially left-leaning (Seattle and New York City) rather than in rural areas that vote Republican (such as the small towns between Syracuse and Ithaca in upstate New York). If our Republican respondents tend to live in small towns or in the outer suburbs of large cities in red states such as Missouri or Texas and our Democrats tend to come from urban areas or from blue states, then partisan differences that we find might be about geography rather than partisanship itself.

In the language of the social sciences, factors such as income, education, and geography that might plausibly explain the differences in health behavior among Democrats and Republicans are known as "confounders." If we want to know whether partisan differences in health behaviors are really about partisanship rather than inadvertently reflecting things such as geography or income that happen to be related to partisanship, we need to adopt a strategy that accounts, or controls, for those differences.

To do this, we use a common statistical technique known as multiple regression (for full details on our methods, see the appendix). This technique helps us determine whether an association such as the one we have uncovered between partisanship and health behaviors is actually explained by other factors that are closely related to partisanship. We know that Democrats have higher levels of education on average and that Republicans have higher incomes, and perhaps they live in different parts of the country and in different kinds of localities. Multiple regression adjusts for these other factors and shows us how Democrats and Republicans who are comparable across all other dimensions (income, education, place of residence, etc.) respond. If we still see differences in behavior after accounting for those differences, we are much confident that it is partisanship that matters.

The overall message from our multiple regression analysis is that the partisan differences we uncovered in figure 3.7 are not explained by any of the sociodemographic or geographic confounders that we have discussed previously. For example, even when accounting for the effect of demographics such as income, education, and gender, Democrats were still about 10 percentage points more likely to avoid gatherings than Republicans and 20 percentage points more likely to seek information about COVID-19.

We also asked this question a different way: "If we had to choose the factors that best predict COVID-19 health behavior, would partisanship be one of them?" Posing the question this way allowed us to use a statistical procedure known as the "lasso" method whereby we can sort through over a hundred variables to select those that best explain health behaviors. We detail the logic of this analysis in the appendix; the result was that partisanship was the best predictor of COVID-19 health behavior of all the factors that we measured.

This is powerful evidence that despite the many ways that Americans differ socially, economically, and geographically, politics matters. Especially when it comes to pro–social health behaviors such as physical distancing, in March there were meaningful partisan differences in health behaviors across Americans that we cannot neatly explain away by other factors.

The Evolution of Partisan Differences over Time

The lockdown measures and stay-at-home orders issued across much of America in March 2020 were difficult for many. While not everyone was equally affected—a *Washington Post* op-ed referred to it as a "white-collar quarantine" where low-income workers were "bearing the brunt of the epidemic"[28]—we know that partisans were already experiencing the pandemic through partisan lenses. And so, just as Americans were hunkering down to face the brunt of the COVID-19 crisis, a deep division emerged over how and when to return to normal. Republicans and Democrats had different appetites for staying at home. According to a Kaiser Family Foundation study, a majority of Democrats (64%) and independents (56%) thought in mid-April that "the worst is yet to come," while 53 percent of Republicans thought "the worst is behind us."[29] As early as March 24, 2020, Trump floated the idea of reopening by Easter (April 12).[30] And many were impatient and sought a return to normal. The $1,200 check from the Coronavirus Aid, Relief, and Economic Security Act would not last long especially for small business owners, and Americans were eager to get back to business.

Driven by the increasing hardship caused by the pandemic and encouraged by Trump's own impatience, some Americans began to mobilize. Protests to "reopen the economy" started to crop up from California to Michigan to Virginia. By early May, 54 percent of respondents to a Gallup poll thought that the greatest threat to America at the time was the coronavirus, while 47 percent answered the economic shutdown.[31] And this divide directly reflected how political parties were talking, with Democrats focused on the virus and Republicans focused on the economy.[32]

As 2020 wore on, many Republican politicians agitated for a return to normal, arguing that the social and economic costs of the shutdown were unsustainable. Wisconsin Republicans in the state legislature even sued the state's top public health official in order to end the pandemic lockdown.[33] Many Americans became less willing to adapt with the pro–social health behaviors that were necessary to manage the pandemic. Worryingly, the pandemic itself began to shift from urban to rural outbreaks, especially in counties that went for Trump in the 2016 election.[34] At the state level, Democratic governors were earlier to shut down, while Republican governors were earlier to open their economies back up, with the notable exceptions of the Republican governors of Ohio, Maryland, and Vermont taking more aggressive measures against the virus.[35] Whereas Republican national leadership had initially downplayed the virus, Republican Party elites soon began mocking those who took it seriously.

During the 2020 campaign, for example, Trump consistently ridiculed candidate Joe Biden, who exercised safety precautions in his presidential campaign including consistently wearing a mask. The Trump campaign also openly flouted prohealth measures during campaign events. Recall from the introduction the events of June 20 in Tulsa, when Trump held an indoor maskless campaign rally. It was so sparsely attended that not only was the arena unfilled, but the outdoor spillover section also went unused. While outsized expectations about crowd size were driven by teenagers and K-pop fans as a prank, low attendance also suggests that Republican supporters were not as comfortable with in-person gatherings as they might seem.

As summer set in, partisan differences grew. By following the same respondents over what was to be an extraordinary seven months, we could see how behaviors evolved. The partisan divide over COVID-19 that began in March 2020 would grow over time, as figure 3.8 shows.

Take, for example, the question of whether one would avoid gatherings. Our first wave captured a roughly 10-percentage-point difference between Democrats, on the one hand, and Republicans

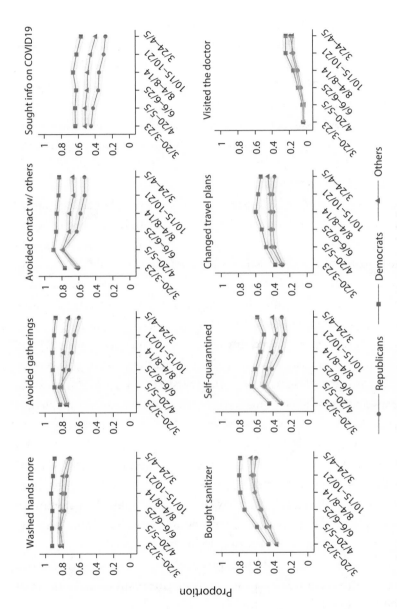

FIGURE 3.8. Partisan health differences across six waves (from March 2020 to April 2021)

and Others. In wave 2, which ran from April 20 to May 5, all three groups became more likely to report having avoided gatherings. So, although a partisan difference remained, all three partisan groups moved in the same direction. But starting in wave 3 (June 6–26), the trend line diverged. About the same proportion of Democrats reported avoiding gatherings, but the proportions of Republicans and Others dropped noticeably. This phenomenon, a partisan divergence in health behavior, reappears in nearly every one of the subplots. And note how enduring those differences were. Even as the overall level of compliance with each of the health measures changed over time, the size of the gap between the Democrats and Republicans almost never shrunk.

Over the course of 2020, Americans' COVID-19 health behavior became more divided as the pandemic wore on. If the seed of partisan differences was planted in early March 2020 with the president's undercutting of the seriousness of the pandemic while Democratic officials urged caution, we can see the reaping of these differences in the summer as states led by Republican governors lifted restrictions more quickly than states led by Democrats. These messaging and policy differences translated into diverging behaviors in the public.

Given the depth of partisan media polarization, one might wonder if these partisan differences are perhaps just a consequence of the sorts of news that Republicans and Democrats consume. On any given day, cable news would cover the pandemic in different substantive ways. Specifically, as one *Washington Post* article writes, "MSNBC was 1.5 times as likely to use the phrase 'protective equipment' as CNN and 2.7 times as likely to do so as Fox News. CNN used the word 'testing' 2.2 times more often than Fox News and 'get test' 1.3 times more than MSNBC."[36] But all coverage was political; both Fox and MSNBC would reference partisans more than health experts.[37]

In figure 3.9, we check this possibility by breaking down the results in figure 3.8 based on whether the respondent reported watching right-wing news in wave 1 of our survey.

It turns out that partisanship explains much more variation in health behavior than does media consumption: Republicans who get their news from right-wing news sources are basically the same

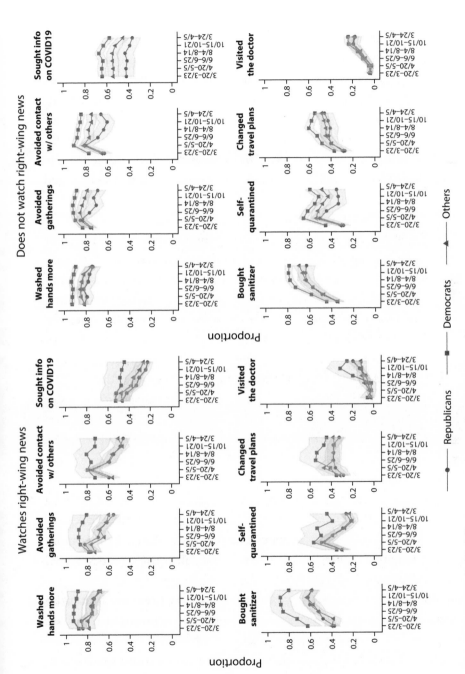

FIGURE 3.9. Partisan health differences across six waves, by news consumption

as Republicans who do not, and the same is true for Democrats. To the extent that there are differences by media consumption it is among those labeled "Others," who are members of neither party. In this group, we find that those who watch right-wing news tend to report fewer pro–social health behaviors than those who do not.

Once again, however, we must ask whether these partisan differences should be attributable to partisanship itself or to the other factors that might be associated with partisanship. For example, stay-at-home orders were lifted in many parts of the United States starting in May, and it might simply be that Republicans tend to live in places that reopened more quickly and more thoroughly than in other places. For Republicans living in rural areas, meeting other people in real life is more rare, meaning they do not need to embrace social distancing measures to the same degree as do Democrats, who tend to live in urban areas where community spread is easy. Using the same multiple regression approach we describe above, we tested whether these differences were due to partisanship itself or to the other factors that might be associated with partisanship and, once again, found that partisanship matters even when accounting for these other factors. We detail these results in the appendix.

Masks as Microcosm

There is no better issue to illustrate the early and enduring partisan differences in pro–social health behavior than the politicization of wearing face masks. Like social distancing, it is one of the more public behaviors that signals an individual's seriousness in the pandemic. But unlike some of the behaviors we already examined, face masks were only recommended by the CDC for public use on April 3 (and as such we did not ask about compliance in the first survey wave). And right out of the gate, mask wearing became the most politicized COVID prevention measure.

We first asked U.S. respondents if they wore a face mask on April 20, nearly three weeks after the CDC endorsed mask wearing. However, there were no masks available for purchase. Masks quickly disappeared off shelves, leading many Americans to pull out their sewing machines to make their own. Sales on the homecraft website Etsy doubled in April.[38]

In our data, we find that almost eight out of ten Democrats reported wearing a mask in early April, compared to six out of ten Republicans. The partisan gap in mask wearing between Republicans and Democrats was 15 percentage points, but mask compliance was high overall. This was some cause for optimism. By May 13, Phillip Bump remarked in the *Washington Post* that "people are more supportive of the necessity of wearing masks than they are of kittens. That's not a sign of an unbroachable partisan divide."[39] And indeed, by June, August, and October we see the gap between Democrats and Republicans narrowing and then stabilizing (figure 3.10).

Not surprisingly, our lasso procedure discussed in the previous section also consistently selects partisanship as a good predictor of mask wearing.

By June 2020 the United States had reached one hundred thousand deaths from COVID-19, and many states that planned reopenings of their economies pushed them back.[40] Amid the summer surge of new infections, the World Health Organization announced that coronavirus was airborne and that the virus could linger in indoor spaces.[41] Over the two survey waves in June and August 2020, we see an uptick in mask wearing among all groups. What should we make of the enduring 10-percentage–point partisan gap in mask wearing that we observe from August 2020 to April 2021? We previewed the politics of mask wearing in chapter 2, where behind-the-scenes efforts to get masks into the hands of Americans were thwarted by Trump. Here, we propose that the public masking choices by elites affected the behavior of ordinary Americans. Republican and Democratic elites exhibited starkly different behavior. When Anthony Fauci, director of the National Institute of Allergy and Infectious Disease, testified before Congress while wearing a mask on May 12, Susan Collins (R-ME) notably did not. Republican senators such as Ted Cruz and Mitch McConnell were spotted in public places without masks while maintaining that they "follow science" and "listen to the experts."[42] And recall the nomination of U.S. Supreme Court justice Amy Coney Barrett attended by dozens of maskless Republicans

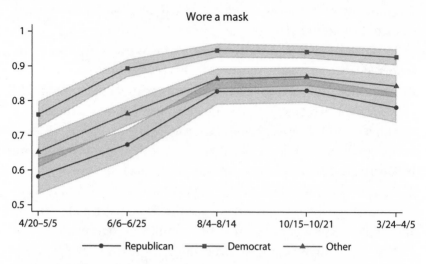

Wore a mask

Republican ——•—— Democrat ——■—— Other ——▲——

FIGURE 3.10. Mask compliance from April 2020 to April 2021, adjusting for confounders

congregating both indoors and in the White House Rose Garden, which ended up being a superspreader event.

This messaging came from the top. Trump frequently flouted mask practices and held dozens of rallies and events characterized by hundreds of maskless participants. He was first seen wearing a mask only on May 21 while touring a factory in Ypsilanti, Michigan, where ventilators, masks, and other medical supplies are made. There is early evidence that some Trump supporters wanted him to wear a mask,[43] but his messaging was ambivalent in May ("I'm choosing not to do it, but some people may want to do it and that's okay") and outright reluctant in July. Trump tweeted a photo of himself in a mask with the words "many people say that it is Patriotic to wear a face mask when you can't socially distance." Not two days after his tweet, Trump was seen at a fundraiser at his Washington, DC, hotel without a mask, which prompted an investigation into COVID protocol compliance at the hotel by local authorities.[44] And in a prominent show of his indifference to public health guidelines, Trump removed his mask in the presence of White House staff and cameras after returning from the hospital while still infectious with COVID-19. The White House had a mask requirement, but Trump did not.[45]

Not all Republicans were as opposed to masking as was Trump. Congresswoman Liz Cheney (R-WY) tweeted a photo of her father, former vice president Dick Cheney, wearing a mask with the message "Dick Cheney says WEAR A MASK. #realmenwearmasks." But prominent promask Republicans were rare, and the contrast to the Democrats is stark. Biden made mask wearing a defining characteristic of his campaign. In his first public appearance with his vice presidential running mate Kamala Harris, both wore masks. Biden also promised to "institute a mask mandate starting immediately." The Democratic National Convention, televised in a revised format to maintain social distancing, featured COVID-19 safety and mask wearing as a cornerstone of its first day's programming. Indeed, at Biden's inauguration masks were worn by every participant, social distancing was maintained on the steps of the Capitol, and the National Mall, typically brimming with crowds of attendees, was filled instead with thousands of American flags. And on his first day in office, Biden signed an executive order to mandate face masks on federal property and in interstate travel.[46]

Despite mounting evidence that masks were effective in mitigating COVID-19[47] and that states with relaxed mask policies had higher incidences of COVID-19 cases,[48] differences in mask-wearing practices have persisted throughout the course of the pandemic so far. We believe that everyday defiance of mask mandates had its roots in the partisan politics of the pandemic, as conservate elites' skepticism and reluctance became a prominent touchpoint in the public debate about the pandemic. Some of the more outlandish protests to mask wearing went viral on social media, involving tantrums in grocery stores and yelling at shop clerks for enforcing store policy. In Orange County, California, chief health officer Nichole Quick was harassed into resignation with death threats for requiring residents to wear masks outside their home when social distancing was not possible. According to a study by The Hill, by the end of July there was high support overall for a national mask mandate (around 82%) but still strong differences by party: 93 percent Democratic support, 85 percent independent support, and 66 percent Republican endorsement.[49] Fast-forward to January 2021, and a similar pattern of agreement is expressed in a YouGov poll, where Biden voters (93%) versus Trump voters (63%) support that members of Congress should be required to wear face masks in the Capitol building.[50] This was the case after reports that several Republican congresspersons refused to wear masks while sheltering in place with colleagues during the January 6 insurrection, resulting in three Democratic members of Congress testing positive for COVID-19 in the immediate aftermath.[51]

The antimask minority was indeed a minority, but they were vocal and persistent and spanned from local grocery stores to public town halls. Opposition was—by definition—a performance. Sometimes these were filmed and put online to go viral, with maskless adults brandishing doctored "medical exemption" cards or having tantrums and being escorted out of a Costco. One Alaska state lawmaker was banned from traveling on Alaska Airlines for life for not complying with its mask requirement.[52] But the politics of mask mandates became so political—and politicized—that by the fall of 2021, despite clear evidence that masks reduce transmission, eight Republican states enacted laws or issued executive orders that prohibited school districts from enacting mask mandates in schools: Arizona, Arkansas, Florida, Iowa, South Carolina, Oklahoma, Texas, and Utah.

How "American" is this partisan division over mask wearing? Partisan differences in mask wearing did decline over time, but gaps persisted. Some argue that Republicans' rejection of mask wearing was driven by their focus on freedom and rugged individualism (as in frontier culture)[53] or toxic masculinity.[54] But at the same time, antimask behavior dotted the globe from Brazil to Germany to Indonesia. According to data collected by Imperial College London, there were stark differences in mask compliance just within Europe. By the end of June, acceptance in Spain was around 92 percent and in Italy at 81 percent, and even in France, where a bus driver was murdered for enforcing a mask policy, compliance was as high as 73 percent.[55] By contrast, only 52 percent of Britons reported wearing a face mask "frequently" or "always," and a staggering 83 percent of Swedes and 85 percent of Finns reported never wearing a mask.[56] Beyond Europe, mask compliance in Hong Kong was as high as

97 percent[57] and as low as 20 percent in Australia.[58] Canada also exhibited high overall compliance.[59]

What makes the United States stand out from even those countries where mask compliance was low is the partisan politics of masking in the United States. Even in a similarly polarized country such as the United Kingdom, mask opposition did not follow partisan lines. In a YouGov survey in early September 2020, a similar share of Conservatives and Labour voters reported wearing a face mask in public places.[60] While the government was at first hesitant to require masks and mask mandates were not ubiquitous in schools or shops, there is not the large partisan difference in mask wearing among British citizens based on partisanship. Masks illustrate how the pandemic in the United States was uniquely American: not because of a specific variant of the virus but instead because of Americans' uniquely partisan response.

Conclusion

We learned two major lessons about pandemic politics from the data that came in over the course of 2020. First, from the very earliest days of the pandemic, there was a clear partisan difference in how Americans were responding to COVID-19. Democrats were more likely to adopt a whole host of behaviors in response to the crisis, from washing hands to social distancing, than were Republicans. Second, these partisan differences endured over the ensuing months. We cannot explain these partisan differences away with reference to other factors such as race, income, education, or anything else that we can measure.

There is more to explore about the partisan differences we have uncovered here. In chapter 4 we turn our attention to the emotional foundations of the pandemic, looking at Americans' emotional responses—feelings of disgust, anger, and also hope—as well as whom Americans blamed for the pandemic in order to delve more deeply into the partisan foundations of pandemic politics in the United States.

4

Who's to Blame?

THE EMOTIONAL RESPONSE TO COVID

The Federal Aviation Administration hadn't been systematically tracking unruly passenger behavior before 2020 when it began receiving an unprecedented number of reports of assaults on flight attendants, noncompliance with standard inflight instruction, and verbal abuse.[1] Passengers were punching and kicking flight staff. People were angry—angry about having to wear a mask, angry at the inconvenience of travel in a pandemic, angry about the lack of responsibility of those around them. Many of these incidents went viral as fellow passengers recorded an adult behaving badly and uploaded it to social media (much like the similar outbursts observed in grocery stores, with adults resisting mask mandates). "We've never before seen aggression and violence on our planes like we have in the past five months," said one flight attendant about the first part of 2021, when Americans started returning to flying in earnest and mask mandates were still in place. By November, the Federal Aviation Administration would record over 5,000 incidents, initiating 970 investigations, compared with 183 investigations in 2020.[2] Another flight attendant was more colorful in her description of the problem: "I'm dealing with a lot of babysitting, which I never counted on doing. . . . The actual children on board behave better than the grown adults do."[3]

Politics is often emotional, and pandemic politics are full of threat, uncertainty, and blame.[4] Who can forget the feeling of anger at hearing one's neighbor refuse to wear a mask or the feeling of sadness watching major life events—weddings, funerals, bar mitzvahs, and Thanksgiving dinner—over Zoom? Although most of us would hope to avoid these kinds of negative emotions, they serve an important function. Emotions alert people to potential harms or rewards in their environment and help them find an appropriate coping mechanism to deal with threats, alleviate uncomfortable feelings, and enhance positive ones.[5] That feeling of sadness at a Zoom Thanksgiving dinner is an emotional manifestation of our social ties, the connections that bind us to our friends and family. That feeling of anger may lead us to avoid those whose inactions place us in danger.

In politics, emotions can come directly from experiences, as with the feeling of disgust at the sight of garbage or sadness at the loss of a loved one. Emotions may also be mediated through social networks or media consumption or from political leaders directly—the feeling of excitement when encountering a charismatic speaker or of anger when seeing media coverage of a policy choice that one opposes. Sometimes our emotions emerge in response to threats that are likely to cause broad harm to the populace, such as disease, war, terrorism, or economic crisis. Individuals usually need little explanation about why people should be concerned about these threats; the 9/11 terror attack in the United States produced an emotional response in all Americans before any politician had time to comment on it.[6] But in other circumstances emotions may be manufactured, or at least harnessed, by political leaders. Leaders do this to create outrage, fear, or disgust in the public, which may spur individuals to adopt policies that these leaders want.[7] Think, for example, of how American politicians play on fears of terrorism to create support for detaining enemy combatants overseas or how images of a so-called migrant caravan are used in discussions of border security. Political leaders also work to tamp down negative emotions and redirect the public toward positive emotions such as hope and optimism when they want to avoid blame or need the public to act collectively.[8]

In this chapter, we show that the emotional reactions of Americans differed by their partisanship from the earliest days of the pandemic and that these differences persisted over time. Republicans expressed fewer negative emotions and felt negative emotions less strongly than their Democratic counterparts. And Republicans were more likely than Democrats to express hope and optimism about the future. In our interpretation, these expressions of emotions come not simply from different experiences in the pandemic (i.e., Republicans were less affected by the virus than Democrats) but also from cues, messaging, and information by party leaders that differed in framing the coronavirus as a threat and what emotions the public should feel. While Democratic Party leaders at the state and national levels, Democratic presidential candidates, and public health professionals rang alarm bells about the threat to public health, President Donald Trump, Republican members of Congress, and conservative media sources downplayed the seriousness of the threats.[9]

To see this argument, take yourself back to the earliest days of the pandemic. Many Americans experienced feelings of confusion and annoyance that quickly evolved into frustration, sadness, and even anger as the pandemic spun out of control and daily lives were upended. Had no American politician or official said anything about the pandemic, emotions would have run high. But now consider the messaging coming from Washington, from state houses, and from the media at that time. Just as the president was downplaying the severity of the pandemic and anticipating a quick return to normal (projecting hope), Americans were confronting empty supermarket shelves and reading news that schools were going online and that major public events were being canceled (producing fear and anxiety).

When a situation is highly uncertain and threatening, people look to the world around them to see whether these stressors will affect them and if so how they might respond.[10] So, a parent will confront news that schools are going virtual by looking for alternatives to regular schooling, and someone with serious health conditions may seek information about working from home. People can cope with stressful situations through psychological means—seeking professional care, confiding in a trusted friend, etc.—or by dealing with the situation that caused the emotion in the first place. Emotion can be the impetus that shakes people out of their routines and fundamentally changes how they work, go to school, and interact with society and the economy.[11]

Emotions can even shake people out of leaning on their identity and predispositions when forming attitudes.[12] This can be a good thing: facing an unexpected threat such as a pandemic, some people might respond to feelings of fright or anxiety by seeking new sources of information in order to make the threat more manageable. But not all emotions can produce such productive responses. For example, anger comes from a sense that there is a threat but is also exemplified by certainty and a sense of who caused the harm in the first place. Angry people are less open to new information and more risk-acceptant than those who are less angry.[13] Positive emotions such as hope and optimism indicate that people experience a situation to be pleasant, consistent with their motives, and perhaps even rewarding.[14] It made perfect sense, then, for Trump to project feelings of optimism and confidence, saying in February that there was a chance that COVID-19 would not spread at all and announcing plans to reopen by Easter.[15] A sense of optimism would encourage Americans not to look at the pandemic as a threat that required a solution. And for those who opposed Trump and his handling of the pandemic, those very same messages may have produced anger.

As with all other aspects of the COVID-19 pandemic, then, this emotional experience was not shared across partisan groups equally. One major means of coping with the threat of the coronavirus was to follow public health guidelines through social distancing, handwashing, masking, etc. So, an American facing worrisome news about the pandemic might spend time online looking to purchase hand sanitizer in bulk or canceling planned family travel. But if people did not want to adopt behaviors such as social distancing and masking or if they did not believe that the pandemic was relevant to their lives, they could cope in a different way: by regulating their emotions, tamping down on negative ones and increasing positive ones.[16] Rather than canceling their vacations, then, Americans might respond to the pandemic by celebrating their vacation with ever greater excitement than normal, sharing stories of their adventures on social media, and studiously avoiding any discussion of the health consequences of the pandemic.

It may seem strange that Americans would respond to a public health crisis by rejecting the recommendations of public health authorities. When health—even life—is on the line, why would people want to change or mute their emotions rather than change their behavior? One obvious answer is that behavioral change is unpleasant. Even people who had risk factors for COVID-19 and perceived themselves to be at risk did not always adopt simple behaviors to mitigate their health risk.

Take masking, for example.[17] Masks are uncomfortable, and they make it very hard to interact with friends and loved ones in a natural way. Almost no one would choose to wear a mask if they didn't have to. But the emotional politics of masking runs deeper than that. The politicization of the pandemic created a view among many Americans that masks were unnecessary, ineffective, and even a sign of totalitarian social control.[18] These messages affected everyday interactions as well. People unconcerned about the virus were less likely to comply with policies such as mask mandates. And when they did express feelings of anger in response to the COVID-19 pandemic, it was often over the mitigation policies rather than the virus itself. In some extreme cases, antimask sentiments led to physical violence against employees trying to uphold these rules, including the murder of a security guard in Michigan.[19]

As we argued in chapter 3, though, masks are just one aspect of the pandemic, albeit it a particularly visible one that has generated emotional reactions in both support and opposition. In this chapter we focus more broadly on the emotional dimensions of the pandemic to outline not only partisan differences in emotional responses but also the role of partisan communication in driving these different responses.

The Emotional Roots of Partisan Health Behavior

In chapter 3, we showed that Republicans and Democrats differed in their health behaviors during the pandemic. Here, we dig more deeply into those behavior differences to show that Republicans and Democrats felt quite differently about what was happening around them. The anger, anxiety, and disgust felt by Democrats—and their worries that they or their loved ones would get sick—encouraged them to adopt pro–social health behaviors as a coping mechanism. Absent these negative emotions and buoyed by feelings of hope, Republicans were less likely to adopt these same behaviors. These emotional differences persisted throughout the last year of the Trump administration, through the very worst of the American COVID-19 pandemic.

One way to see this is to look at how worried Americans were about various aspects of the pandemic at different points in 2020. In the early days of the pandemic, the media paid a lot of attention to scarcity of health products such as hand sanitizer and surgical masks as well as basic home goods such as toilet paper, yeast for baking, and aluminum foil. At the same time, Americans began to consider that the pandemic would truly disrupt their lives. And of course, Americans worried about the virus itself, whether they or their friends and loved ones would fall victim to it.

In each wave of our survey, we asked Americans about a wide variety of worries. We asked respondents questions about how worried they were about different aspects of the pandemic on a scale of "Not at all" to "Very." We assign these scores a value from 1–4 and then take the average of these values by party and each survey wave to capture average levels of worry across Americans and across time. Specifically, we asked how worried respondents were about the three social impacts of the virus: the economic impact, the disruption of normal life, and schools closing. We also asked about two health worries: how worried they were about getting sick themselves and how worried they were about friends and family getting sick.

Figure 4.1 shows the average level of worry for respondents by their partisan identity. These figures do not account for other

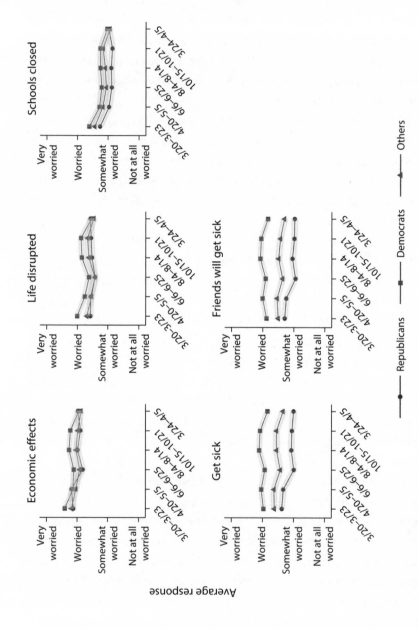

FIGURE 4.1. Worries across six waves (from March 2020 to April 2021)

demographics, but as we demonstrated in chapter 3, even accounting for education, employment, COVID cases in the respondent's
zip code, and other social and political factors does not alter these
patterns.

There are two main takeaways from Figure 4.1. First, the top three
figures show that there were high levels of worry on average about
the social disruptions from COVID-19. We see that in general Democrats were always more worried about the pandemic's social impacts
than Republicans, but the difference across parties is rather small.
Average levels of worry did not change very much except in the case
of worries about schools being closed, which for most Americans
happened between wave 1 and wave 2, so it was no longer something
to worry about; it was something to cope with.

Second, the bottom two figures show that there was significantly
more variation and disagreement in worries across the parties over
the health effects of the virus. Here we see a large difference. Republicans were substantially less worried about getting sick than were
Democrats, a difference that only grew over the course of the pandemic. In those figures, we see the psychological foundations of partisan differences in health behaviors. It stands to reason that if you
are worried about the virus, you will be more likely to take actions to
protect yourself such as self-quarantining and avoiding gatherings. By
contrast, those who are less worried about the pandemic would be
less likely to feel the need to take any individual actions that would
contain its spread. Figure 4.1 thus helps us to explain why, as we saw in
chapter 3, Republicans were less likely than Democrats and indepen-
dents/nonpartisans to adopt pro–social health behaviors. This was
not only true at the start of the pandemic, when the virus was more
concentrated in urban areas and in blue states but also grew throughout the course of the pandemic under the Trump administration
even as red states began to see huge numbers of hospitalizations and
deaths. The partisan gap in worries about COVID-19's health impacts
only began to shrink in the final wave of our survey once Joe Biden
was inaugurated and after three months of mass vaccination. And
these partisan gaps are not a product of different media habits: patterns are generally the same among right-wing news watchers and

those who consume news from other sources, although Republicans and Others who watch right-wing news are even less worried about getting sick than are Republicans and Others who do not.

Worries about the consequences of the pandemic were just one emotional response. Many Americans also experienced feelings of anger, sadness, and even disgust in response to the pandemic. In our survey, we asked respondents about five important feelings—anger, disgust, anxiety, sadness, and hope—and whether they had felt each when they thought about the U.S. government's response to the outbreak. This allowed us to see what emotional reaction people had to not just the virus itself but also, more specifically, the government's handling of the crisis. Figure 4.2 shows the percentage of respondents of each partisan group who answered that they felt these emotions at each wave of the survey.

The partisan divide in emotional responses is particularly striking, and we see the strong role of elite cues where we observe a reversal in wave 6 under President Biden. Throughout the final year of Trump's presidency, Democrats reported feeling more negative emotions, while Republicans expressed the positive emotion of hope more strongly. Seven out of ten Democrats reported feelings of anger, disgust, and sadness at the pandemic in late March, and this proportion grew over time. Levels of anxiety were high among Democrats throughout Trump's last year in office. As for hope? It was low among Democrats at the outset and fell over time nevertheless, just until Trump was replaced by Biden.

Republicans, by contrast, expressed very low levels of anger and disgust in March 2020. Feelings of sadness and anxiety among Republicans were more common but not by much. These numbers rose a bit over the first three waves, only to decline once again by late summer and into the fall. Republicans, though, remained far more hopeful through the course of the pandemic than did Democrats, even if their levels of hope did decline over the last survey wave. What really led Republicans to lose hope in the government's handling of the COVID-19 pandemic was the inauguration of Biden.

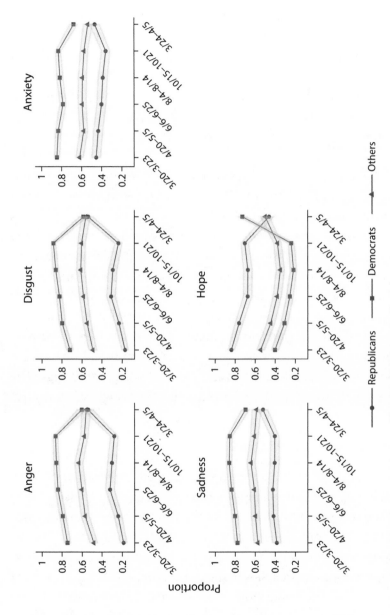

FIGURE 4.2. Emotions across six waves (from March 2020 to April 2021)

Republicans and Democrats, in sum, reported entirely different emotional responses to the pandemic. Republicans felt very hopeful at the outset of the pandemic, whereas Democrats experienced a range of negative emotions from anger to disgust. Although we do see some movement—rising anger, declining hope—across all Americans, these changes over time never even come close to erasing the stark partisan differences that we see. The only thing that seems to change what Americans think about the COVID-19 pandemic is the election of a new president from a different political party, as sure a sign as any of the essentially partisan character of the COVID-19 pandemic in the United States.

These emotional reactions surely help to explain partisan differences in health behaviors. And they also translate into politics in another way, by shaping which government actors Americans blame for poor pandemic performance and who they credit for doing well. Americans who were not worried about the consequences of the pandemic for their health and who expressed hope in the face of crushing adversity were exactly those Americans who were less likely to adopt strict measures to contain the spread of the pandemic. Likewise, those who felt fearful, anxious, and angry were those who sought to contain the crisis by adopting difficult and unpleasant responses such as self-quarantining and avoiding gatherings. The difference between these two groups of Americans? Partisanship.

Who Was to Blame?

Given that partisanship so strongly governed emotions and health behaviors in the pandemic, it is not surprising that it also guided which actors the public blamed for the country's poor performance in the earliest part of the pandemic.

When considering how the public evaluates government performance, most approaches to the politics of accountability expect that voters will consider how governments perform and will punish or reward them accordingly. These approaches usually assume that the public can evaluate how well government serves the public even when people have very little information about what the government is actually doing.[20] However, a strand of research in political science has argued that factors other than policy performance matter in how the public perceives of how well government is doing. If this is true, then citizens do not evaluate governments based on their performance in office because they don't know how, they make mistakes, or they care more about other things than performance itself.

As evidence of the weakness of public evaluation of government performance, political scientists have shown that voters punish incumbents for issues over which they have little control (e.g., shark attacks and bad weather), misattributing their own unhappy circumstances to government action or inaction.[21] In making attributions of credit and blame, people tend to ascribe positive outcomes more easily to their own groups and negative outcomes to outgroups, a "group serving bias."[22] Think about sports rivalries: Red Sox fans blame their losses on the Yankee players having cheated (a negative outcome from the outgroup), and Yankees fans will attribute their wins to their own skill and determination (a positive outcome for the ingroup).

No group in politics is more salient and important than the party. Partisan bias affects both who voters give credit to for successes and who they blame for failures. Partisans will attribute a successful economy to the president of their own party but to other actors when their party is not in power.[23] In a study of Hurricane Katrina, for example, researchers found partisan rationalization of blame in a natural disaster, showing that Democrats were almost twice as likely to blame Republican officials for the deaths from the hurricane when that information was presented in a partisan manner rather than simply describing what the official's job responsibility was.[24] In other words, simply referring to Louisiana governor Kathleen Blanco as "Louisiana governor Kathleen Blanco (Democrat)" increases the likelihood that Republicans blamed her for the devastation of Hurricane Katrina.

The American political system may also make it difficult to apportion blame properly even when people want to. Responses to major disasters such as the coronavirus pandemic involve the coordination of multiple federal agencies, leadership from the White House, state health departments, and governors, not to mention local authorities.[25] When things go wrong—when there aren't enough tests, contact tracing is inadequate, schools do not have enough resources to upgrade ventilation systems, and there is not enough personal protective equipment for frontline health workers or ventilators for hospitals—it is not always clear to voters which actors, among many, are most to blame.

To see how Americans apportioned blame in the context of such a complex political system, we asked respondents in waves 1 (March 2020) and 3 (June 2020) of the survey to evaluate who was most responsible for the lack of U.S. preparedness for the pandemic. Respondents saw this question: "Public health officials warn that the United States was not fully prepared for a coronavirus outbreak. Who do you think is most to blame for this lack of preparedness?" We then asked respondents to rank four actors with the names displayed in random order: President Donald Trump, former president Barack Obama, the Centers for Disease Control and Prevention, and state health agencies. We included Obama in the list so that respondents could signal that the previous administration had not done enough on pandemic preparedness even though the Trump administration had been in office for three years by that time. In wave 3, we randomized whether respondents saw "Barack Obama" or "Democrats in Congress" to test whether people who said "Obama" in wave 1 were signaling a blame of Democrats as a party or Obama as a president who previously faced the H1N1 and Ebola crises.

Figure 4.3 shows the percentage of respondents who rank each of the actors they saw as the "most blameworthy" by the respondent's partisan identity (we use the label "Barack Obama" to denote both those who saw "Barack Obama" and those who saw "Democrats in Congress").

Two big trends emerged from the data. First, Democrats and people who identify as independent or nonpartisan (the Other category) blamed Trump for the lack of preparedness more than any other actor. Their blame of Trump grew over the survey waves: in

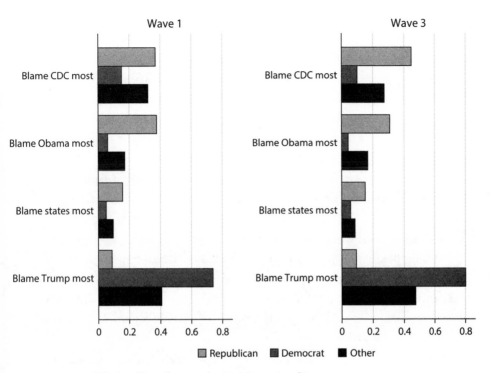

FIGURE 4.3. Who is to blame for poor planning? By partisanship

wave 1 in March, a little over 70 percent of Democrats put the primary blame on Trump for the poor COVID-19 response, and by June that had grown to 80 percent. Independents were more likely to spread their blame around than Democrats, but a plurality of them ranked Trump number one for blame, with 40 percent of those in the Other category blaming Trump the most in March, rising to 45 percent by June. Respondents in the Other category ranked the Centers for Disease Control and Prevention (CDC) as the second most blameworthy institution in both survey waves.

The second trend was that Republicans put the least blame on Trump of all actors they ranked, less than either Democrats or Others. Republicans are most likely to put blame on the CDC; almost 40 percent of Republicans in March 2020 and 43 percent in June blamed the CDC for failure to prepare. In March, equal numbers of Republicans blamed former president Obama for poor planning as blamed the CDC, which was about four times as great as the number of respondents who blamed Trump, who shared their partisan identity. By June, Republicans' rankings of culpability were unchanged; they still ranked Trump as the least blameworthy and the CDC as deserving of the most responsibility. We find similar results when we look at differences in blame according to intended vote choice (Trump, Biden, or Other) instead of partisan affiliation (Republican, Democrat, or Other).

To take stock so far, we have seen that our survey respondents viewed the same set of circumstances—a countrywide lockdown, an economy in freefall, and soaring death rates across the states— but responded in very different ways. There was wide disagreement among partisan groups about which part of the government should be held responsible. Republicans and Trump voters looked for any- one other than the president to blame, whereas Democrats and non- partisans/independents put the most responsibility on Trump and the CDC for failure to prepare.

Consistent with our discussion of the politics of accountability above, knowing who or what to blame after a disaster such as a pan- demic is important for democracy so that voters can decide how to sanction actors they believe are not living up to their obligations or acting in the best interests of the country. When the public feels pain from deaths or destruction that can be at least tangentially linked to government policy, they do hold government responsible—but they blame leaders of the other party rather than leaders of their own.[26] If the threat is external, such as a terrorist attack, or if a leader is successful in framing the threat as external—as Trump attempted to do by consistently bringing up China and using a series of pejora- tive, racialized epithets to describe the virus—incumbent leaders can sometimes deflect blame.[27]

This is more than just an intellectual curiosity. Wide partisan gaps in blame attribution suggest that the public may inadvertently pun- ish actors who are not clearly responsible for tasks such as, in this case, having a pandemic playbook or distributing federal reserves of personal protective equipment efficiently.[28] Partisan bias in blame attribution means that people do not use the same criteria to judge presidents of their own party as they do members of the other party. Indeed, they may actually shift how they view conditions on the ground on issues as wide ranging as the economy, war, and foreign policy to comport with their partisan identity.[29] In the COVID-19 case, this produced a partisan feedback effect in blame attribution whereby Republicans declined to blame Trump for mishandling the pandemic, which led them to believe that the pandemic was not as serious in the first place, further hardening their belief that Trump was not to blame in the first place. And the same occurs in reverse for Democrats. Democrats' high levels of anger and Republicans' extremely low levels are reflected in which actors they blame for the poor performance on keeping Americans safe from COVID-19. Republicans, more hopeful than angry about the pandemic response, put little blame on Trump, the actor Democrats deemed the most responsible and culpable for the disaster. Democrats, worried about their own health and angry about the government response, put the blame squarely on the president.

Given these dynamics, partisans became ever more divided precisely because they disagree about what the pandemic meant. And without a common belief about what constitutes good policy making or what sorts of behaviors are deserving of sanction, bipartisan responses to policies—good or bad—are impossible. Without bipartisan consensus on at least some policies, it is hard to see how democratic policies could produce political accountability. Partisan politicians, knowing this, have little reason not to play to their base whenever possible.

Figure 4.4 shows these relationships between anger, anxiety, hope, and blame directly. Each graph compares those who blame each group the most by whether they report feeling anger, anxiety, and hope.

Among the respondents who expressed anger over the government's handling of the pandemic, almost 70 percent blamed Trump the most in both waves of the survey. Among those who expressed no anger, they were more likely to blame the CDC for poor performance. Hopeful respondents put the most blame on the CDC, consistent with what we found above: that Republicans expressed

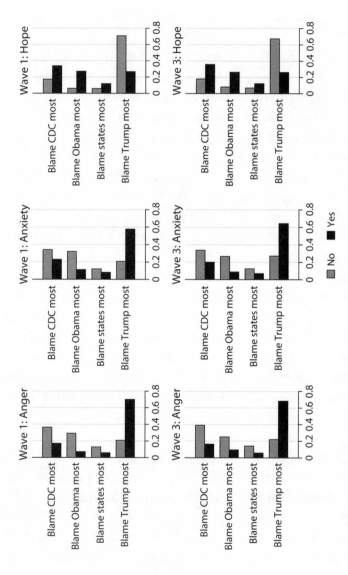

FIGURE 4.4. Who is to blame for poor planning? By respondent emotion

higher levels of hope and were more likely to blame the CDC or Obama than Trump.

Who Deserved Credit?

While there is a great deal of difference in who the public blames for the government response to the pandemic, there is more agreement on which people they give credit to for their actions. In wave 2 of our survey (April 2020), we asked respondents to evaluate not just who was to blame for what was clearly now a national crisis but also who should get credit for helping Americans *during* the COVID pandemic. Respondents could say that an actor deserved none at all, very little, some, or a great deal. Respondents were given the following choices to rate: Trump, state health agencies, state governors, doctors, essential workers (grocery store workers, bus drivers, janitors, etc.), and Dr. Anthony Fauci (director of the National Institute of Allergy and Infectious Diseases).

Figure 4.5 shows the percentage of all respondents who fall in each category of credit. Majorities gave some or a great deal of credit to state actors—governors and health departments—for their performance. And large majorities also answered that doctors, essential workers, and Dr. Fauci deserve a "great deal" of credit. (Fauci, an early hero of the U.S. pandemic response, would later become a central villain among conservative media and the political right. Tucker Carlson on Fox News would refer to him as "the guy who created Covid," among other pejoratives. Florida governor Ron DeSantis would sell merchandise that said "Don't Fauci My Florida." Trump attempted to fire Fauci numerous times, retweeting a message as early as April 13 that ended with "Time to #FireFauci." And by the winter of 2021 several Republican members of the House and Senate would call for Fauci to be jailed.)

Trump was the only actor on the list who was judged as not deserving credit from a majority of respondents. Approximately 60 percent of respondents judged Trump as worthy of "very little" or "none at all."

We know how strongly divided respondents were by partisanship based on their emotional reactions and their evaluations of blame for

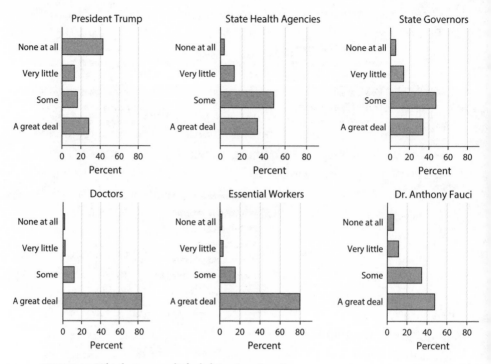

FIGURE 4.5. Who deserves credit for helping Americans?

the pandemic, but it appears that there was a clearer shared reality on which actors were helping people in the pandemic. If we divide up respondents by their partisanship, the same story emerges: there was wide agreement across parties that doctors, essential workers, Fauci, governors, and state health agencies were deserving of high praise from most respondents. The one actor where there was a clear partisan difference in evaluating was Trump. Voters who preferred Trump said that he deserved a similar amount of credit as doctors and essential workers for helping people with the pandemic, but Biden and third-party voters gave Trump very little credit on average for helping the American public. This also revealed a degree of cognitive dissonance for Republicans; one would not think that doctors and essential workers merit the lion's share of credit if one also believes that the pandemic is not a serious threat. The fact that Republicans also credited Trump might explain this finding if they

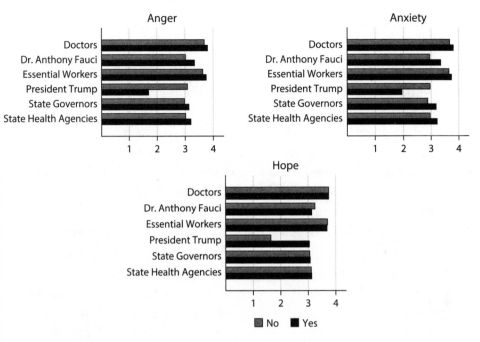

FIGURE 4.6. Who deserves credit? By respondent emotion

believed that the pandemic was not much of a threat because he had led a successful public health responses.

Emotions, particularly anger and hope, strongly determined which actors the public blamed for a lack of preparedness for COVID. Did emotions matter for how much credit people gave government officials for helping? Figure 4.6 shows the average level of credit respondents gave to the same actors by whether they felt anger, anxiety, or hope about government's handling of the pandemic. For the most part, feeling either a negative or a positive emotion did not correlate with how creditworthy people rate most actors. The exception to this pattern is ratings of how much credit Trump should get for his handling of the pandemic. These findings are a mirror image to the blame findings: those people who express anger or anxiety give Trump very little credit, while those who express hope give significantly more credit to the president's handling of the pandemic.

Conclusion

The COVID-19 pandemic was an emotional time, perhaps the greatest understatement in the history of social science. In theory, few political scenarios are more threatening for the public and for political leaders than an unknown pathogen capable of killing otherwise healthy people making its way around the globe with little respect for borders. The regular tools of policy making and keeping the public safe were inadequate against a crisis that not only was sickening Americans but also crashed entire industries such as travel, entertainment, and dining, leaving the whole economy upended.

Unsurprisingly, there was a great deal of negative emotion about the pandemic—anger and disgust at the government's poor performance and worry about getting sick and life being disrupted—and these negative feelings have been sustained over the course of many months. We have shown, though, that these negative feelings about public health and the government response to the pandemic were stronger among Democrats than Republicans at the outset of the pandemic and stayed stronger over time. Democrats worried more than Republicans, and in particular they worried about getting sick. Republicans were hopeful, expressing less worry about becoming ill and fewer negative emotions about the early chaotic and ineffective government response to the pandemic.

Most of the time, people respond to shock events such as a pandemic in a standard fashion. They assess whether there is something wrong, how relevant this threat or opportunity is to them, how certain they are of the cause, and whether there is someone or something responsible for the threats. The emotions that they feel, in turn, help to shape their responses to the event in terms of both self-protecting behavior and whom they blame for the event. But in the COVID-19 pandemic, partisanship intervened in this process. Partisanship affected both the emotional response and how people apportioned credit and blame for the handling of the pandemic. Something as basic as our emotional response to the pandemic was essentially biased by partisan identity. Democrats and Republicans alike saw the same death rates and government response but blamed different actors for these outcomes and even felt differently about them. We showed in chapter 3 how partisanship shaped health behavior, and in what follows we will investigate the implications for public policy in response to the pandemic.

For the millions of Americans who suffered hardship and loss during the COVID-19 pandemic, it is deeply troubling to know that at a very basic level, so many of their fellow Americans experienced the pandemic entirely differently. It is not just that their experiences were different but also that their emotional responses were different. For many Democrats and others consumed by anxiety about the pandemic, the idea that many Republicans and others were simply not that worried about it is jarring. For Republicans and others who maintained hope that the pandemic would be brief and that reopening would be feasible after just a couple of weeks, the notion that millions of Americans were settling in for months—even years—of reduced activity was unsettling. These partisan emotional responses eroded any possibility of bipartisan comity, a truly American response to the pandemic in which all Americans feel themselves to be in the crisis together. Americans like to believe that wars, economic crises, and other moments of national hardship bring us all together. But the feelings of anger, anxiety, and hope prompted by the COVID-19 pandemic divided Americans in partisan terms rather than uniting them.

5

What Your Country Can Do for You

THE PARTISAN SPLIT IN POLICY

Cars lined up around the block outside of Dodger Stadium in downtown Los Angeles (LA), with wait times to get inside exceeding three hours. This wasn't a playoff game, though. Dodger Stadium was made into one of LA County's first mass coronavirus drive-up testing sites in March 2020, and these were people waiting to get a COVID test. All had already been screened and made appointments using an LA city web portal. At first, these tests were only available to individual exhibiting symptoms, first responders, and caregivers. One couple, who were both feeling sick and had been waiting for over two hours, expressed frustration with the system: "We're both here to be tested. She's worse than I am. We didn't expect this. . . . I'm losing faith. I'm getting ready just to leave. This is ridiculous."[1]

Scaling up mass testing was slow; there weren't enough tests, and there weren't enough appointment slots. Some surrounding counties, such as Riverside and Orange, were also ramping up tests, but others, such as San Bernadino, had yet to start. And there weren't enough staff; the National Guard and firefighters were collecting nasal swabs alongside health care professionals. It was dire enough that California governor Gavin Newsom was asking retired health care workers to come back. And even someone who managed to get tested for coronavirus in those early days would see massive delays in getting the results. A commercial lab in Orange County increased testing fivefold, and people in the county were waiting a week or more for test results during which time they were likely spreading the virus to others. There was also a question of who would pay. As the president of the American Clinical Laboratory Association wrote in a letter to congressional leaders, while the Donald Trump administration promised free COVID-19 testing for Americans, "Laboratories should not bear the cost of 'free' testing."[2] By March 2020, LA County had given up on testing as a means of "containing" the coronavirus outbreak.[3]

Eventually, Americans would be able to buy rapid antigen COVID tests for at-home use. There was free testing at some sites across the country, including CVS and Rite Aid pharmacies, and some cities and schools made tests freely available to their residents, but Americans had to pay for the convenience of an at-home test: a two-test pack manufactured by Abbott Pharmaceutical cost $23.99. Meanwhile, Britons could buy them for a pound or get them delivered to their home free of charge. In Germany, tests were free until October 2021 (phased out as part of a scheme to encourage vaccination), and in France an at-home test cost the same as a cup of coffee. Unlike European models, the Food and Drug Administration (FDA) only ever approved two companies to manufacture at-home tests, which necessarily constrained supply and drove up prices. Moreover, fewer Americans were testing over the summer of 2021, as vaccines were widely available, so Abbott scaled back production.[4] Thus, by the time kids were heading back to school in the fall and cases started rising again, there were no tests to be found. At the end of October, President Joe Biden—using funds from the American Rescue Plan—would direct the National Institutes of Health to help speed up the authorization process for new tests to enter the market.[5]

This chapter pivots from the question of what Americans did in response to the pandemic—how individuals behaved (chapter 3) and felt (chapter 4) in response to the pandemic—to ask what Americans thought the government should do. What kind of policies should the government enact during the pandemic? What kind of authority should the government have? What factors shaped Americans' attitudes toward unprecedented policies rolled out during the pandemic, such as providing free COVID-19 tests, expanded unemployment insurance, and rent relief? Should the federal government or state governments take responsibility for managing the resources and response to COVID-19? How long would government intervention be necessary? The answers to these questions reveal the extent to which divides over government responses to the pandemic would mirror the behavioral responses and emotional reactions we have uncovered so far.

Unsurprisingly, partisanship drove policy attitudes. How Americans thought about government performance and responsibility were primarily determined by their partisan identities during the pandemic. Republicans wanted quick reopening and fewer regulations, while Democrats sought more caution and a greater role for government in ensuring public health and managing the pandemic. And as we show later in this chapter, at least part of this partisan gap is the consequence of Republicans' and Democrats' different beliefs about how long the pandemic would last and for how long an active government response to it would be necessary.

In analyzing how Americans believed the government ought to respond to the COVID-19 pandemic, we confront some key questions in American politics. One central axis of debate is individual liberty versus state authority: although many Americans cherish their freedom from government interference in most aspects of their daily lives, the COVID-19 pandemic forced them to weigh that freedom against the benefits of the kind of swift and comprehensive public health response that only a government can provide. In the context of very low levels of trust in government, a particular feature of modern American politics, these questions get at the core of the relationship between citizens and their government.

A secondary debate involves how a government should respond to a pandemic. Should a government mobilize the National Guard to coordinate the pandemic response? Should the federal government or the states take the lead? Should the federal government implement contact tracing in response to confirmed diagnoses, or should it implement more aggressive policies (as did countries such as Singapore) to monitor people's movements? Amid all of this, the question of partisanship generated interesting tensions as well, because giving authority to the federal government would mean for most Democrats empowering a Republican administration whose actions they generally opposed. The conundrum for Republicans— commonly viewed as more skeptical of federal authority than Democrats—is that their party controlled the federal bureaucracy.

As we saw with the case of health behaviors, partisan differences on policy attitudes emerged early in the pandemic and persisted over time. That Americans were so divided so early over government responses to the pandemic is a worrying sign of how partisanship shapes public life even in the face of a truly unprecedented crisis. The persistence of partisan differences over health policy, moreover, runs contrary to many expectations that a severe public health crisis would eventually bring Americans together as the devastating toll that the pandemic had on Americans of all backgrounds became clear. A more united American mass public might have presented a bipartisan case for concerted government action to combat the pandemic, but in its absence government responses to the pandemic became just one more partisan issue.

But, again, partisan disagreements over government responses to the pandemic were not inevitable. As we argued in chapter 2, we believe that a committed federal government response led by the Trump administration could have produced a different outcome. Democrats wanted to support a strong pandemic response, and Republicans wanted to support their president. Bipartisan approaches could have increased national unity by truly encouraging Americans to pull together and rally around the flag, much like what has happened in national emergencies and crises of the past. But that is not what happened.

COVID Testing

Diagnostic testing was one of the most vital steps for mitigating the spread of COVID and also proved to be one of the more elusive steps for the United States in the early days of the pandemic. The Centers for Disease Control and Prevention (CDC) decided not to adopt a German-developed test used by the World Health Organization and instead create its own. On February 4, 2020, when the CDC received "emergency use authorization" from the FDA to distribute its test widely, it only sent out around two hundred tests nationwide.[6] When some of these tests started to report inconclusive results, revealed later to be the result of manufacturing errors, this created an estimated delay of six weeks. Moreover, bureaucratic red tape from the FDA prohibited states, hospitals, and private labs from developing their own tests.

On February 28—forty-seven days after the Chinese distributed the virus's genetic sequence[7]—the CDC announced that the contamination issue with its test was fixed and that it was ramping up for mass rollout, and the next day the FDA relaxed its rules to allow for COVID-19 tests to be developed in-house. But February was a lost month, and these delays enabled the virus to spread and establish a toehold across communities in America. Citing the *Washington Post,* "As late as Feb. 27, only 203 specimen tests had been run out of state labs; another 3,125 had been run out of the CDC."[8]

Developing a COVID-19 test was a problem, as was distributing tests on a scale that could enable mass testing. The CDC had to get tests to the states, where mass testing sites had to be constructed de novo. With demand far outweighing supply, by early March the United States was still only testing those who had been to China, had been exposed to someone who tested positive for COVID, or were experiencing symptoms. The lack of widespread test availability, for both the symptomatic and asymptomatic, ultimately meant that the death toll was undercounted, as only confirmed cases of COVID were included in the official tally. And as we knew at the time and know all too well now, testing asymptomatic people is essential to mapping, tracing, and ultimately containing the spread of COVID-19.

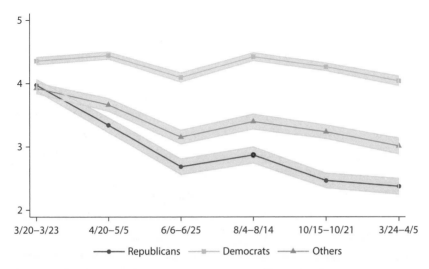

FIGURE 5.1. "We have enough coronavirus tests in my state," by partisanship

What were citizens thinking? Factually, we know there were not enough tests. Newspapers were also reporting on the difficulties facing Americans who needed a test. A *New York Times* headline on March 12 states "Sick People across the U.S. Say They Are Being Denied the Coronavirus Test."[9] But did all Americans agree that there were not enough tests? We asked respondents in all six waves of our survey whether they agreed that there were not enough tests to see if Americans shared a basic set of beliefs about the pandemic itself and, indirectly, to probe whether Americans might expect different responses from their government. Figure 5.1 presents average levels of agreement on a scale of 1 (strongly disagree, meaning that there were enough tests) to 5 (strongly agree, meaning that there were not enough tests).

In March, a majority of respondents—regardless of party—held that there were not enough tests. Republicans, though, were significantly less likely to agree that there were not enough tests. Moving into April 2020, this gap began to widen: even as Americans of all partisan orientations moved toward the position that there were enough tests, Republicans moved faster than did Democrats. This shift in Republican opinions about testing capacity coincides with

Trump's attempt to counter critiques over availability from public health experts: "There have been some very partisan voices in the media who have spread false and misleading information about our testing capacity."[10]

By June as testing capacities were expanded and bottlenecks in distribution were addressed, both Republicans and Democrats expressed more confidence that testing capacity was sufficient, but differences in party positions were still quite large. This partisan gap grew further in August, coinciding with the second wave of COVID-19. In sum, we see a wide and consistent partisan gap in beliefs about testing availability that persists throughout the final year of the Trump administration. The partisan gap only truly narrowed in wave 6 (April 2021). By then, with a new president in office and over twenty-one million vaccines having been allocated in the United States,[11] Democrats' beliefs about testing availability finally began to approach those of Republicans and nonpartisans. There was no wave 7, but we can imagine that had we asked this question again in September of 2021, the same Americans who are vaccinated would be the very same expressing concern about the availability of COVID tests, given the rise in breakthrough cases from the novel delta variant, and with unvaccinated kids going back to school.

Did attitudes about test availability vary by age? Given the disproportionate impact of COVID-19 on the 65+ cohort during the first wave, we might expect older citizens—who were more vulnerable to the pandemic—to be more concerned about test availability. Figure 5.2 shows confidence in test availability by partisanship and age cohort.

Unsurprisingly, older Americans were more concerned about the pandemic than younger Americans. But surprisingly, the gaps between Democrats and Republicans are larger among seniors than they are among any other age group. This tells us that just as Democratic seniors were the most concerned about test availability, Republican seniors were the most confident in test availability.

In chapter 6, we examine attitudes toward other COVID-19 policies as they relate to the economy and welfare, including making

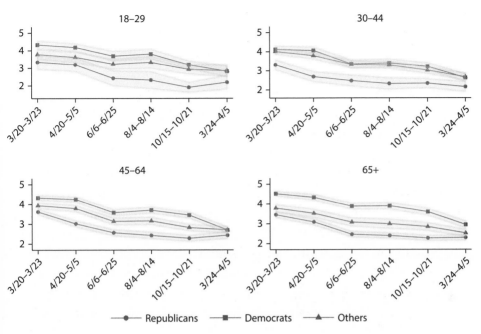

FIGURE 5.2. "We have enough coronavirus tests in my state," by partisanship and age

COVID tests free for all Americans, waiving insurance costs for treating COVID-19, and proving paid leave for individuals diagnosed with COVID-19. But this first policy—beliefs about whether there are enough tests available—gave us an early window into partisanship and policy attitudes over time. Americans did not share common beliefs about core facts about the pandemic. From this baseline, it will not be surprising that Americans disagreed about what to do about it.

Federal Authority

There are many other things that governments can do besides distributing tests. Viewed relative to other advanced democracies, in fact, making sure that tests were available to everyone who needs them was a very low bar. We now move from the question of government capacity to government authority: instead of asking how the federal government was doing (and whether that was sufficient or not), we asked what Americans thought the federal government should do? This taps into fundamental questions that have long divided American parties about how much authority to give to the federal government.

In the context of a divided Congress, a divisive president, and an unprecedented pandemic, though, the partisan politics of granting more authority to the federal government are complicated. On the one hand, partisan consideration should predict that Democrats would want to give a president of the opposing party as few powers as possible. On the other hand, Democrats wanted the government to do something in response to the pandemic and for the pandemic to be taken seriously. Republicans, for their part, might have preferred a more limited role for government, consistent with conservative principles in American politics. But at the same time, they might have preferred that their president be given the authority to respond to the pandemic on the belief that only by acting quickly and decisively can the president bring the pandemic to an end. And given the general low-trust environment in which policies are made, even minimal government steps might be opposed. But our survey revealed that Democrats' reluctance to grant Trump more powers was outweighed by their desire for the government to do something in response to the pandemic. Republicans, by contrast, generally preferred government inaction.

To disentangle the partisan politics of COVID-19, we begin by looking at responses to a general question of lockdown enforcement. We asked individuals in June whether "authorities in my state should strictly enforce lockdown measures" or "not enforce lockdown measures," with a sliding scale to indicate a respondent's position between 1 (strictly enforce) and 9 (not enforce). This question not only measures support or opposition to lockdown measures but also explicitly forces respondents to gauge how involved their state government should be in enforcing lockdown measures. Around the world, there was wide variation in how stay-at-home orders were designed and enforced. For instance, on the more restrictive end of the spectrum, for nearly two months beginning in March 2020

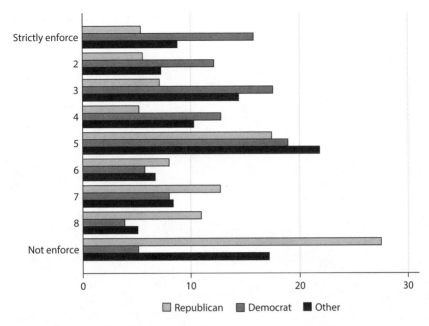

FIGURE 5.3. Support for enforcement of lockdown measures, by partisanship

France required all residents to obtain permission for any travel outside of the home and were fined if individuals were found outside of their allowed perimeter.

Figure 5.3 presents support for enforcing lockdowns by partisanship. We see a clear partisan divide in support for enforcement of lockdown: Democrats wanted the governments to exercise stronger enforcement of lockdown measures, and Republicans did not.

While Republican attitudes here may also be tapping into general antigovernment sentiments rather than something particular to the COVID-19 pandemic, these differences reveal the deep partisan divide in how Americans were thinking about enforcing lockdowns in June 2020. A plurality of Republican respondents adamantly opposed any government effort to impose a lockdown whatsoever. Democrats were slightly less extreme in their willingness to embrace lockdown measures, but most Democrats were nevertheless mildly to strongly supportive of lockdown measures. As we discuss below,

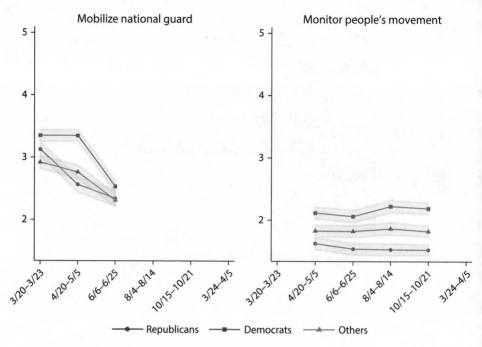

FIGURE 5.4. Support for state authority in implementing quarantines

this difference in tolerance for lockdown measures reflects different expectations about the likely course of the pandemic.

Related to the general issue of lockdowns and their enforcement, we also asked citizens about their support for two very specific policies about how to control the pandemic: mobilizing the National Guard to enforce quarantines and the government monitoring people's movements. Respondents answered these questions on a scale of 1 (strongly disagree) to 5 (strongly agree). Republicans tend to have greater confidence in the military[12] and digital surveillance measures[13] yet also tend to oppose federal or state interference in their private lives. Democrats, by contrast, are less supportive of the military but more comfortable with using the coercive capacity of the state the protect public health.

Figure 5.4 shows how these policy views evolved over time, with the caveat that we did not ask each of these questions in every survey wave.

When it comes to mobilizing the National Guard, which state governors did discretionarily from time to time to distribute personal protective equipment and provide patient care, partisan differences in policy attitudes were very small in March 2020. The divide increases dramatically in wave 2, driven by changes in Republicans and independents/nonpartisans who became much less supportive of deploying the National Guard to enforce quarantines. April was also the time when Trump began intimidating state governors in an effort to push them to open their economies up once again, a point we expand on below. By June, as economic and social life began to thaw, all groups expressed fairly low support for enforcing a quarantine. With the question of enforcing a quarantine no longer salient for most Americans, we stopped asking this question in wave 3.

Monitoring people's movements, by contrast, proved to be a widely unpopular view across all Americans, Democrats and Republicans alike. This opposition to monitoring people's movements may be motivated by privacy concerns that are shared by Americans of all partisan orientations. Yet even given this low level of support for monitoring people's movements, there is a substantial partisan gap that persists over time: Democrats are much more likely to support the monitoring of movement than are Republicans, probably on the belief that the objective of controlling the pandemic outweighs concerns about privacy. These results align with a Pew Research Center study conducted in April 2020 that shows only modest agreement that "if the government tracked people's locations through their cellphone during the coronavirus outbreak it would help a lot/a little in limiting the spread of the virus." Thirty-one percent of Republicans agreed with this statement, while 45 percent of Democrats and 42 percent of independents agreed.[14]

This general opposition to monitoring people's movement notwithstanding, the nearly complete lack of systematic and coordinated contact tracing made the United States an outlier among advanced industrialized countries. Elsewhere we saw a variety of contact tracing practices. Israel used cellphone location data, while Singapore employed a smartphone app, relying on a voluntary location-tracking system whereby individuals scanned a quick-response code when entering a taxi or shop. Taiwan's location-tracking phone app was mandatory and was used to enforce quarantines, and citizens who strayed beyond their lockdown range were notified by text to contact police immediately or incur a hefty fine. In advanced democracies, concerns about privacy rights make citizens more hesitant about app-based contact tracing,[15] but a study in France showed that people with higher trust in government were more willing to download a contact-tracing app.[16]

There are many reasons why the United States fared so poorly during the early stages of the pandemic, with staggering death tolls and uncontrolled spread, not the least of which was the insufficient number of tests and the patchwork U.S. health care system. But privacy concerns[17] and distrust of government[18] from both parties likely discouraged the federal government from pushing for a more aggressive contact tracing system. In August 2020, an article about contact tracing titled "The Most American COVID-19 Failure Yet" appeared in *The Atlantic*.[19]

To probe these issues more fully, we asked a second version of this monitoring question to see if we could tease apart the idea of the government monitoring movement (knowing enough about people's movements to track their activities, whom they meet, and so forth) and the explicit implementation of a government-run contact tracing program. We asked this question in August 2020 (wave 4). This timing is important: August 2020 was far enough into the pandemic that mass testing and mobile apps were widely available and could be distributed at scale. August 2020 was also the middle of the second wave of the pandemic, after a summer of loosened regulations and the country letting down its guard.

Figure 5.5 compares our results for these two items, revealing very different levels of support for the two different approaches to monitoring and contact tracing. On the right, we replicate the results from figure 5.3 (wave 4 only); on the left, we see the item that explicitly asks about contact tracing. Americans are broadly opposed to monitoring people's movement, but they do support contact tracing, especially Democrats.

This level of support for contact tracing among Democrats is notable. We might have expected low trust in government among

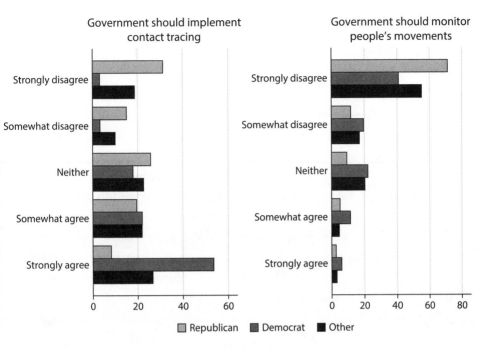

FIGURE 5.5. Comparing contact tracing and monitoring movement

Democrats to lead them to oppose policies that empower the government in this way. But in the context of the pandemic, Democrats were motivated to do something to combat the spread of COVID-19, and their desire for the government to "do something" outweighed their distrust of Trump's administration and their antipathy toward Republicans.

In the end, there were many things that the federal government could have done to mitigate the impact of the COVID-19 pandemic. So far in this chapter, we have looked at two of the most important: mass testing and strategies to monitor (and thus control) the spread of COVID-19. The delay in mass testing and the total failure to adopt contact tracing directly contributed to unnecessary loss of life. In fact, White House coronavirus response coordinator Dr. Deborah Birx, once the Biden administration had taken over, stated in an interview with CNN that "I look at it this way. The first time, we have an excuse. There were about 100,000 deaths that came from that original surge. All of the rest of them, in my mind, could have been mitigated or decreased substantially if we took the lessons we had learned from that moment."[20]

Cancel Everything?

As Trump sought to project an image of "politics as usual" to assuage economic uncertainty at the beginning of the pandemic, events were beyond his control. On March 6, the University of Washington in Seattle announced that it was moving all classes online. On March 11, the National Basketball Association suspended its season after Utah Jazz players tested positive for COVID. This was soon followed by Major League Baseball and the National Hockey League. On March 12, Broadway shut its doors. St. Patrick's Day parades nationwide were canceled. The Coachella Valley Music Festival was canceled. The 2020 Summer Olympics in Tokyo was canceled, the first time that an Olympics were canceled since World War II. Taylor Swift and Harry Styles canceled sold-out world tours. And if something couldn't be canceled, it moved online. All of these changes took place before Trump declared a national state of emergency on March 13.

These mass cancellations created de facto lockdowns throughout the United States, even in states that did not issue official stay-at-home orders. This was what Mounk described in his *Atlantic* column "Cancel Everything," which included "extreme social distancing" in the form of mass cancellation of events, from sports to universities to presidential campaigns.[21] "This administration is unlikely to do these things well or quickly," he wrote. "Hence, the responsibility for social distancing now falls on decision makers at every level of society."

Mounk's argument reminds us that when we consider policy options in response to COVID-19, we have to include those that were outside of the government's authority. How much did individuals support "canceling everything"? This idea shifts from thinking explicitly about what government should do to more general views about how society as a whole ought to respond to COVID-19. As Mounk indicates, this captures what individuals and businesses should do in the absence of government leadership.

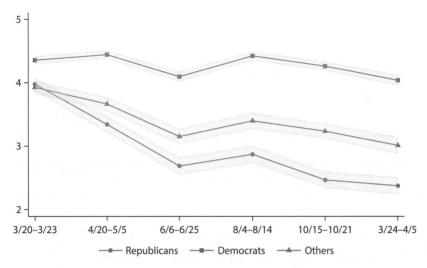

FIGURE 5.6. Support for canceling everything

To capture Americans' views about these issues, over the course of our survey we asked individuals whether they supported banning public events. In figure 5.6, we map support for banning public events among Democrats, Republicans, and Others across all six waves. Respondents indicated their support for banning events on a scale from 1 "Strongly disagree" to 5 "Strongly agree."

In March 2020 at the outset of the pandemic, there was relatively strong support for "canceling everything" among all Americans. This aligns with an early consensus whereby, as the saying goes, "we're all in this together."[22] Schools went virtual in red states and blue states alike, and late-night TV shows started broadcasting from home.

By April, however, there were the beginnings of the sort of partisan divergence that we have detected in so many other aspects of the pandemic. For Democrats, support for canceling everything remained consistently high throughout the pandemic, persisting even into wave 6 under the Biden administration. For Republicans, support for canceling everything dropped precipitously in April and June. The steep drop-off in support for canceling everything in mid-April happened just as protests started to crop up across the country to "reopen the economy." From Minnesota to Utah and California to

Michigan, Trump lambasted Democratic governors for their strong measures to control the spread of the virus ("the cure can't be worse than the problem itself"). And as one Utah citizen put it, "Quarantine is for sick people; you lock sick people away. . . . But when you lock healthy people away, that's tyranny."[23] April 12 was also the date that Trump, who liked the idea of packed churches on Easter Sunday, had previously announced as his target for a return to normal.

The closeness of Democrats and Republicans in early March 2020 occurred during that window of opportunity that we have discussed previously, where a unifying message might have kept these groups closer together. But the Trump White House was not so inclined. As Democratic presidential nominees Biden and Bernie Sanders moved their campaigns online, Trump continued to hold in-person rallies, some of which proved to be COVID-19 superspreader events.[24] Republican opposition to canceling or adapting events reflected Trump's eagerness, shared by the Republican Party leadership, to project confidence and get the economy going again. Many Americans were genuinely hurting from the economic shutdown, and surely many Americans found the onetime Coronavirus Aid, Relief, and Economic Security (CARES) Act stimulus of $1,200 per adult to be insufficient. And although it can be difficult to recall those months, March and April were a time of confusion and uncertainty. How much of the opposition to cancellation might be driven by optimism, eagerness, fatigue, or all of the above?

To get a sense of Americans' views about the likely course of the pandemic—and thereby understand Americans' feelings of optimism toward reopening and their expectations for the coming months—we asked in wave 2 of our survey "When will American businesses be able to resume normal business operations?" Figure 5.7 shows the results.

Republicans were quite confident that businesses would reopen by May or June, an optimistic perspective that is consistent with the feelings of hope that we identified in chapter 4. And many Democrats and independents believed that businesses could reopen by June as well. But a large proportion of Democrats did not share this optimism. Democratic respondents reported either a readiness to reopen soon (by June or July) or at a later date after the summer

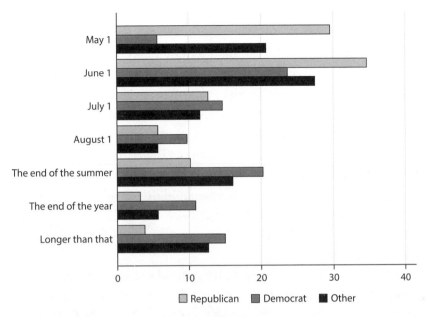

FIGURE 5.7. Prospects for reopening businesses, April 2020

("end of the summer," "end of the year," "longer than that"). These responses may reflect Democrats' fundamental pessimism about the president's ability to coordinate a safe reopening or their general unwillingness to prioritize the economy over human life. Whatever the reason, Republicans were far more optimistic about reopening early and likely were thinking about reopening as a worthwhile policy choice even given the risks to vulnerable Americans. In late March Dan Patrick, Texas's Republican lieutenant governor, said on Tucker Carlson, "Let's get back to living. Let's be smart about it. And those of us who are 70-plus, we'll take care of ourselves, but don't sacrifice the country. . . . Our biggest gift we give to our country and our children and our grandchildren is the legacy of our country, and right now, that is at risk. . . . I think we can get back to work."[25]

Schools: Back in Session?

Perhaps nothing was more destabilizing to American families than school-age children learning from home. The pandemic forced a "near-total shutdown" whereby almost every school switched to virtual learning in March 2020,[26] with tens of millions of American children remaining online for some or all of the 2020–2021 school year. School closing and reopening policies were generally made by local school district and county officials, and experiences varied widely even within a single geographical area. In southern California, you could drive south one hundred miles along Pacific Coast Highway, from Long Beach in Los Angeles County, where first graders attended school virtually, to Newport Beach in Orange County, with in-person first grade, to La Jolla in San Diego County, where first grade was virtual again. Or you could drive twenty miles from downtown Cleveland, where schools were virtual for the 2020–2021 school year, to find hybrid and in-person models in neighboring counties.

The politics of schooling laid bare some of the more difficult trade-offs about the pandemic. The epidemiological data are clear that young people are far less likely to be seriously affected by COVID-19 than are adults. But young people live with adults, in many cases with grandparents or other extended family members who are at elevated risk to COVID-19, and schools could be prime sites for transmission among even low-risk youths. Unsurprisingly, the public debate on the question of how to reopen schools was divisive. Emily Oster, an economist at Brown University, urged schools and childcare centers to reopen.[27] Her essays focused on the economic implications of prolonged virtual schooling: the health risk to children was low, and parents needed to get back to work. This position faced stiff opposition from teachers' unions that felt schools that were not taking necessary safety precautions and also from public health experts who observed that Oster's advice seemed to address the conditions of upper-middle-class suburban white families, even though Black and Hispanic children were at much higher risk of COVID.[28]

But how did ordinary Americans think about these risks? We can answer this question in a couple of ways using data from our survey. In waves 1–2, from the spring of 2020, we asked our respondents how much they agreed with the statement that schools should be closed in response to the pandemic. The fourth wave of our survey, which we fielded in August 2020, coincided with the beginning of

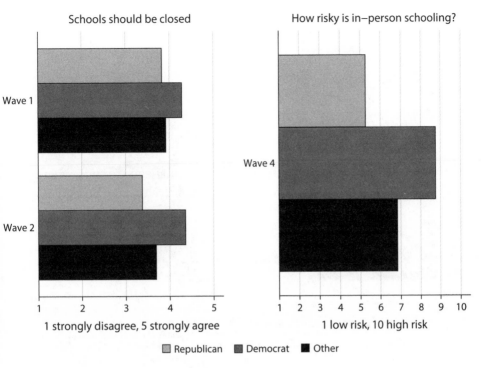

FIGURE 5.8. School opening and safety, by party

the regular school year across the United States and therefore presented us with an ideal opportunity to look at Americans' attitudes about in-person school. In this wave, we asked people to rate the riskiness of sending children on a scale of 1 (low risk) to 10 (high risk). In figure 5.8 we display our results, broken down by partisan affiliation of the respondent.

When we look at views on school closures from the earliest months of the pandemic, there was fairly strong support (especially in wave 1) for school closures regardless of respondents' partisan identities. The gap widened in wave 2 between Democrats who favor school closures and Republicans who are becoming more eager to reopen schools. Turning to wave 4, we see that partisanship plays a central role in respondents' views about just how risky in-person schooling is. For some context, the average Democratic score for the riskiness of in-person schooling (8.8 on a scale of 1–10) was higher

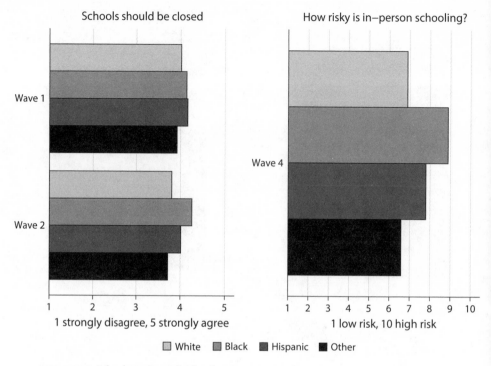

Schools should be closed

How risky is in–person schooling?

Wave 1

Wave 4

Wave 2

1 strongly disagree, 5 strongly agree

1 low risk, 10 high risk

☐ White   ◼ Black   ◼ Hispanic   ◼ Other

FIGURE 5.9. School opening and safety, by race

than the average Democratic score for the riskiness of eating indoors (8.2) and the same as attending a social gathering (8.8). Among Republicans, the score for the riskiness of in-person schooling was 5.3, lower than eating indoors (5.7) or attending a social gathering (5.6). We can explain these differences by noting that Republicans in our data were far more likely to believe that children are at low risk from COVID-19 (an average 3.7 on a scale of 1–5) than are Democrats, who average just 1.5.

We also can examine the role of inequality in shaping beliefs about school closures in our data. To our surprise, we do not find many differences across income levels in our survey. On the margins we see very limited evidence that higher-income Americans viewed in-person schooling to be a bit less risky in wave 4 than did lower-income Americans, but that is it. Racial inequality, though, affected views about the pandemic and schooling quite a bit (figure 5.9).

Black Americans were significantly more supportive of school closures beginning in wave 2 than were white Americans and also believed that in-person schooling was riskier than did white Americans in wave 4. Some of these racial differences come down to partisanship, but even accounting for the fact that Black Americans in our survey are more likely to be Democrats, we can see the uneven racial dimensions of school closures in American politics.

These racial and partisan dimensions of schooling during the pandemic are themselves rather unsurprising: there are few areas of American life in which race and partisanship are more fundamental than in the context of American schooling. But for the purposes of our argument, they reinforce just how much Americans' understanding of the pandemic itself had come to be viewed through a partisan lens and how important it is to think through the different experiences that Black Americans had with the COVID-19 pandemic. Our findings comport with research that finds local partisanship drove reopening, with Republican-leaning districts more likely to reopen than Democratic-leaning ones.[29] Even if Americans mostly agreed that COVID-19 was particularly deadly for older and immunocompromised adults, Democrats still saw COVID-19 as more dangerous than did Republicans. Once again, partisanship has become a guiding force for helping Americans understand the very nature of the COVID-19 pandemic.

What Is the Right Amount of Regulation?

Another way to see how partisanship shaped COVID-19 policy attitudes is to look at the general question of how much the government should regulate everyday life during the pandemic. In other words, rather than asking how much Americans support particular policies, we shift focus to the overall policy environment. Thinking about the overall policy environment gets at some of the central questions about government authority versus individual liberty that we posed in the introduction to this chapter. It also gets to questions about the concentration of government authority in the federal government versus the states, for American federalism gives the states authority over

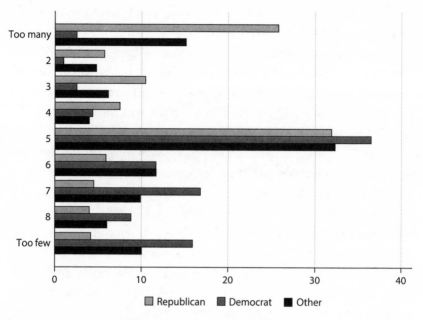

FIGURE 5.10. Attitudes on COVID-19 regulations, by partisanship

managing much of the policy response to the pandemic, and state governments varied substantially in how aggressively they implemented policies to contain the spread of COVID-19 among their populations.

We asked in June whether individuals thought that "my state has declared too many" or "too few" regulations, with a sliding scale to indicate a respondent's position between 1 (too many regulations) and 9 (too few). Using the language of "my state" was important, as it invited our respondents to think about more localized efforts, such as mask mandates in stores and parks, social distancing practices, and indoor capacity caps at local businesses and restaurants rather than policies and the partisan rhetoric coming from Washington. Figure 5.10 displays differences in beliefs by partisanship.

Policy attitudes are once again strongly associated with partisan identity. Twenty-five percent of all Republicans gave the strongest possible answer, that their state declared too many regulations; very few Democrats held this view. Democrats were not quite as extreme, but nevertheless 16 percent of Democrats provided the strongest possible response that their state had too few regulations. Relatively few Republicans held this view. This partisan difference likely reflects more basic differences in Republican and Democratic views about government authority versus individual liberty.

But the most common response across parties was in the middle of the scale, reflecting a view that the number of regulations was "just right." Although this bipartisan stance is reassuring, the clumping of responses at the middle of the scale might also simply reflect respondents' uncertainty, leading them to choose the middle value to avoid taking a strong position either way. It may also be that thinking about state politics does not produce the same kind of fidelity or motivated reasoning as questions that ask respondents to think about Trump directly. Although each of these interpretations of bipartisan moderation about the state policy environment are plausible, we emphasize that Democrats and Republicans were far more polarized about federal policies than they were about state policies, reflecting the preexisting condition of a sharply divided national political environment driven by Trump's own leadership style.

But once again, we face a tricky problem disentangling views about regulations during the pandemic from respondents' views about regulation and government authority more generally. It could be that Americans are generally opposed to government interference in their daily lives, but that in the extraordinary context of an unprecedented global pandemic they are willing to tolerate state regulations. It could also be that individuals with authoritarian leanings support more authority for the government in all areas. To differentiate between views about regulation in general and regulations more specific to COVID-19, we also asked whether individuals agree that "our society needs tougher government and stricter laws." We can use this to see if the same respondents who think that society needs a strong government are also those who think that there are not enough COVID-19 regulations and whether this relationship varies according to partisanship.

Figure 5.11 shows the correlation between support for COVID restrictions and whether a respondent agrees or disagrees that

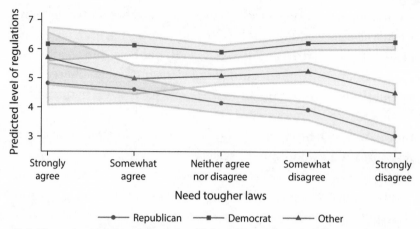

Note: To construct this figure, we used multiple regression to calculate the predicted level of belief that the state has implemented too many or not enough laws (the 9-point scale described previously) based on a respondent's partisanship and a host of demographic and geographic variables such as income, state of residence, and urban or rural county. We then array this next to respondents' level of agreement with the general position that society needs tougher laws.

FIGURE 5.11. Support for more COVID-19 restrictions and tougher laws

society needs tougher laws, separating out respondents by their partisan affiliation.

The results of this analysis are revealing. Democrats appear fairly evenly distributed in their views on tough laws. That is, many Democrats endorse the view that society needs tougher laws, and many other Democrats strongly disagreed with this position. But regardless of their views on that general question, Democrats across the board strongly believed that their state implemented too few regulations in response to COVID-19. Among Democrats, then, the unprecedented COVID-19 pandemic appeared to outweigh any disagreement with the position that society needs tougher laws. Not so among Republicans. Republicans who strongly agreed that there should be tougher laws rate the level of COVID-19 regulations in their state as neither too many nor too few. But those Republicans who strongly oppose tougher laws also tend to believe that their state has too many COVID-19 regulations.

The implication of this analysis is that among Democrats, attitudes about COVID-19 regulations is unrelated to beliefs about the strength of government. This means that policy needs of the COVID-19 pandemic could override any opposition to strong government control held by Democrats. Recall from above that one of the key dilemmas for Democrats was that giving the federal government more authority to respond to the pandemic means giving more authority to their partisan opponents. By and large, however, even those Democrats who were most likely to be suspicious of government authority were willing to tolerate more of it in the service of an effective COVID-19 response.

By contrast, among Republicans attitudes about government strength and COVID policy making are closely related. Put another way, Republicans who support limited government in general also support limited COVID policies specifically. Republicans, though, were in a different position, one that might have complicated a more unified and aggressive response to the pandemic by the Trump administration. There were some Republicans who did indeed support tougher laws as a general matter. Although they tended to support lower levels of state regulation than did Democrats who held similar views, these differences are relatively small. But those Republicans who disagree that there should be tougher laws also opposed COVID-19 regulations by the states.

The presence of this group of Republicans—who, unlike Democrats, were not willing to suspend their beliefs about government intervention in the context of the COVID-19 pandemic—might have made it difficult for the Trump administration to mount a more aggressive response to the pandemic. While we do believe that the Trump administration missed a key opportunity to mobilize bipartisan support for a comprehensive strategy to manage the COVID-19 pandemic, the more libertarian wing of his party would have probably balked in any case.

Who Should Do Something?

Among many unprecedented elements of Trump's management of the COVID-19 pandemic, one particularly notable governance issue is that of responsibility for managing the pandemic. With one hand

Trump foisted decision making and implementation onto the states, and with the other he claimed, in this dangerous phrase, that "when somebody is President of the United States, the authority is total. The governors know that."[30]

As a legal and constitutional matter, state governors are primarily responsible for ensuring public safety in their states. Although state constitutions vary in the specific authorities granted to the governor versus state legislatures, governors generally have the authority to implement stay-at-home orders and to guide the process of reopening the economy. The Trump administration interpreted this responsibility expansively, leaving it to the states to acquire personal protective equipment and medical devices such as ventilators. Yet Trump also believed that he could mobilize his base to pressure Democratic governors to open their economies, knowing that lockdown measures and stay-at-home orders would have deleterious effects on local economies in key battleground states, hurting his reelection chances. Trump infamously tweeted "LIBERATE MINNESOTA!," "LIBERATE VIRGINIA!," and "LIBERATE MICHIGAN!," the last of which brought a mob of gun-toting Trump supporters to the state Capitol in Lansing, Michigan. This, as we mention in chapter 6, not only established health and economic measures as policy tradeoffs but also elevated the idea of individual choice above collective responsibility.

Trump's political strategy was a savvy one. He made the states take responsibility for the lack of preparedness or organization at the federal level. Governors learned quickly not to depend on the federal government for emergency supplies and logistical support. New York, for instance, received only 1 out of every 5 ventilators it had requested and received surgical masks instead of the requested and more coveted N95s.[31] In the absence of a national procurement scheme, New York would have to outbid other states for critical supplies and seek contracts directly for suppliers in China.[32] LA County would receive 170 ventilators as part of a federal aid package directly from the federal stockpile, but they were broken.[33] Kentucky governor Andy Beshear would report that not only was his state not supplied with enough personal protection equipment by the federal government, like every other state, but that he also lost outright to Federal Emergency Management Agency in bidding wars: "The federal government says 'states, you need to go find your supply chain' and then the federal government ends up buying from that supply chain."[34]

But what of the views of ordinary Americans watching state governments scramble to manage the pandemic in a tense battle between federal and state authority? National politics played an important role in shaping local policy making during the pandemic,[35] and this might have also affected ordinary Americans' views about state versus federal authority. Indeed, at the county level, statistical analysis of mobility data shows that state government leaders' recommendations were more effective in Democratic-leaning counties than in Republican-leaning counties, even as Republican-issued stay-at-home orders had larger effects in Democratic-leaning counties than Republican-leaning counties.[36] It may also be the case that Democrats felt more comfortable investing power in their state government and health agency, especially if they live in a blue state.

To tease out Americans' views about state versus federal responses to the COVID-19 pandemic, we included a survey experiment in waves 4 (August) and 5 (October) of our survey. We included these later in the pandemic, with the assumption that citizens would have become habituated to the differences between state and federal authority by this time but specifically to more localized governance. By then, Americans had received almost half a year of state and local health authority messaging in which regulations would vary city to city and county to county. The county level would report COVID caseloads and hospital bed availability but also mask requirements and whether schools would open. This, we believed, enabled citizens to discern meaningful difference in terms of who was in charge.

The details of how survey experiments work can be found in the appendix; here, we focus on the basic idea. We asked two questions about policy that differ on one detail only, varying that detail randomly across respondents. First, we asked whether the federal government, the state government, or "we" (the control), "should provide additional tax cuts and loans to businesses." Second, we

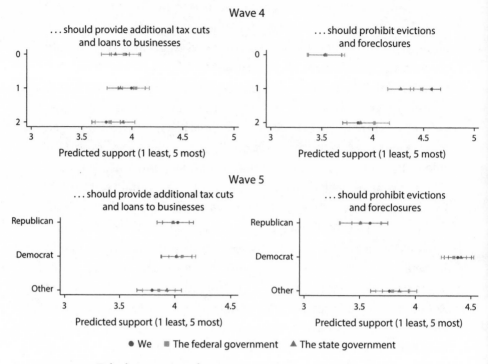

FIGURE 5.12. Federal versus state preferences

asked whether the federal government, the state government, or "we" "should prohibit evictions and foreclosures." Both of these policies were instrumental to controlling the social and economic costs of the pandemic. The latter was especially salient during the summer, when Trump pushed Congress to extend the expiring eviction ban put in place by the CARES Act prior to its August recess.[37]

Figure 5.12 presents the findings. To read this figure, note that each marker (circle, diamond, and square) is the average level of support for a policy implemented by the federal government (square), state governments (triangle), or the control condition (circle).

Regardless of the policy or the wave in which we ask about it, figure 5.12 shows that the level of government responsible for a policy does not affect support for that policy. There are no statistically significant differences by partisanship between support for either policies based on whether the federal or state government (or control) is responsible. However, we do find—unsurprisingly—that there are strong partisan differences in support for policies that would prohibit evictions and foreclosures. Democrats strongly favor eviction and foreclosure protections at a significantly higher rate than Republicans. Rather more interestingly, we find that support for businesses via tax cuts and loans is broadly popular across partisans of all affiliations. Regardless of what party a respondent is a member of and what level of government is responsible for it, Americans favored policies that supported businesses during the pandemic.

Conclusion

Our analysis in this chapter has revealed that Americans were divided by partisanship on almost every policy related to the COVID-19 pandemic, from how the government is doing to how much authority the government should have to what the government should do to respond to the pandemic. These findings are consistent with the evidence that we have provided in previous chapters about how partisanship shaped the COVID-19 pandemic. Democrats were more likely than Republicans to adjust their behaviors and worry about the pandemic and its effects, and as a result they wanted their government to do something about it. Republicans experienced the pandemic differently and objected to many of the policies designed to contain it.

Stepping back, though, this chapter presents us with one of the more surprising aspects of the politics of the COVID-19 pandemic in the United States. Rather than Trump's Republican copartisans supporting an active federal government response to the pandemic, it was Democrats who were most supportive of such a response. This, we believe, can ultimately be explained by—and despite—Trump's polarizing presidential style. One of the most distinctive features of the Trump administration was the president's lack of interest in governing. Not only did he gut the bureaucracies that may have capably spearheaded a full-on attempt to minimize the first wave, but he also shifted policy responsibility to the states when he found it to be politically convenient to do so. Consistent with the idea that ingroup partisans "follow the leader" (in this case, Republicans) and outgroup partisans reject presidential cues (in this case, Democrats),[38] we see Republicans following Trump's efforts to reopen the economy and downplay the pandemic, while Democrats demand more closure, more testing, and greater caution.

And it is *despite Trump's* leadership style because Democrats would typically want to reduce federal government powers when the other party is in power (and likewise for Republicans), but Democrats (as we saw in chapter 4) were exhibiting emotions that made them fearful, eager for information and (policy) control. They would have supported strong polices, such as enforced stay-at-home mandates and contact tracing, had strong policies been offered. This may have led to a different conversation that the country ultimately did not have, though other countries (such as New Zealand) did: how much emergency power should an executive have before a line is crossed from protection to authoritarianism?

The findings in this chapter help us make sense of how major ideological debates in American politics—about the role of government in everyday life, about who should lead government responses to crises such as a public health emergency—affected and were affected by the pandemic. There are advocates for privacy and liberty among both the Democratic Party and the Republican Party, and in the context of a highly polarized two-party presidential system, Democrats had every reason to be suspicious of giving even more authority to a federal government led by their partisan rivals. Yet Democrats would have tolerated a much more aggressive response to the COVID-19 pandemic by the Trump administration—they may even have welcomed it. Republicans, however, were much more suspicious of government action to combat the pandemic both at the federal level and within the states, even with a Republican president at the helm. With Americans deeply polarized and partisanship an important driver of public opinion on COVID-19, we now can make sense of one of the more baffling aspects of the Trump presidency: that the position of the governing party was to not govern a way out of the pandemic.

6

The Cost of a Pandemic

COVID-19 AND THE AMERICAN ECONOMY

The COVID-19 pandemic was more than just a shock to Americans' everyday lives—their ability to see friends and family, send their children to school, and go to the movies or watch their favorite team play in person. It was also an unprecedented shock to their economic lives. Tens of millions of American workers found themselves working from home on a full- or part-time basis. Tens of millions of Americans found themselves suddenly unemployed. And the Federal Reserve estimated that there were roughly two hundred thousand extra small businesses closures because of the pandemic in the first year alone.[1] On June 1, 2021, Vice President Kamala Harris characterized this figure on MSNBC as "one-third of our small businesses." While the federal Paycheck Protection Program provided billions of dollars in relief to some businesses to pay employees and fulfill contracts, others were not so fortunate. California experienced the greatest hit, with some forty thousand small businesses closed by September 2020.[2] Many of these small business owners would join antilockdown protests or rally behind the campaign to recall California governor Gavin Newsom in September 2021, frustrated with the untenable effects of shutdowns, claiming that "he's broken the back of small-business owners and put many of them out of business for the rest of their lives."[3]

Simply put, COVID-19's effects on the U.S. economy were sudden and devastating. Even those Americans who were fortunate enough to keep their jobs found themselves thrust into the sharpest economic recession in modern American history. In this chapter we examine the economic consequences of the COVID-19 pandemic as well as the political debate around them. For President Donald Trump, who had campaigned on his success as a businessman and promised to deliver a roaring economy and good jobs, the massive economic toll of the COVID-19 pandemic was nothing less than a frontal assault on his reelection campaign. By contrast, for congressional Democrats and others who opposed Trump, the very fact of Americans' economic vulnerability highlighted issues such as precarity, inequality, and the gendered and racialized dimensions of American employment. The 2020 presidential election campaign saw both Trump and Democratic nominee Joe Biden campaigning consistently on their ability to not just manage the pandemic but also jump-start the economy once again. Upon his inauguration, President Biden immediately announced the American Rescue Plan, a $1.9 billion health care and economic support package that represented his big push to rescue the American economy from the throes of crisis.[4]

We tell the story of the economic consequences of the pandemic—and their implications for partisan politics—by first digging more deeply into what COVID-19 did to the American economy, as captured in official statistics as well as in our own survey data. We then explore the American public's views on two interrelated policy questions: what ought to be done about COVID-19's immediate costs for citizens and employers, and what should the government do more broadly to support the American economy in the time of an unprecedent global pandemic? It will not be a surprise to see that the pandemic had devastating economic consequences. But perhaps unexpectedly, COVID-19 was an especially gendered pandemic, hitting women's employment harder than men's in a pattern never seen in previous American economic crises. We also find that the negative effects of the pandemic were felt more by Democrats than Republicans. These differences foreshadow a predictable partisan debate about the economic measures needed to respond to the crisis but with a unique twist for the Trump era: Republicans became the party who believed that protectionism would best serve an American economy in crisis, and Democrats moved to embrace free trade.

Trends in Unemployment

On March 19, 2020, the Labor Department released its periodic updates on the nation's employment numbers. The numbers were stunning: the previous week 281,000 Americans had filed for unemployment.[5] As staggering as these numbers are, it is hard to make sense of their magnitude. To see just how sharp and severe the effects of COVID-19 were on everyday Americans, we can look to trends in unemployment rates across the country, comparing the COVID-19 pandemic to the 2007–2009 Great Recession. Figure 6.1 shows how these trends look based on official data from the U.S. Bureau of Labor Statistics.[6]

The spike in unemployment that accompanies the COVID-19 pandemic far surpasses the surge in unemployment from the 2007–2009 financial crisis. Also visible is the rapid recovery in unemployment rates after the initial spike. Whereas the post–financial crisis recovery in unemployment was long and slow, unemployment rebounded quickly in 2020, before the pandemic had run its course.

Viewed in the comparative perspective, the U.S. COVID-19 unemployment shock looks even more exceptional. In figure 6.2 we compare the United States with five other large and prosperous democracies to illustrate just how unemployment in each country responded to the COVID-19 pandemic.

Each of these states fared better in containing the spread and death toll of COVID-19 than did the United States,[7] and they also were able to contain much more effectively the effects of the COVID-19 pandemic on unemployment. In normal times, unemployment rates in the United States are enviably low. But during the pandemic,

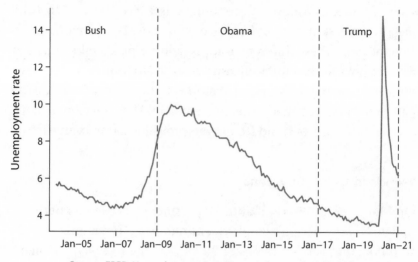

Source: FRED, Unemployment Rate (Percent, Seasonally Adjusted)

FIGURE 6.1. U.S. unemployment rate, 2004–2021

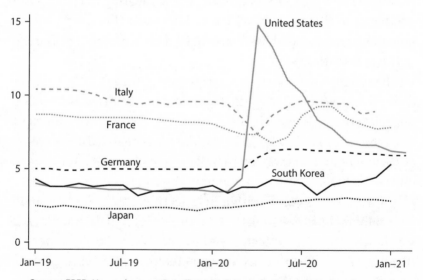

Source: FRED, Unemployment Rate (Percent, Seasonally Adjusted, Various Countries)

FIGURE 6.2. Comparing unemployment shocks, selected economies

the United States stands out as perhaps uniquely unable to manage the economic fallout from a pandemic, whereas other advanced industrial democracies saw unemployment rise either marginally or in some cases not at all. This was possible because these states were able to respond swiftly to the threat of mass unemployment by shifting to policies such as *Kurzarbeit* (short work) in Germany that allowed firms to pay their employees a large portion of their prepandemic salaries using government support.[8] Such policies socialized the costs of the economic response to the pandemic and in doing so protected jobs.

Not surprisingly, the policy-making environments in these countries also made it easier for them to contain the immediate effects of the pandemic. Universal health care made COVID-19 testing easy to roll out on a mass scale at no cost, whereas it took an act of Congress to ensure that Americans would not be charged by their insurance plans for COVID-19 testing. Whereas other advanced economies focused their efforts in the summer of 2020 on testing, tracing, and treating while their citizens waited for a vaccine, Americans lamented the slow rollout of the Paycheck Protection Program and politicians bickered about the need for a fiscal stimulus.[9]

One important theme of this book is that the experience of the COVID-19 pandemic has been highly uneven by race, a topic that we will address in further detail in chapter 8. But as a preview and to illustrate the racialized economic consequences of the COVID-19 pandemic, figure 6.3 uses the same official sources to break down trends in unemployment by race.

These figures paint an entirely different story that what we saw in figure 6.1. Unemployment among Black and Latino Americans reached almost 20 percent at the height of the COVID-19 pandemic, meaning that almost one out of five members of these two communities was looking for work but unable to find it. The effects of the pandemic on white and Asian communities were indeed severe but more muted. And with the benefit of a bit of historical context, we also can see that the unemployment consequences of the financial crisis of 2007–2009 were just as severe for Black Americans as was the COVID-19 pandemic. These unequal experiences of America's

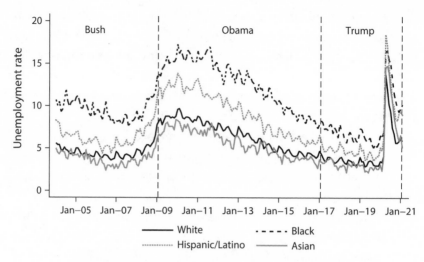

Source: FRED, Unemployment Rate (Percent, Seasonally Adjusted)

FIGURE 6.3. U.S. unemployment rates by race, 2004–2021

racial and ethnic minorities in the American employment market reflect exactly the preexisting conditions (from chapter 1) that have made the pandemic so devastating.

When we break out unemployment trends by gender, yet another nuanced picture emerges, as we show in figure 6.4.

Comparing the 2007–2009 financial crisis to the COVID-19 pandemic, we see that in terms of unemployment, the COVID-19 pandemic disproportionately affected women rather than men, with a 2.5 percent gap in the peak unemployment rates in mid-2020. The 2007–2009 financial crisis, by contrast, disproportionately affected men rather than women, as is normal among U.S. recessions.

Explanations for the unusual gender gap in unemployment during the COVID-19 pandemic are many. In the 2007–2009 financial crisis, men suffered greater unemployment than women because the crisis affected sectors such as construction, manufacturing, and real estate in which men were overrepresented relative to women.[10] The COVID-19 pandemic was different. Women were disproportionately employed in the health care sector, which ought to have insulated them from the unemployment shock due to the rising demand for

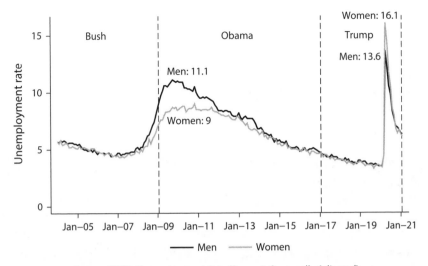

Source: FRED, Unemployment Rate (Percent, Seasonally Adjusted)

FIGURE 6.4. U.S. unemployment by gender, 2004–2011

health care. Indeed, one in three jobs held by women was classified as essential work.[11] But any such insulation was overwhelmed by the dramatic drop in demand in the restaurant and hospitality sectors, in which women are overrepresented relative to men. Even more perniciously, the sudden closure of U.S. schools and the immediate need for childcare forced many women out of the labor market on a temporary basis.[12] These figures together meant that many women's labor shifted from the formal sector to the household just as many of the sectors in which women are most commonly employed faced sharp contractions.[13]

These official data give us a lot of detail about the severity of the unemployment shock of COVID-19 as well as how it has been unequally experienced by race/ethnicity and gender. Other research bolsters these findings: the effects of the COVID-19 pandemic were unequally experienced based on race, gender, income, and job security, with those who work under irregular arrangements and with lower incomes and more precarious employment suffering more than high-income Americans in stable jobs.[14] However, these numbers do not tell us much about the mechanics of what was happening to Americans: what happened to their wages, their ability to pay rent, or their need for various forms of public and private welfare assistance. They also do not allow us to look at differences among Americans according to political factors such as partisanship. Fortunately, our survey data give us just the data that we need to examine these questions more fully.

Unemployment and Economic Precarity: A Detailed View

The first question to investigate is whether Americans experiences with unemployment differed by partisan affiliation. We investigate this question in figure 6.5 the figures that follow it based on our surveys. We also plot 95 percent confidence intervals in gray that allow us to visualize whether differences across the Americans in our sample are statistically significant.

Our data show very clearly that there was a substantial partisan gap in the percentage of unemployment at the very beginning of the pandemic and that this gap persisted as the crisis worsened. Uniformly, we find that Democrats and nonpartisans experienced higher levels of unemployment than did Republicans. Unemployment rates rose between March and June 2020 for all three groups and then declined for all three groups over the rest of the year as the economy stabilized to the new "normal" of the pandemic. By October we no longer see statistically significant differences by partisanship among our respondents in this graph, although we suspect that these differences would be both statistically significant and substantively meaningful if we were able to interview the entire U.S. workforce. The wave 6 (April 2021) data reveal a surprise jump in unemployment specifically among independents/nonpartisans in the data, even as unemployment rates continue to fall for Democrats and especially Republicans. We have no explanation for this surprise finding, although it could reflect independents who have decided to reenter the labor force and are experiencing job search frictions.

Although the numbers in figure 6.5 are simple averages delineated by partisan affiliation, we can also show that these partisan differences

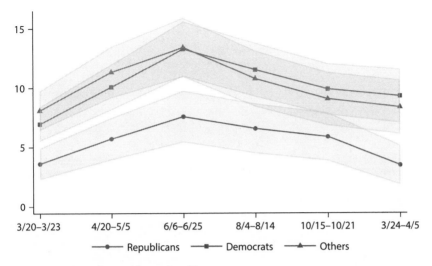

FIGURE 6.5. Unemployment by partisanship

in unemployment were not simply a function of racial differences in unemployment that happen to also overlap with partisanship. In other words, even accounting for respondents' race, age, education, and other demographics, we found persistently higher levels of unemployment among Democrats and Others than among Republicans. The most likely explanation for this difference is that Americans of different political backgrounds tend to work in different sorts of occupations. Although we do not have fine-grained measures of our survey respondents' occupational profiles, it is likely that Democrats more commonly work in positions that are subject to layoffs during the pandemic, such as lower-wage service-sector positions. Republicans, by contrast, may be more likely to be self-employed. Such differences would mean that even though partisanship itself did not cause Democrats and Republicans to have different employment experiences during the pandemic, partisans nevertheless experienced the pandemic differently.

To what extent should we attribute this sharp rise in unemployment to COVID-19 itself? It is difficult to know the extent to which we can blame any individual's unemployment on a specific cause, but we asked our survey respondents—in waves 2–6—about the

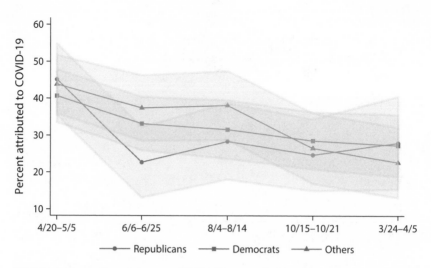

FIGURE 6.6. Causes of unemployment, COVID-19 versus other

conditions of their unemployment, whether they attributed it to COVID-19 or to some other factor independent of the pandemic. The proportion of our respondents who report that their unemployment was due to COVID-19, by partisanship, appears in figure 6.6.

There were no partisan differences in whether COVID-19 was the cause of unemployment (at least in the eyes of our survey respondents). We also found a modest downward trend in how often our respondents attributed their unemployment to COVID-19 over time, although once again there was an upward spike in wave 6 (April–May 2021) among independents/nonpartisans. With the caveat that survey respondents might not have a very good understanding about why they are unemployed, we conclude from these figures that although unemployment spiked for all Americans during the crisis, its effects on unemployment were particularly strongly felt by Democrats and nonpartisans. Substantial proportions of all Americans who were unemployed attributed this condition to the direct effects of COVID-19 itself.

But how else did the pandemic affect Americans' economic situation? Our survey data allows us to see beyond labor statistics to how Americans' economic lives were shaped by the pandemic. In waves 2–6 of our survey, we asked our respondents whether any of the following had happened to them or anyone in their immediate family in the preceding months: lost their job, worked at reduced pay, applied for unemployment, visited a food pantry, been unable to pay rent, or sought assistance from a charity. These items give us a fuller picture of the economic precarity facing Americans than do employment figures alone.

We found that roughly 20 percent of Americans reported that they or someone in their family had lost their job and that close to 25 percent of Americans reported that they had applied for unemployment and worked at reduced pay. These figures do not change much until April 2021 under the Biden administration and with the vaccine rollout well under way. This gives us a sense of the durable effects of the pandemic that differs from the message of a "quick rebound" that we saw in the overall trends in unemployment above. If we focused only on unemployment, we would be missing the more subtle ways in which Americans' economic situations were affected by the pandemic and also just how long-lasting these effects were. For example, our data tell us that 8 percent of Americans in our sample report visiting a food pantry in June 2020. Feeding America (a nonprofit organization) reported that during the pandemic more than forty-five million Americans experienced food insecurity during the pandemic in 2020, including fifteen million children.[15]

Our data also show that these more subtle and enduring economic consequences of the pandemic were experienced unequally. Black and Latino/a respondents to our surveys were more likely to report having difficulty in paying rent or having resorted to food pantries and charities to support themselves and their families during the pandemic. This finding remained true even when accounting for age, education, urban-rural status, and other demographic factors. Perhaps even more surprisingly, though, we also find that economic precarity varied by partisanship, as we show in figure 6.7.

The broad pattern is that Democrats consistently faced higher levels of each of these forms of economic precarity than did Republicans; and in general nonpartisans were in between Republicans

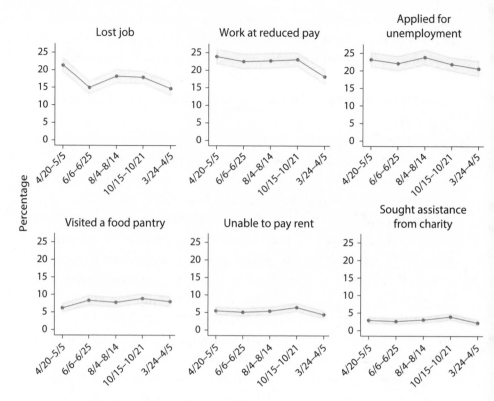

FIGURE 6.7. Economic precarity, by partisanship

and Democrats. All these partisan differences remained when we account for factors such as geography, income, and education.

To sum up what we have learned so far, official unemployment statistics and our own survey data together paint a singular picture of a sharp economic contraction that led to a massive spike in unemployment. But the burdens of the COVID-19 recession were unequally felt across America's racial and ethnic groups, and unlike in previous American recessions, unemployment disproportionately fell on women rather than men. These economic effects spilled over into a host of pocketbook issues that shaped Americans' economic lives even among those who managed to keep their jobs. We also saw partisan differences in economic precarity during the COVID-19 pandemic, mirrored by partisan disagreement in Washington about the role of the government in addressing these concerns.

We can put these numbers in context by thinking back to our discussion of the different emotional reactions that Democrats and Republicans reported throughout the course of the pandemic. As we described in chapter 4, Democrats reported greater anxiety and more worries about the effects of the pandemic than did Republicans. Our data suggest that Democrats' economic experiences were worse than Republicans', which can partially explain observed differences in emotional responses to the pandemic. As we speculated earlier in this chapter, one reason is that Republicans and Democrats work in different sorts of occupations, which created different types of vulnerability to an abrupt economic slowdown such as that associated with the COVID-19 pandemic. It could also be that some Democrats, concerned as they were by the pandemic, opted to leave their jobs in hopes of protecting themselves from exposure to the coronavirus. Other possible explanations for these differences abound, but all in all, our data show conclusive evidence that the economic lives of Democrats and Republicans were differentially affected by the COVID-19 pandemic.

These partisan differences in the economic effects of the pandemic help to explain some otherwise odd features of the policy debate. For example, just as the need for food relief became particularly urgent, the Supplemental Nutritional Assistance Program (SNAP) known as "food stamps" became subject to partisan bickering, with Republicans in Congress reluctant to expand the assistance available to families in need and Democrats demanding greater benefits to combat the unprecedented rise in food insecurity.[16] In the end SNAP benefits were extended, but the states (which are responsible for administering SNAP) created a range of complexities and conditions that varied across the country. Some states such as Florida temporarily implemented work requirements even after the U.S. Department of Agriculture, which oversees the program, had suspended those requirements.[17] The Trump administration pressed forward with plans to cut SNAP benefits through October 2020, only to have its plans halted by a federal judge just three weeks before the November 2020 presidential election.[18]

The Policy Debate

Almost as soon as the severity of the pandemic became clear, Americans began to anticipate its economic consequences. For Trump, facing reelection with a highly divided electorate and a strong record of job growth, any economic contraction was a singular threat to his political survival. Already by March 9, 2020, he was publicly advocating for an economic stimulus to ease the costs of the pandemic.[19] His complaints about the Federal Reserve's monetary policy stance had begun in late February, when he began to argue that the Fed should keep interest rates as low as possible in order to encourage businesses to spend.[20] In the end, Trump's wishes were fulfilled: the Federal Reserve pushed interest rates close to zero in mid-March, and by the end of the month Congress had passed a huge stimulus package known as the Coronavirus Aid, Relief, and Economic Security (CARES) Act, which directed onetime cash payments to millions of Americans while also creating key programs such as the Paycheck Protection Program.

The economic policy responses to COVID-19 fell into two groups. The first were direct measures to ease the economic consequences of managing COVID-19 itself. For example, one persistent problem facing businesses was whether to keep workers at home or not. Businesses risked costly interruptions to their work if they kept employees home, but it was only possible to contain the spread of COVID-19 by encouraging sick or exposed workers to stay home. A policy of compensating firms for the losses due to the coronavirus—much as the Paycheck Protection Program did[21]—encouraged their workers to stay home when they were sick or exposed. In doing so, the policy sought to ease the burdens facing productive firms, allowing them to survive the pandemic, while also safeguarding public health. But of course, such policies are costly and subject to gaming or exploitation by unproductive or uncompetitive firms. The Paycheck Protection Program, for example, generated significant public backlash when it emerged that large firms such as Shake Shack were benefiting from provisions meant to protect small businesses.[22] Other policies that could address the economic implications of the pandemic itself included policies to make COVID-19 tests free to all who needed them, to waive the costs of treatment to anyone affected by the virus, and to provide paid leave to workers who had to remain at home due to sickness or exposure. Many of these policies were ultimately folded into the CARES Act.[23]

Such policies could do more than just protect Americans' jobs; they could also play a central role in controlling the pandemic's spread. In a widely reported story from mid-April, workers in the poultry and meatpacking industries described that they were provided with insufficient protection in cramped and sweaty conditions.[24] And without any ability to support themselves if they were to stay home, workers faced the perverse incentive to come to work even when they suspected that they had contracted COVID-19. Worse still, some businesses incentivized workers to come to work even when sick with promises of extra pay and even rib eyes for coming to work during the early lockdown period.[25] In such a context, economic support to workers is a policy that could yield downstream benefits for containing the virus.

Paying firms to pay workers to stay at home was a policy many countries adopted. In Canada, workers whose incomes were affected by the pandemic were eligible for CAD$2,000 a month for up to six months. And both countries' policies were in excess of what the United States would offer. Germany, as mentioned, adopted a policy of short-work whereby affected companies received government subsidies to reduce employee work hours and wages to avoid mass layoffs. Similar approaches were taken in France and Spain. The United States proposed no such workshare approach. Another set of policies addressed the broader macroeconomic consequences of the COVID-19 pandemic for trade and investment. These included policies such as lowering interest rates to support the economic recovery as well as policies such as increasing trade or, alternatively, imposing import taxes to protect American industry in the face of the recession. Trade issues are of particular interest because they interacted with the resurgence of nativist protectionism in the modern Republican Party and because the Trump administration was so eager to blame COVID-19 on China, referring to it with racist terms such as

"China virus" and "kung flu." China itself faced a massive decline in exports in the first quarter of 2020 on the heels of the pandemic,[26] and the question of whether the United States should impose new restrictions on Chinese imports or should instead embrace imports of much-needed goods proved a novel axis of partisan conflict in 2020.[27]

In wave 1 of our survey—right after the CARES Act was signed into law by Trump—we asked our respondents about each of these policies, asking them how much they agreed that the U.S. government should implement each of them. Responses could range from 1 (strongly disagree) to 5 (strongly agree). We were careful to ensure that the questions that we asked cued our respondents to think about the economic implications of these policies for the United States and that respondents understood that these were policies that would need to be adopted by "the government." Had we not done so, respondents might not have understood that we expected these to each be actions taken by the government and on behalf of all Americans. They might have then responded with answers that reflected abstract preferences that are divorced from politics (everyone, we presume, would prefer that testing be free) or that were specific to their own position (respondents may not favor a government policy that affects everyone equally). The full question wordings appear in table 6.1.

Note as well that the three economic recovery survey items make an explicit case that these policies would be broadly good for the American economy without explicitly raising the downsides of such policies, such as the risk of inflation following lower interest rates or the effects of import taxes on consumer prices.

In figure 6.8 we plot the average level of support for each of these policies across all our survey respondents, dividing policies by whether they are COVID-19–focused versus more general economic policies.

Very clearly, Americans were generally supportive of an activist economic policy stance, in terms of policies that both tackle the economic implications of COVID-19 care and are designed to address economic recovery in the medium term. The adage often heard in Washington, D.C., during the Great Recession—that just like there

TABLE 6.1. Economy policy survey items

COVID-19 Response

Free COVID-19 testing	The government should make all testing for coronavirus free for all Americans.
Waive treatment costs	The government should waive insurance costs and hospital fees for treating coronavirus.
Paid leave	The government should grant paid leave to anyone diagnosed with coronavirus to encourage them to stay home until they are fully healthy.
Compensate firms	The government should provide bailouts, or financial compensation, to American companies to recover losses from coronavirus.

Economic Recovery

Increase trade	The United States must strengthen its economic ties and increase trade with other countries in order to strengthen our economy.
Import taxes	The United States must increase taxes on foreign imports in order to stimulate the growth of our own domestic industry.
Lower interest rates	The United States should keep interest rates as low as possible, which will encourage more spending and will support the American economy.

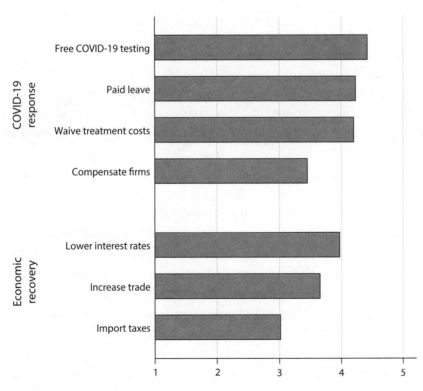

FIGURE 6.8. Economic policy responses, March 2020

are no atheists in foxholes, there are no libertarians during economic crises[28]—seems to apply quite well to the COVID-19 pandemic.

It would not be surprising to find that there are partisan differences in these policy preferences, however. Economic policy has long been a central axis of policy disagreement between Democrats and Republicans and between liberals and conservatives. Since the 1930s Democrats generally have favored more activist and interventionist economic policies, whereas Republicans have opposed government intervention in the economy. This can be tied to a broader ideological divide between noninterventionist conservatives and libertarians, on one hand, and interventionist liberals and progressives, on the other.[29] For most of the past century, moreover, these policy bundles have described American trade policy, with Republicans broadly known as the party of free trade and low tariffs and Democrats as the party of protectionism in the service of so-called fair trade.

When we break down these policy responses by partisanship and ideology in figure 6.9, we find that these differences are borne out in the data with a couple of notable exceptions.

Look first at the COVID-19 response policies. Democrats were noticeably more supportive than Republicans of policies that supported workers by lowering the economic implications of COVID-19 care: free testing, waiving the costs of treatment, and supporting paid leave for those who are ill or vulnerable. When it comes to compensating firms for their losses, however, Republicans were slightly *more* supportive than Democrats (and the same is true when comparing conservatives to liberals). It seems that in the realm of COVID-related economic policy, partisan attitudes were driven in some part by the direct beneficiaries of the policy in questions, with Republicans more likely to support policies that target businesses and Democrats more like to favor policies that support workers. But these partisan differences—which accord with our general understanding of parties' general ideological tendencies—are relatively small. The more important finding is how popular all these policies are.

Policies related to economic recovery show some surprises and starker partisan divides. Republicans (and conservatives) in March 2020 were much more supportive of import taxes and much

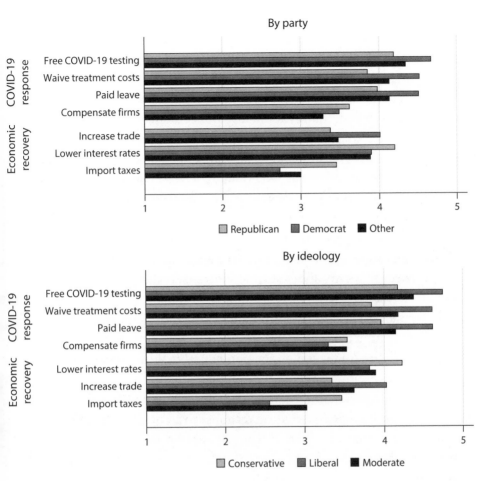

FIGURE 6.9. Economic policy responses, wave 1, by partisanship

less supportive of free trade than were Democrats (and liberals). Republicans and conservatives also expressed more support for lowering interest rates than did Democrats and liberals. The parties' policy preferences here seem to have flipped from the regular patterns of twentieth-century U.S. politics. What is going on?

The likely answer is Trump, whose campaign and presidency captured the nativist vote in ways that Republican presidents had rarely done in the past.[30] His open disdain for free trade and vocal support for protecting American firms and workers from foreign competition produced a reaction among Democrats, who found themselves more willing to embrace free trade as a result. In the context of the early pandemic, with the economic implications of nationwide lockdowns firmly on the minds of politicians and voters alike, policy preferences had already come to reflect Trump's highly charged anti-internationalist rhetoric. So too were Republicans more supportive of an accommodating monetary policy stance of lower interest rates to encourage Americans to spend, thus keeping the economy moving.[31] These partisan policy positions—unusual in the context of recent U.S. political history—certainly predate the pandemic as part of the preexisting conditions associated with Trump. But they took on new meaning and urgency in the context of an economic crisis.

These initial partisan differences would prove remarkably durable over the course of the pandemic, so durable in fact that we stopped asking respondents about several of these economic policies after wave 2 in late April because we found such stability in responses. We nevertheless tracked responses about free testing, paid sick leave, and increasing trade over the entirety of our panel, so we can illustrate in figure 6.10 just how stark and durable those partisan differences in economic policy responses were.

Democrats remained consistently more supportive of free testing, paid leave, and free trade in response to COVID-19 than Republicans or nonpartisans. As with health behaviors and other policies, we find that Republican support for free testing and paid leave trends even more negative over time, increasing the magnitude of partisan differences over time. This continued divergence in opinions once again reflects the sheer divisiveness of the COVID-19 pandemic, characterized by ever greater polarization of attitudes rather than the kind of bipartisan common cause familiar from past moments of national crisis.

What of the racialized and gendered dynamics of economic policy preferences in response to COVID-19? In figure 6.11, we divided respondents up by their race and ethnicity (left panel) and gender (right panel).

The plots that trace out policy preferences by race and ethnicity reveal no simple pattern in the racialized policy responses to COVID-19. In general, Black and Latina/o respondents were more

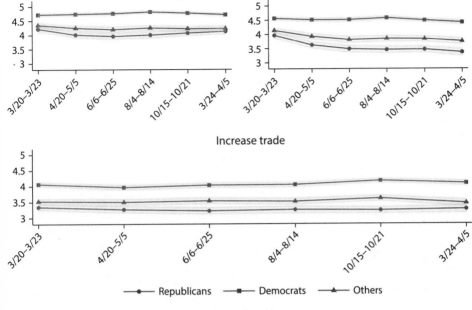

FIGURE 6.10. Economic policy responses, by partisanship

supportive of free testing and paid leave than white respondents, but differences are modest (and are most notable in wave 3, in early summer). The consistently lower support for paid leave among Americans who do not identify as white, Black, or Latina/o is particularly striking; this group includes Asian Americans as well as mixed-race, Native American, and other respondents. There is no consistent racial or ethnic pattern at all in support for free trade. Notably, when we use multiple regression analysis to test for racial differences in economic policy preferences over time when controlling for factors such as partisanship, age, and geography, we find no evidence whatsoever of racial and ethnic differences.

The gendered patterns of economic policy responses in response to COVID-19, by contrast, are striking. Women were consistently and substantially more supportive of free testing and paid leave than men, and yet women were generally less supportive of free trade. Our finding that women were generally more opposed to free trade than men is consistent with established research of American public

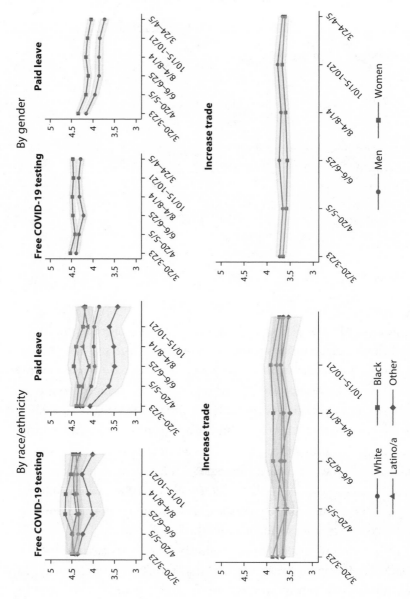

FIGURE 6.11. Economic policy preferences, by race and gender

opinion toward free trade, which has found that women are consistently less supportive of free trade in "normal times" as well.[32] In comprehensive statistical tests that control for partisanship as well as geographic and demographic differences, these gendered differences remain strong and statistically significant—even in the case of free trade. These results on gendered economic policy preferences in response to COVID-19 make good sense considering the discussion above about the novel gendered effects of the pandemic. With American women disproportionately bearing the economic costs of COVID-19 and transitioning away from formal employment and into household labor, policies such as paid leave and free testing— even though they would not themselves reverse the gendered labor market effects of COVID-19—were particularly salient for them.

Conclusion

It is no surprise that the COVID-19 pandemic caused a major economic recession. Unemployment claims in early and mid-2020 were some of the highest ever on record, bringing American economic growth to a sudden halt after a decade of steady economic recovery under Presidents Obama and Trump. Like many past recessions, the effects on unemployment were particularly felt by Black and Latina/o Americans. Unlike most past recessions, the unemployment effects were also disproportionately felt by women compared to men. Accompanying the rise in unemployment was a stark rise in economic precarity, exposing the long-standing weaknesses of the American welfare state and the racialization of poverty and inequality in the United States.

Digging more deeply into our survey data also gives us important insights into the politics of the pandemic economy. Americans broadly supported an activist response, including the measures in the CARES Act, but the partisan disagreement in Washington about how to respond to the crisis was mirrored by partisan differences in how Americans wanted to respond to the crisis. Taken together, our analysis in this chapter once again illustrates a key dynamic of the politics of COVID-19 in the United States: partisan

differences in economic policy responses to the pandemic were clear
in the earliest days of the pandemic and persisted—sometimes even
growing—over time. But in this chapter we see a new twist on the
policy debate, driven by Trump's repudiation of many of the key
platforms of the modern Republican Party. The Democrats' move
to embrace free trade and the Republicans' new fondness for tariffs were not themselves caused by the COVID-19, but as Americans pondered how a government response to the economic crisis
unleashed by the pandemic might look, partisanship helped to drive
respondents' preferences. The one area in which we find the strongest bipartisan consensus is simply around the general idea that the
government ought to respond to the economic dislocation caused by
the pandemic; it is in the details where partisan differences emerge.

And once again as we have argued in this book, it need not have
been this way. A comparative perspective on America's pandemic
response reveals just how our preexisting conditions—structural
inequalities, partisan polarization, and a wobbly health care system—
have made the crisis more difficult to manage than it otherwise
might have been. In other advanced industrial democracies such as
Germany and South Korea, strong and interventionist states play
a more active role in managing their economies than does America's patchwork welfare state. Of course, concerns about the long-
term costs of COVID-19 stimulus packages were not unique to the
United States. In the words of German finance minister Olaf Scholz,
"Naturally it's important that we return to normal times at some
point, with normal income and expenditure. . . . But now it's about
stabilizing the economy. That we did this [stimulus] quickly and
on a large scale contributed to Germany coming through the crisis
much better than many others.[33] Still, when viewed in comparative
perspective, America's ineffective policy responses, the dramatic
rise in economic precarity, the interaction between the COVID-19
and America's long-standing inequalities, and the partisan rancor
associated with all of it reveal the depths of pandemic politics in
the United States.

7

Do Not Enter

COVID-19 AND THE POLITICS OF IMMIGRATION

From the day he descended the escalator in Trump Tower to announce his candidacy for president, one of Donald Trump's signature political issues was curbing immigration. And throughout his presidency, his immigration policies were the sources of controversy and criticism. These ranged from the Muslim ban a week after his inauguration to his administration's practice of child separation, which coincided with a significant reduction in illegal crossings and asylum claims at the U.S.-Mexican border. In 2017, President Trump's "Buy American and Hire American" initiative sought to severely limit the entry of new foreign workers (H1-Bs).[1] The Trump administration cut the U.S. refugee resettlement to its lowest intake in the program's history. And Stephen Miller, the president's chief adviser on immigration, frequently advocated for Trump to use his expansive public health powers to curb immigration. In 2018 as migrant caravans headed north to the U.S. border, the *New York Times* reported that "Mr. Miller looked for evidence that they carried illnesses."[2]

In this context, it is not surprising that Trump's first real action against the pandemic was to shut the border. On January 31, 2020,

Trump issued an executive order establishing a travel ban from China. The administration extended restrictions to Iran (February 29), Western Europe (March 12),[3] and the U.S.-Canadian border (March 19). In closing the U.S.-Canadian border to nonessential travel, this brought the total number of countries affected by the U.S. entry ban to thirty-eight. Travel restrictions were later extended to countries such as Brazil (May 24, 2020) and, much later, India (May 4, 2021). Entry to the United States for European citizens did not resume until November 2021. Later that month as the new omicron variant of coronavirus began to spread, new travel restrictions were imposed against South Africa, where it was first detected, as well as Botswana, Eswatini, Lesotho, Malawi, Mozambique, Namibia, and Zimbabwe.

Trump repeatedly referenced the "China ban" as his greatest pandemic achievement. As early as February 28, 2020, he boasted on Twitter, referring to himself in third person, that coronavirus was spreading "very slowly in the U.S. because President Trump closed our border, and ended flights VERY EARLY" (though recall from chapter 2 that what was actually "slow spread" was in reality a dearth of testing for positive cases). By May, Trump was tweeting about his China ban nearly every day. He would say, for instance, "we're the ones that gave the great response, and we're the ones that kept China out of here. . . . If I didn't do that early call on China—and nobody wanted that to happen. Everybody thought it was just unnecessary to do it."[4]

In fact, limiting travel restrictions during pandemics is something that most states do. Australia, Japan, Italy, and Russia had already announced similar plans by the time Trump announced his. And by March 19, 2020, 127 countries had some form of no-entry policy in place.[5] Travel restrictions and quarantines had been used in other recent instances, such as the HIV/AIDS epidemic in the 1980s and the H5N1 avian flu outbreak in 2006.[6] But it is a fraught policy filled with trade-offs.

Diseases such as COVID-19 spread through human contact and interaction, meaning that human mobility truly is the mechanism through which the virus spread around the world. Strict travel bans can contain the spread of the virus, but anything short of full containment means that travel restrictions are at best a tool for slowing down the spread of a virus and new variants.[7] Screening of passengers may miss asymptomatic carriers or symptoms that gestate for longer periods. Both of these describe the presentation patterns of COVID-19, which then requires any entry allowance to be paired with long mandatory quarantine periods. But while island states such as New Zealand and Taiwan were able to successfully restrict the spread of COVID-19 by fully closing their borders and had the staff and capacity to implement quarantines, other states could only achieve containment by forceful border control, such as Vietnam, which prohibited even the return of its own citizens from abroad. This is one trade-off: free movement for control.

A second trade-off of travel bans is that in cutting off the movement of people, a state is also curbing the free flow of goods and services. Not only are there are trade implications to border closure, but states could also cut off the flow of vital supplies and services that they need for fighting a disease. For instance, Germany was initially a vocal proponent of keeping the Schengen area borders open—as they always were—in the early days of the pandemic. This enabled German hospitals to take in Italian patients when northern Italy was slammed with its coronavirus outbreak, with the minister president of North Rhine–Westphalia stating that "we need solidarity across borders in Europe. . . . We want to preserve the European spirit."[8] Borders would eventually be closed to all of Germany's neighbors as part of a sweeping shutdown. But it also meant that later when Germany had its own uptick in cases in the fourth wave (November 2021), it could rely on Italian hospitals to reciprocate.[9]

The United States faced these same trade-offs in its decision to close borders. But due to some of the preexisting U.S. conditions, the repercussions of the travel ban would manifest in unique ways. First, the United States has a long legacy not only of racial inequality but also specifically of targeting immigrant communities and racial minorities as scapegoats during public health emergencies.[10] In the 1800s, Chinese immigrants in the United States and Canada were frequently targeted as sources of disease, a pattern that repeated in the early 2000s with the SARS pandemic. Similar allegations have followed West Africans around the world during the Ebola outbreak and in countless other cases. Sadly, such biases against migrants as vectors of disease or infection frequently emerge where migrants already face discrimination. This was true for COVID as well: the pandemic arrived in the United States at a moment when immigrants and racial minorities were already being blamed for various social and economic ills.

The second thing that differentiated U.S. travel restrictions from other countries was, in fact, ironic: for a president who so proudly "built walls," the implementation of U.S. border restrictions was very leaky. As we showed in chapter 2, thousands who were technically subject to restrictions traveled into the country as the pandemic unfolded, and few were quarantined or contact-traced. Despite Trump's grandstanding on this one policy as a singular achievement, the gap between policy and practice was enormous. By focusing on the policy, he obfuscated facts on the ground.

Last, because international travel restrictions were so poorly enforced, the borders that would ultimately prove to be most consequential for slowing the spread of the virus were not the international ones but rather the domestic borders that exist between U.S. states. Freedom of movement within the United States meant that once people passed through immigration, where border control could exercise a modicum of health supervision, they were free to move throughout the country. While there were attempts to limit interstate travel in the early days of the pandemic—Hawaii and Rhode Island required travelers to self-quarantine, and mayors in cities near Cleveland, Ohio, were asking snowbirds not to return from Florida—there was no enforcement mechanisms or contact tracing.[11] Other large countries implemented domestic border controls, such as Australia's ban on travel between the states of Victoria and New South Wales (which was only lifted, and only for those fully vaccinated, in November 2021).[12] But with no such interstate travel bans within the United States, however, people continued to travel within the country. While these figures were certainly lower than previous years, they were not negligible. As we saw in chapter 3, many Americans changed their travel plans, but most did not.

In this chapter, we examine public attitudes to immigration policy during the COVID pandemic. Immigration is one of the most polarizing issues in contemporary American politics. Democrats are more supportive of immigration than Republicans across a range of issues, from establishing pathways to citizenship to incorporating linguistic and cultural diversity into conceptions of national identity. By contrast, Republicans typically express more support for the "law and order" aspects of immigration policy, such as deporting undocumented migrants and building a wall along the U.S.-Mexican border. But would there be consensus when it came to border closure in response to a public health emergency? And would support vary over time as the pandemic became a fact of life?

We looked at several immigration policy measures adopted or proposed during the pandemic in the United States: immigration bans, halting international air travel, quarantining foreigners, interstate travel bans, and repatriation of Americans abroad. Across each of these policy issues, we found that partisanship continued to drive and divide Americans' attitudes. Republicans became even more restrictive on immigration policy than they perhaps would have been otherwise, an outcome that we attribute to elite partisan cues and ingroup bias. We also find that Democrats worked to signal even more inclusiveness than their baseline preferences for an open immigration stance would otherwise suggest. We think this is because immigration was such a signature issue for Trump before the pandemic, making it hard for Democrats to signal support for COVID measures that would risk suggesting support for some of Trump's more divisive policies.

This reinforces an important message for dealing with health emergencies: they do not happen in a vacuum. Not only did relevant preexisting conditions shape the kind of pandemic that the United States would have, but the existing political landscape also shaped what kinds of policies could and could not garner mass public support. Some of America's handicaps were structural and inherited, but some were fresh and a consequence of politics.

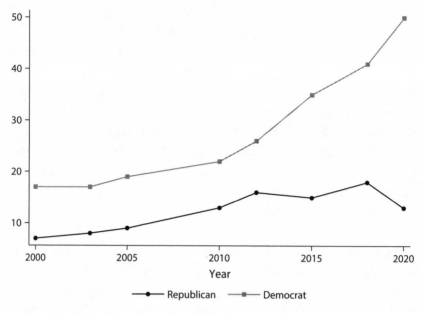

FIGURE 7.1. Preferences for increasing immigration, by partisanship

Immigration Attitudes Were Partisan before the Pandemic

Immigration attitudes have always had a partisan dimension. Democrats are more in favor of legal pathways for undocumented migrants than Republicans, Republicans are more in favor of increasing deportation for undocumented migrants than Democrats, and Democrats generally favor taking in refugees from violent contexts.[13] The size of this difference, however, has changed over time. Figure 7.1 uses data from Gallup to illustrate how support for increasing immigration has also differed between Democrats and Republicans.[14] This gap was roughly stable in size during the George W. Bush administration, with both Democrats and Republicans becoming slightly more favorable toward increasing immigration (the vast majority of Americans during this period, regardless of party, wanted immigration to stay the same or to decrease). During the Barack Obama years, though, the partisan gap in willingness to welcome migrants grew in size, only to explode during the Trump presidency.

Partisanship, naturally, is not the only personal characteristic that explains Americans' views toward immigration. Around the world, individuals who hold biased stereotypes about racial and ethnic outgroups are also more opposed to immigration; in the United States, this is particularly true among those who harbor prejudice against Latinos.[15] As large-scale immigration inevitably alters the racial and ethnic composition of the United States—a long-term process that is even older than the United States itself—immigration attitudes may be part of a larger "white backlash"[16] in which negative media portrayals of Latino immigration create support for ethnocentric attitudes.[17]

For this reason, before we examine specific attitudes about immigration policy during COVID-19, we also need to know about individual immigration attitudes in general. In wave 1 we asked our respondents three questions that tapped into immigration attitudes: whether they agreed or disagreed that (1) immigrants enrich the cultural life of the United States (or not), (2) whether immigration should be increased (or decreased), and (3) whether immigrants strengthen the economy (or not). Higher values indicate more support for immigration across all questions. We also asked the first two items a year later (in wave 6). A summary of the results by party appears in figure 7.2.

These results revealed persistent partisan differences in immigration attitudes. First, Democrats were reliably more supportive of immigration—that it enriches cultural life, that it should be increased, and that it strengthens the economy—compared to Republicans, with independents/nonpartisans falling somewhere in the middle. Second, immigration attitudes were stable over time. Not only were average levels of support consistent over time, but so were gaps between Democrats and Republicans. And in other results, we found that these patterns held among both right-wing news consumers and those who did not get their news from right-wing news sources, although anti-immigrant sentiments were on the whole more negative among the former than the latter. This pattern is consistent with existing research, which has shown that immigration attitudes are relatively stable over of time and cross-nationally.[18] Nonetheless, immigration attitudes do often move toward support for greater restriction in

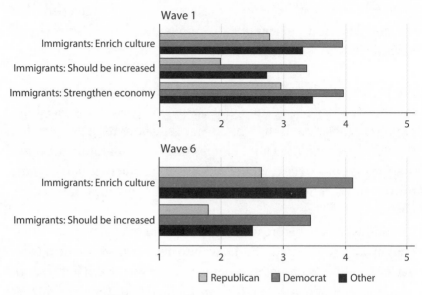

FIGURE 7.2. Immigration attitudes, by partisanship

response to major events such as economic crises,[19] terrorism,[20] immigration "caravans,"[21] and, certainly, pandemics.[22] We suspect that by the time wave 1 of our survey was fielded, starting March 20, 2020, public opinion had already begun to shift in favor of greater border controls and immigration restrictions.

Close the Borders

Consistent with his persistent efforts to build a wall at the southern border, Trump eagerly embraced border control and touted it as a central part of his governance strategy. Wasting no time in making explicit his views about the link between pandemic and immigration, in a February 28 rally in South Carolina, Trump even connected the initial spread of the coronavirus to failed (Democratic) immigration policy: "Whether it's the virus that we're talking about, or the many other public health threats, the Democrat policy of open borders is a direct threat to the health and wellbeing of all Americans."[23] Reflecting upon his February 2 travel "ban" from China, Trump boasted that "I cut off China very early. And if I didn't, we would have a chart that you wouldn't believe." Trump would continue to reference the China ban as his go-to talking point and greatest achievement in defense of his administration's early pandemic response.

Like so many aspects of the Trump administration, however, it was the public image of border closure and control that was key to his political strategy. The reality was entirely different. As a *Washington Post* headline put it, "Trump's 'Early' Travel 'Bans' Weren't Early, Weren't Bans and Didn't Work."[24] Compared to countries such as Australia and Singapore that implemented aggressive measures to restrict entry, Trump's was hardly a ban at all. It temporarily barred entry by foreign nationals who had traveled in China within the previous fourteen days and included several exemptions, such as allowances for conationals and legal permanent residents and family members, various visa holders, and residents of Hong Kong and Macau. The Associated Press reported that over 8,000 Chinese and foreign nationals based in China were able to enter the United States in the first three months after the "ban" was imposed.[25] A *New York Times* story found that at least 40,000 travelers arrived from China on over 1,300 direct flights to the United States in the two months after the restrictions were put into place; between January 1 and April 1, the total number of travelers entering the United States from China was 430,000.[26] And even had Trump's so-called ban been implemented rigorously, it would have had limited effect, because COVID-19 spreads among American citizens abroad too. The choice to restrict entry from foreign nationals only plainly reveals the anti-immigrant foundations of Trump's signature border control measures.

Beyond the headlines, the Trump administration was also working to substantively restrict immigration. With COVID-19 as a pretext, 2020 proved to be a productive year for Trump and his immigration czar, Stephen Miller, to crack down on migration. Nearly twenty policy changes affected tourists, refugees, asylum seekers, foreign workers, and international students. These policies ranged from the border restriction known as Title 42 policy, which disallowed the entry of noncitizens in the name of public health, and bans on entry for asylum seekers and suspension of refugee resettlement to postponement of immigration hearings, restricting access to the

Diversity Immigrant Visa Program lottery for certain nationals, and suspension of green card issuance abroad and, for some, renewals within the United States. In combination with the global effects of the pandemic, these strict measures fed a precipitous decline in immigration to the United States.

Some of these emergency restrictions were justified on public health grounds, but policies kept getting renewed, with justifications that changed over time. First viewed as a public health problem, where immigration was "halted" and "banned" to contain the virus, immigration was subsequently viewed as a problem for American economic recovery. We see these different framing devices in the changing rationales for limiting immigration. As Trump tweeted in late April to justify suspending immigration, "We must first take care of the American worker." This messaging pivot and sentiment was supported by key Trump allies in the Senate such as Tom Cotton, who claimed that "given the extreme lack of available jobs for American job seekers as portions of our economy begin to reopen, it defies common sense to admit additional foreign guest workers to compete for such limited employment."[27]

When public health experts recommended removing immigration restrictions for vulnerable categories such as unaccompanied minors and refugees,[28] Trump, the Centers for Disease Control and Prevention, and the Department of Health and Human Service held the party line. Well into the summer months of 2020 as rules eased to admit entry for agricultural workers,[29] the Department of Homeland Security and the Department of Justice were still using public health concerns to justify closing the border to "mitigate the risk of a deadly communicable disease being brought to the United States, or being further spread within the country."[30] When refugee resettlement ultimately resumed in late July 2020, intake was at a historical low, with fewer than twelve thousand refugees resettled in the United States in 2020.

Having painted a landscape of the political context of migration control, we can return to the question of what Americans thought about border closure. Consistent with the themes in this book, when we take a broad view of support for banning entry into the United

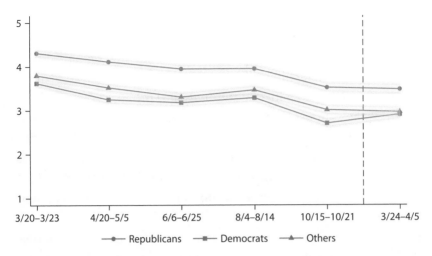

FIGURE 7.3. Support for entry ban

States—a general mitigation strategy against the spread of COVID-19—we find that partisanship strongly predicts immigration policy attitudes. We asked our respondents in each of these waves how much they support an entry ban, with the possible answers ranging from 1 (strongly oppose) to 5 (strongly support). In figure 7.3, we present the average answer across partisan groups.

Republicans start off strongly in favor of entry bans in wave 1, with 58 percent of all Republican respondents saying that they strongly support an entry ban, compared to 37 percent of Democrats. Over the course of the early pandemic average support for entry bans declined among all Americans, but the partisan gap remained stable.

The level of support for entry bans and the differences between parties remained broadly similar before and after the November election, illustrating the relative stability of immigration policy attitudes by partisanship, irrespective of who the president is. Not all policies show this kind of partisan stability. When it comes to the dangers of government spending, for example, we know that Republicans tend to be much more concerned about the deficit when Democrats hold the White House. Democrats tend to be much more in favor of the filibuster when they are the minority party in the Senate than when they hold the majority in the Senate and want to pass legislation.

These are cases in which partisan opinions are flexible, but at this moment in American politics, partisan positions on immigration seem to be far more durable and more fundamental than positions on issues such as the filibuster.

This fact leaves us with a subtle analytical problem, though. How much of the support that we identified above for entry bans—and partisan differences in that support—is driven by preexisting, anti-immigrant attitudes? Will someone who holds anti-immigrant views always be in support of entry bans, or, more interestingly, might someone who typically holds proimmigration views move to support hard borders during a national crisis? Knowing the answer to this question is important because it helps us to understand whether the pandemic itself has increased xenophobia and anti-immigrant attitudes.

To answer this, we looked at how support for an entry ban lines up with one's general attitude toward immigration. To determine this, we combined our questions about general attitudes toward immigration (from figure 7.2) into a single number that we call an anti-immigrant attitudes (AIA) index. A high AIA score means that a person, in aggregate, holds more xenophobic attitudes (e.g., believes that immigration should be decreased and that immigration contributes negatively to the economy and/or cultural life). A low AIA score corresponds with more proimmigration attitudes. Figure 7.4 shows how partisanship and anti-immigrant attitudes, measured by the AIA index, interact with support for entry bans.

Looking first at the plot on the left, we see among those who score low on AIA that partisanship played a strong role in explaining support for entry bans, even though support for entry bans was lower among these respondents than among those who score high on our AIA index. Democrats and independents/nonpartisans were significantly less likely to support entry bans than were Republicans throughout the pandemic, just until wave 6 under the Joe Biden administration.

Looking to the plot on the right, a different picture emerges. Among high AIA respondents, there was no significant difference in support for entry bans between Democrats and Republicans. Even

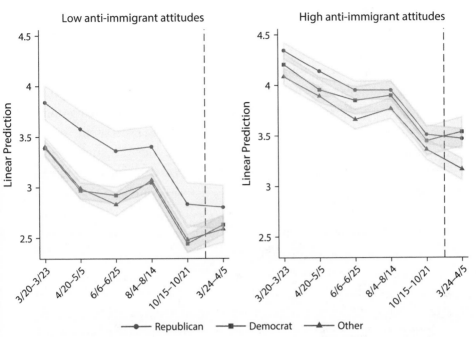

Note: For purposes of exposition, we classify all respondents as either high AIA (anti-immigrant) or low AIA (pro-immigrant) based on whether their AIA score is higher or lower than the median value of AIA among all respondents.

FIGURE 7.4. Entry ban, by partisanship and anti-immigrant attitudes

after the election of Biden, coinciding with the increased vaccination rates at home and exploding caseloads abroad in places such as India, there was relatively strong support for entry bans among Democrats and Republicans alike. Partisanship, in other words, is only related to support for an entry ban among those respondents who were more receptive to immigrants in the first place.

Why did support for entry bans decline over time, a pattern we see across individuals regardless of immigration attitudes and partisanship? For one, Americans may have simply tired of the pandemic. For another, the fact that entry bans turned out not to be bans at all may have also undercut what was initially strong policy support. That is, evidence over time showed the travel ban to be ineffective, and enthusiasm inevitably waned. It could also be that broad concerns about the state of the economy, identified in previous chapters, led Americans of all partisan stripes to soften their support for entry bans, where barriers to human mobility also mean disruptions to the movement of goods and services. But more broadly, the administration's messaging on border closure as a COVID-19 mitigation strategy was unsupported by policies that would make it successful, such as contact tracing and isolation/quarantine that could complement essential travel. This became evident by the summer as "bans" continued but COVID-19 spread unabated. As Marc Lipsitch, a Harvard epidemiologist, observed during a *PBS NewsHour* interview in July 2020, "while the border controls probably did buy us a little bit of time, we frittered that time away by not building up our defense. And now with the high rate of COVID-19 cases in the country, continued border restrictions likely will not make a big difference."[31]

We also suspect that partisan elite messaging played an important role in explaining the patterns over time in figure 7.4. To support an entry ban—for whatever rationale—would be to support Trump, a position that strong Democrats would be instinctively against. Low support for an entry ban may not reflect an individual's attitudes about immigration or COVID policy per se but rather a rejection of Trump and his policies, increasingly tied over time to his rhetoric on border closures and entry bans.

Taken together, though, these findings help us to make sense of how partisanship interacted with anti-immigration sentiment during the course of the pandemic. On a broad level, anti-immigrant attitudes appeared to be more enduring than were attitudes about how immigration policy might be used to combat the pandemic. And among those with high levels of animosity toward immigrants, partisanship does not seem to explain policy preferences. But at the same time, policy preferences were more responsive to ongoing events than are anti-immigrant attitudes. That is why support for entry bans declined over the course of the pandemic, even though we consistently find that it is higher among Republicans and those with high AIA scores. This subtle distinction between policy preferences (which seem easier to move in response to events) and more fundamental political attitudes (which are harder to move) speaks more generally to one of our broader arguments in this book: that a different set of messages from the Trump administration might have produced a different policy environment.

Discrimination by Nationality

Entry bans, at least as we have described them so far, are blanket policies that would apply to all travelers coming from anywhere to the United States. But as we know, entry bans are frequently targeted toward entrants from specific countries. Trump's supposed ban on entry from China applied to travelers entering the country on flights that originated in China but not from other foreign airports. And bans on flights from Europe did not target all travelers but instead targeted specifically those who are not U.S. citizens or did not hold the proper visa. Given these policy details and the discretion available to U.S. policy makers to implement bans that targeted people by nationality, we can investigate such policies to see if they might reflect particular forms of racism or xenophobia in their targeting of entrants from particular types of countries.

We do this using a survey experiment that is similar in form to our survey experiment on federal versus state authorities in chapter 5. Specifically, we can compare who supports entry bans (and who does not) according to the country of origin of the people targeted by the entry ban. It could be, for example, that even a low-AIA respondent who is generally favorable toward immigration is willing to support entry bans against travels from certain countries in the context of a COVID-19 outbreak in those countries. And a high-AIA respondent who harbors generally xenophobic attitudes may just believe that we should stop all immigration, regardless of country of origin.

The United States under President Trump (and President Biden) adopted an approach to entry bans in which only some immigrants are perceived to present a public health risk. Specifically, bans are designed to target travelers from countries with high case counts or new variant types, who are more likely to bring COVID-19 into the United States than are travelers from countries with low case counts. At the beginning of the pandemic, American news was preoccupied with coverage of the spiraling pandemic in China and Italy. In northern Italy quarantine began on February 22, accompanied by school closures, the cancellation of religious services, and the suspension of local transit.

But of course, even though the outbreaks in China and Italy grabbed the headlines, the COVID-19 outbreak was a global problem. As the American media focused on COVID in Italy and China, other countries began to grapple with their own crises. The United Kingdom, for example, was in a desperate situation. In an emergency COVID meeting at Downing Street on March 13, Dominic Cummings, chief adviser to Prime Minister Boris Johnson, scribbled on a whiteboard a series of questions and observations. These ranged from observation number 1, "No vaccine in 2020," to the ominous and unanswered question number 6, "Who do we not save?" The United Kingdom was added to the Trump administration's COVID-19 travel ban on March 16. Around this time, the Johnson-led Conservative government started holding daily televised press conferences and canceling public events.

But as figure 7.5 shows, Americans were looking at Italy and China, not the United Kingdom, during the first wave of the pandemic. This figure shows data from Google Trends, which capture the relative frequency of searches within the United States for China, Italy, and the United Kingdom in the first four months of 2020.[32]

We see very clearly the spike in attention to China and Italy, relative to the United Kingdom, just as we launched the first wave of our survey. Did Americans, then, have views about who *should* be banned based on their sense of threat in the belief that China and Italy were hotspots but (erroneously) that the United Kingdom was not? Or did perhaps the racial background of the target matter, in which case Italians and Britons would be treated similarly (despite different levels of attention to the mass outbreak in their countries), with Chinese treated differently?

To answer these questions, in wave 1 when we asked about entry bans, we randomly alternated the target of the entry ban to be China, Italy, and the United Kingdom. Specifically, we asked whether a respondent agreed or disagreed (on a 5-point scale) that

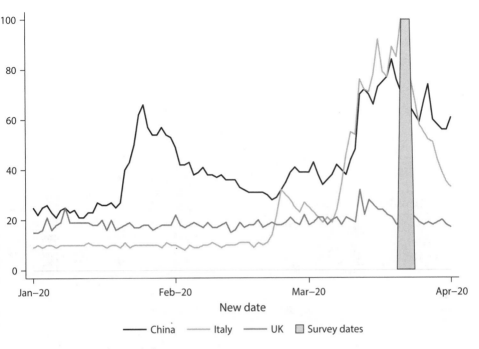

FIGURE 7.5. Google Trends data

"The United States must continue to ban the entry of citizens of [China/Italy/Great Britain] into the United States." Respondents were randomly assigned to receive one of the three countries. This kind of experimental analysis is often termed "racial priming," as the use of each term can "prime" respondents to reveal their attitudes toward each group, enabling us to evaluate the role they play in policy evaluation.[33]

We show the results of this analysis in figure 7.6.

Among high-AIA Republicans and Democrats alike, we see the strongest support for entry bans regardless of the group to which it is applied. Both Democrats and Republicans supported bans against Italians, and for Democrats that support is higher compared to the other national origins. There was no statistical difference for xenophobic Democrats between support for banning Britons and Chinese. Republicans supported bans from China and Italy but to a lesser extent than they did bans from the United Kingdom. In all,

Should we ban entry of people who are . . .

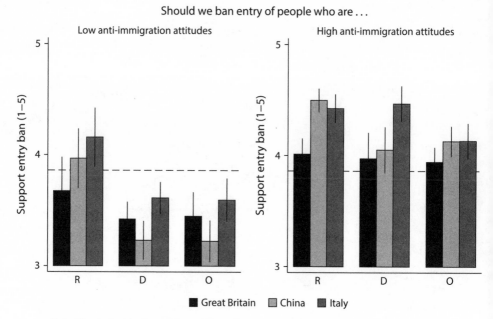

Note: The dashed horizontal line is the mean response across all respondents in the sample.

FIGURE 7.6. Ban entry, by partisanship and immigrant attitudes, March 2020

among those respondents with the highest level of anti-immigrant attitudes, neither Democrats nor Republicans followed a simple racial heuristic of targeting Chinese more than Europeans. Rather, the United Kingdom was always favored relative to Italy, and China was less penalized among Democrats only.

Among low-AIA respondents, however, partisanship clearly mattered. Republicans were more strongly in favor of entry bans regardless of which group they are applied to, echoing our findings from figure 7.4. Democrats expressed lower support for entry bans applied toward any national origin group, and independents/nonpartisans expressed a similar hesitance. Importantly, low-AIA Democrats and independents/unaffiliated were most reluctant to apply entry bans to China. Once again, we see that Americans' views on entry bans cannot be explained by simple racial attitudes. If anything, we view the pattern of results as indicating that low-AIA Democrats were compensating for the Trump administration's anti-Chinese rhetoric by becoming particularly opposed to entry bans applied to China.

The results in figure 7.6 capture the situation in March 2020. But as the pandemic wore on, hotspots around the world changed. China and Europe (along with Iran) were central concerns for international travel in March and April, but by summer the COVID-19 pandemic had spread elsewhere. Brazil, as it ascended its first wave, was added to the U.S. entry ban list on May 24 (figure 7.7).

This evolution allowed us to compare entry ban support against a different national origin. In a similar experiment, we asked for agreement/disagreement on the same item as before but replaced Italy with Brazil: "The United States must continue to ban the entry of citizens of [China/Brazil/Great Britain] into the United States." We asked this question four times, in June (wave 3), August (wave 4), October (wave 5), and March 2021 (wave 6), which allows us to follow support for entry bans by country of origin over time.

In figure 7.8 we plot the results of this experiment, distinguishing the effects of national origin by partisanship.

Among Republicans, the highest level of support for an entry ban is when it is applied to China. Thinking back on results from March in figure 7.6, these results suggest that if immigration policy during the COVID-19 pandemic did not start off racialized, it certainly became racialized over time. Support for an entry ban from Brazil was consistently second among Republicans, with support for an entry ban from the United Kingdom significantly lower among Republicans throughout.

The pattern for Democrats is entirely different. Support for an entry ban from Brazil is consistently higher than support for entry bans from either China or the United Kingdom throughout the pandemic, peaking in August to coincide with the zenith of Brazil's first wave. Support for an entry ban from Brazil is higher among Democrats than Republicans at any point. Interestingly, we see the lowest support among Democrats for an entry ban from China, with a marked divergence in trends in wave 6. We suspect that this reflects Democrats' signaling of their opposition to the racialization of the pandemic by Republicans—including the sizable uptick in

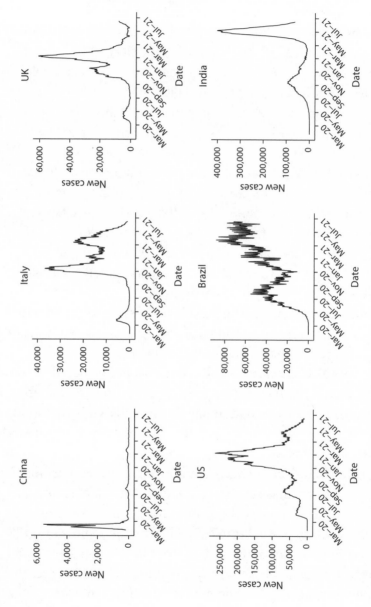

FIGURE 7.7. COVID-19 cases and deaths in Brazil, China, India, Italy, the United Kingdom, and the United States

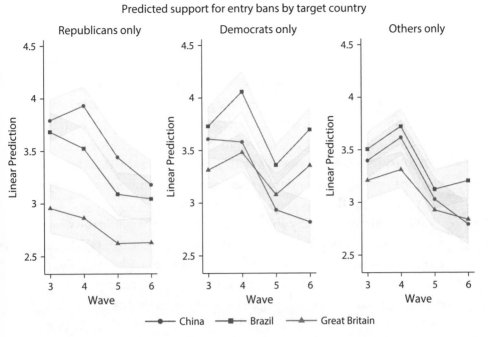

Predicted support for entry bans by target country

FIGURE 7.8. Ban entry, by partisanship and immigrant attitudes, June 2020–March 2021

anti–Asian American and Pacific Islander hate crimes in the United States. Among nonpartisans, still another pattern emerges: there is generally no difference in support for entry bans regardless of their target.

Broader Immigration Policy Debates

An entry ban was not the only immigration policy put into place in response to COVID-19. It wasn't even the most controversial. During the first wave of the pandemic in the United States, several states implemented policies that put conditions on interstate travel that— while not quite matching the firm restrictions implemented by Australia's states and not enforced rigorously—did seek to slow the virus's spread.[34] Many states required fourteen-day self-quarantining for out-of-state travelers, depending on their state of origin. For example, in March 2020 Florida governor Ron DeSantis ordered travelers from

New York, New Jersey, and Connecticut to self-quarantine for two weeks, leaving travelers from all other states unaffected. Chicago Department of Public Health commissioner Allison Arwady issued a similar order for travelers from states with surging cases in July 2020 (e.g., Alabama, Arizona, Louisiana, Nevada, Utah). And some states, such as Indiana, never implemented any travel restrictions. And while some states could issue and meaningfully enforce quarantines (Hawaii), others could not or would not. As New Jersey governor Phil Murphy stated, "I say this with a heavy heart, I would love to be able to stop people and turn them around at our borders. . . . We can't. That's not the way the United States works."[35]

What did citizens think about state-level travel bans and the wider menu of policies as emergency measures in response to COVID-19? Here we zoom out to consider a variety of other immigration policies that were nominally used or considered during the pandemic: halting all international travel, imposing entry restrictions at the U.S.-Mexican border, quarantining Chinese citizens in the United States (including Chinese Americans), implementing interstate (domestic) travel bans, and rescuing/repatriating American citizens abroad. We asked about support for these policy items in March and April 2020, so we can observe levels of both support and change during the first wave of the pandemic.

Figure 7.9 shows average support—on a five-point scale ranging from strongly oppose (1) to strongly support (5)—for these immigration policy items, distinguishing as always by respondents' partisan affiliations.

Some of these policies (such as U.S.-Mexican border controls) are mainstays of the Republican Party platform, and unsurprisingly, support for this policy shows strong division by partisanship. But the other policies in figure 7.9, such as halting all international air travel, are novel emergency policy measures. For these, we saw only small differences according to partisanship. Republicans only barely support halting all international travel and quarantining Chinese citizens in the United States more than Democrats and independents do, and there was no difference in attitudes on repatriating American citizens abroad at all.

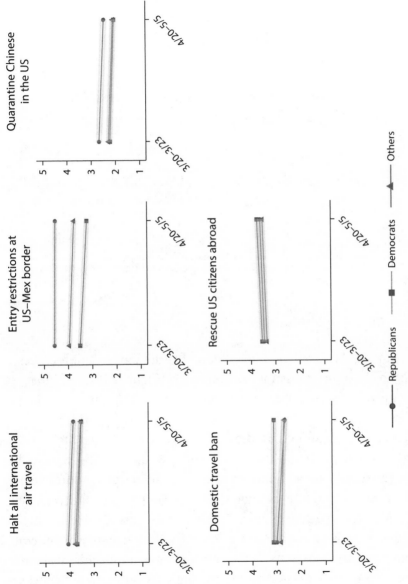

FIGURE 7.9. Public attitudes on immigration policies, by partisanship

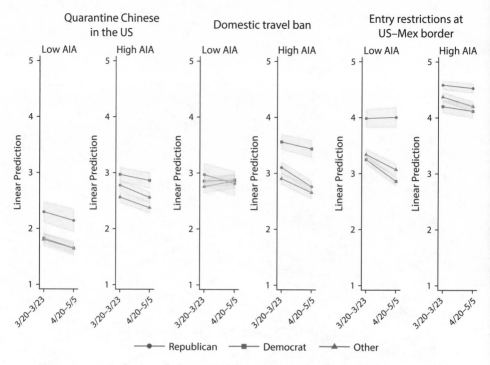

FIGURE 7.10. Attitudes toward select immigration policies, by partisanship and AIA

Among those policy items that do feature partisan differences, what role do anti-immigrant attitudes play? Figure 7.10 differentiates between low-AIA and high-AIA respondents, as before.

Among low-AIA respondents, we see strong partisan differences in support for quarantining Chinese in the United States and implementing entry restrictions at the U.S.-Mexican border (with diverging trajectories). But there are no such partisan differences in support for a domestic travel ban, and support was fairly evenly divided. This suggests that low-AIA respondents did not yet have solid opinions about domestic travel bans. Had state and federal authorities so desired, they could muster mass support for or against closing interstate borders, imposing highway temperature checks, and otherwise limiting travel within the country.

Among high-AIA respondents, by contrast, partisan differences were opposite from what one might expect: high-AIA Democrats express greater support for quarantining Chinese in the United States, whereas high-AIA Republicans express greater support for entry restrictions at the U.S.-Mexican border than do Democrats but only marginally. High-AIA Democrats also supported domestic travel bans more than did high-AIA Republicans and independents/ nonpartisans. While we have limited information about what might motivate this finding about high-AIA Democrats, it could be that these Democrats had a general appetite for a strong government response to managing COVID-19.

Conclusion

COVID-19 transformed U.S. immigration policy at a time when immigration policy was more politicized than it had ever been in recent history. The COVID-19 pandemic provided cover for Trump to enact some of the harshest restrictions in recent history. Federal emergency measures of early March 2020 were extended into the summer, with deleterious effects on both immigration numbers and federal government practices. And while immigration control was a broadly popular policy, the administration squandered an opportunity to unify and protect Americans. Restrictions were poorly implemented, politicized, and left unsupported by related policies that can make immigration control work to mitigate the spread of the pandemic. Trump's policies were successful at lowering immigration, which was his main policy objective; they were largely ineffective at doing anything else.

Our survey data help us to make sense of the politics of immigration policy as a tool for managing the pandemic. More so than other issue areas that we have addressed in previous chapters, when it comes to immigration policy, we found that partisanship mattered in subtle ways that depended on respondents' general orientation and predispositions toward immigrants. And although the immigration policy debate was highly racialized by the Trump administration's anti-Chinese rhetoric, Americans' views toward policies such as entry bans did not follow a simple racial logic. Rather, the survey evidence that we amassed told us that general concern about the pandemic in specific national contexts mattered at least as much as racial cues. Notably, for those non-Republicans who held strong pro-immigrant positions, we detected a form of solidarity with Chinese as the undeserved targets of Trump's ire. We also saw how low-AIA Democrats may have worried that support for prohealth measures such as an immigration ban could be misconstrued as support for Trump's xenophobic policy agenda, which only deepened under the cover of the pandemic. And we saw high-AIA Democrats supporting restrictive immigration measures, such as domestic quarantining and closing the U.S.-Mexican border, suggesting where emergency times could find rallying points.

Put another way, what we learned in sum is that emergency travel policies were made in the context of latent public attitudes that support control and prohibit nuance. But perhaps the real legacy of a continued focus on border control, coupled with racist elite commentary about the "Chinese virus," may have been that it pivoted attention toward the border and away from mitigation efforts that may have slowed the spread of the virus in the United States, such as domestic travel restrictions, quarantining, and contact tracing.

8

The Burdens of Inequality

RACE AND THE COVID-19 PANDEMIC

In March 2020 Michigan was under a state of emergency because of the coronavirus pandemic, but the buses in Detroit were still running. Essential workers needed to get to work, people needed to shop for groceries or go to the doctor, and residents without a car had little choice but to take the bus. Detroit is a poor city: more than 50 percent of its residents live below the poverty line. The city has a legacy of residential segregation that has left predominantly Black neighborhoods with fewer resources and higher crime rates than predominantly white neighborhoods.[1] Black residents are also more likely than white residents to live in dense neighborhoods with fewer hospitals and pharmacies and are more likely to be public transit riders than white residents.[2]

One bus driver named Jason Hargrove went to work in March 2020 despite the risks posed by the coronavirus. At the time, bus drivers were not provided with personal protective equipment, and passengers were not socially distanced or masked. On March 21, Mr. Hargrove posted a Facebook video criticizing a rider for coughing in the bus without covering her mouth, noting that she was putting everyone at risk. He pleaded with people in the public to take the virus seriously, saying "'I feel violated. I feel violated for the folks that was on the bus when this happened,' he said, adding: 'To those who are watching, this—this is real.'"[3] On April 3, the Centers for Disease Control and Prevention (CDC) started recommending that the public consider wearing cloth masks in public. This recommendation came too late to help Mr. Hargrove, who died of COVID-19 on April 1, 2020.

What happened to Mr. Hargrove is emblematic of what would happen time and again across the United States over the coming months. Hargrove was a Black man working as a frontline worker during the early days of the pandemic in a city with clear racial inequality in housing, employment, infrastructure, and access to health care. Minority communities suffered early and disproportionately from the virus as well as from the economic fallout from the pandemic. Communities of color were also slower to get the vaccines aimed at ending the pandemic. As Brookings Institution fellow and sociology professor Rashawn Ray wrote in April 2020, "When America catches a cold, Black people get the flu. Well, when America catches coronavirus, Black people die."[4]

So far in this book, we have focused on how Americans' responses to the pandemic were shaped by their partisan identities. With over eight hundred thousand Americans dead from COVID-19 in December 2021, no part of our nation was spared from the pandemic. But we know all too well that other identities, particularly race and ethnicity, mattered a great deal in how people experienced the pandemic. We saw this in chapter 5, when we looked at race and schooling during COVID-19, and again in chapter 6, when we explored the racial dynamics of unemployment during COVID-19. Here we examine more closely how America's racial and ethnic minorities suffered disproportionately from the COVID-19 pandemic.

Racial Disparities in American Public Health

Individual partisan identity goes only so far in explaining the impact of the COVID-19 pandemic on communities of color in the United States. The reason is because there is less variation in partisan identification among communities of color than there is among white Americans. In the 2020 presidential race, 43 percent of whites voted for Democrats compared to 92 percent of Black voters, 59 percent of Latino voters, and 72 percent of Asian voters.[5] But partisanship did affect Americans of color through the partisanship of their state governments and through the types of social policy pursued by those governors prior to and during the pandemic.

COVID-19 was particularly devastating for minoritized communities. As of March 2021, American Public Media estimated that 1 in 390 Native Americans, 1 in 555 Black Americans, and 1 in 680 Latinos had died from COVID-19.[6] By the end of 2021, Black deaths occurred at 1.4 times the rate of whites.[7] A study of twenty-three states found that Native Americans were twice as likely to contract COVID-19 and four times as likely to die as whites due to factors such as more multigenerational housing, more limited access to running water, more reliance on shared transportation, and more underlying health conditions that increase the fatality of the virus.[8] These deaths are tragedies for individual families and represent cultural losses for entire communities as well. In Native American communities, the loss of elders from COVID-19 also meant a loss knowledge of traditions, languages, and customs.[9]

Health inequality was one of the preexisting conditions that we discussed in chapter 1, and it is particularly acute along racial lines. These conditions are structural—from hand sanitizer dispensers and pulse oximeter readers (a tool used to estimate blood oxygenation, which was vital for determining compromised breathing due to COVID-19) being unable to detect Black skin with the accuracy of white skin[10]—and also behavioral, whereby patients receive unequal treatment while in care.[11] These political and social conditions interacted with the disease conditions to produce distinctly worse outcomes for minorities.[12]

At the beginning of the pandemic, Black and Latino Americans were less likely to be insured and have access to primary care physicians than their white counterparts and more likely have more chronic conditions such as hypertension, obesity, and diabetes.[13] In 2018, Black Americans had a life expectancy four years shorter than whites.[14] Communities of color are more likely than white communities to be exposed to environmental pollution, making Black, Latino, and Asian Americans more vulnerable to respiratory illnesses,[15] a comorbidity that led to worse outcomes for COVID patients. Native American communities also face persistent inequality in health outcomes due to overlapping structural issues such as poverty, policy neglect from state governments, inadequate funding of the Indian Health Services, and underemployment.[16]

We can see race-based health inequalities in our survey data as well. In wave 1 of the survey (March 2020), we asked respondents about background health conditions. First, we asked respondents to rate their general health on a 5-point scale from "poor" to "excellent." Figure 8.1 shows the percentage of respondents in each category by the racial and ethnic identity: (non-Hispanic) white, Black, Hispanic or Latino/a, and an "other" category that contains respondents who identify as Asian American, Native American, or multiracial.[17]

A plurality of respondents (48%) assessed their own health as either "very good" or "excellent," but that varied by the racial identity of respondents, with 48 percent of white respondents reporting very good or excellent health compared to 43 percent of Black respondents. On the other end of the spectrum, 13 percent of white respondents reported "fair" health compared to 15 percent of Black respondents and 15 percent of Latino respondents. These differences were not large, but they are meaningful. A back-of-the-envelope calculation suggests that if the rates of feeling in "good or excellent" health were equal across races in our survey, this would imply that two million more Black Americans would feel healthy.[18]

We can also examine trust in key health institutions in our survey respondents, this time drawing from wave 6 of our survey, which was fielded in late March 2021 and for which we deliberately collected additional data from communities of color. The racial differences in trust were modest but still plainly evident in the data (figure 8.2).

White Americans were more trusting of doctors and hospitals than were Black Americans, although when it comes to schools and the health care system more generally, there are basically no differences by race. Yet even acknowledging these differences, we see

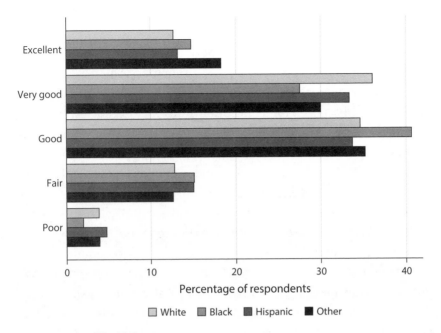

FIGURE 8.1. Overall health, by race

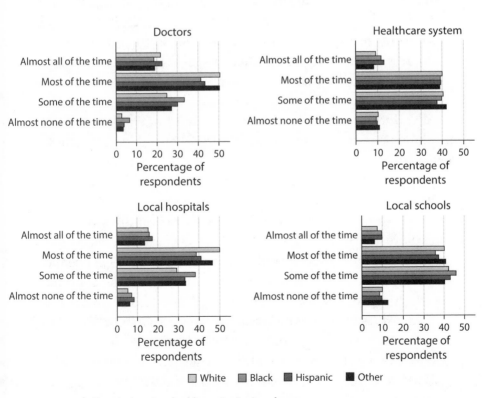

FIGURE 8.2. Trust in American health care institutions, by race

in figure 8.2 a summary of the general issue facing all Americans when it comes to health care: by and large, most Americans simply do not trust health care institutions. Our description in chapter 1 of the wobbly, unreliable, and oftentimes incoherent U.S. health care system as a preexisting condition is one that most Americans would share.

Moreover, health care *coverage* is also uneven by race, only exacerbating the preexisting conditions that is poor health care infrastructure. Among our respondents, 18 percent of Black respondents and 20 percent of Latino respondents—one in five—had no health insurance, compared to only 9 percent of white respondents and 10 percent of respondents in the "other" category. Underlying economic disadvantage and income inequality also made the pandemic more serious in minority communities, as we described in detail in chapter 6. Racial minorities were particularly affected by job losses, with attendant consequences for access to affordable health care. And due to the employment-based health care system in the United States and the disproportionate job losses among nonwhite Americans, this meant that approximately one million Asian Americans, two million Black Americans, and three million Latinos lost their health insurance in 2020.[19]

Even if we put aside the sudden rise of unemployment for communities of color during the COVID-19 pandemic, structural inequalities in economic conditions sustain racial differences in health outcomes. State and local income inequality is associated with higher levels of mortality and poor health for minority groups and whites alike.[20] Cities with a higher portion of Black residents and those with lower levels of public services have generally higher levels of mortality.[21] As a result, during the COVID-19 pandemic, income inequality put poorer citizens at more risk of infection and death than people who were able to work from home, live in less crowded housing, and had access to private transportation. Counties with higher degrees of income inequality had higher incidences of COVID-19 as well as more deaths.[22] And these forces interacted with racial differences in employment to put Black and Latino Americans at particular risk during the pandemic, who were more likely to work in essential sectors of the economy—transportation, retail, agriculture, food service, and health care—where telework or social distancing was not an option.

Incarceration and congregate living conditions also increased the risk of COVID-19 exposure and illness, and these experiences vary significantly by race. More than 2 million adults are in prison, and more than 40,000 are in immigration detention.[23] Black Americans are incarcerated at a rate that is 5.1 times higher than whites at the state level, and the rate for Latinos is 1.4 times that of whites.[24] Prisons, jails, and immigration detention facilities are often crowded, with inadequate ventilation and limitations on hygiene. Incarcerated individuals are also likely to have comorbidities, high levels of stress, and limited capacity for social distancing, all factors that can make them uniquely vulnerable to the coronavirus. As a consequence, prisons were the sites of some of the worst COVID-19 outbreaks in the United States. By January 2021 there were more than 510,000 positive cases in prisons, and more than 2,200 prisoners and staff had died from COVID-19.[25]

The narrative we have provided so far in this section risks portraying the COVID-19 pandemic's racialized consequences as the unfortunate consequences of income, employment patterns, and incarceration that happen to be correlated with race. But we know that policy making itself during the COVID-19 pandemic reinforced racial differences in health outcomes. Here the structural preconditions that we discussed in chapter 2 are most insidious. Mitigation measures such as widespread testing, isolation, and distribution of personal protective equipment were more slowly implemented in communities with more minority residents.[26] Mass testing centers were not always set up in places easily accessible to low-income neighborhoods or those without good transportation options. As testing sites spread into neighborhoods around the country, those in mostly Black and Latino neighborhoods served more people, had longer lines, and were more likely to run out of tests than ones in nearby white neighborhoods. In the early response to the pandemic, public health messaging aimed for more universal messaging about how individuals could keep themselves safe, but much of this messaging was deemed confusing, untrustworthy, or irrelevant in minority as well as low-income and rural communities.[27]

Race and the COVID-19 Pandemic

When we began our survey, we suspected that one way in which COVID-19 might have uneven racial consequences would be because Americans would look at the early hotspots and conclude that COVID-19 was primarily an urban problem. To the extent that urban areas are also those with larger minority communities, "urban" might then serve (as it often does in American discourse) as a code word for "race." When we asked Americans to what extent they saw COVID-19 as primarily a problem for urban or densely populated areas, though, we found mixed evidence, as shown in figure 8.3.

As expected, from the first time we asked this question in wave 2, Republicans were far more likely than Democrats to consider COVID-19 an urban problem. But racial differences were muted. Although Black Americans always were least likely to believe that COVID-19 would be primarily an urban problem, these differences do not amount to much substantively. To see the implicitly racialized politics of COVID-19 as an urban problem, we really do need to focus on partisanship itself and Republicans' beliefs about COVID-19.

Starting in April 2020, we asked survey respondents to tell us whether they had COVID-19 at some point, whether confirmed by a medical test or not. Figure 8.4 shows us the percentage of respondents who reported having a case of COVID-19 by the race of the respondent.

In the public as a whole, the percentage of respondents who had fallen victim to COVID-19 was very low in the first few waves of the survey, only to grow over time, with the most growth among Latino and Black respondents. In wave 6 of our survey, we expanded the sample dramatically to include a new sample of nonwhite respondents: 450 Black respondents, 450 Asian American respondents, and 450 Latino respondents. If we include those new respondents, the percentage of all respondents who had COVID-19 rises to 13 percent in wave 6.

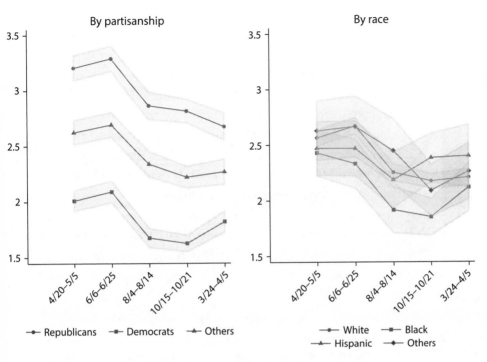

FIGURE 8.3. COVID-19 is an urban problem, by partisanship and race

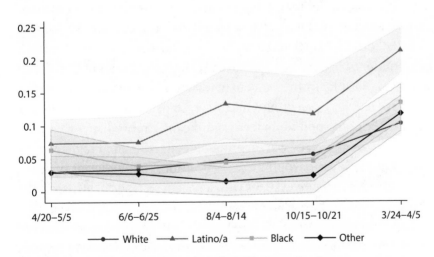

FIGURE 8.4. Proportion of respondents who had COVID-19 over time, by race

One puzzling feature of figure 8.4 is decreasing levels of COVID-19 between waves 2 and 3 of our survey for Black respondents and between waves 4 and 5 for Latino/a respondents. To explain this, recall that some of our respondents dropped out between each survey wave, so evidently those Latinos who dropped out of our survey at this stage were disproportionately those who had contracted COVID-19. The same phenomenon explains decreasing rates of COVID-19 infections between waves 2 and 3 for Black Americans. In these numbers, then, we can see a bit of evidence of just how disruptive COVID-19 is for people's daily lives.

But the main takeaway from figure 8.4 is the unequal incidence of COVID-19 by race. Starting in the spring of 2020, Black and Latino respondents were more likely than white respondents or respondents of other races to report having had COVID-19, and those gaps grew over time. Latino respondents reported the highest level of coronavirus cases of any group from April 2020 onward, and the gap between Latino respondents and other groups grew over time. By the time of the April 2021 wave, 21 percent of Latino respondents reported having had the virus at some point, double the rate of white respondents and significantly higher than the 13 percent of Black respondents who report having had the virus. Respondents in the "other" racial category had similar disease rates to Black respondents. From April 2020 to a year later their rates of COVID-19 jumped fourfold, from 3 percent in wave 2 of the survey to 12 percent in wave 6. Even as all groups had increasing rates of COVID-19 over time, Latino respondents were significantly more likely to report cases across all survey waves, probably reflecting their higher likelihood of working in frontline work positions, higher levels of being uninsured, and living in states with less generous social welfare policies. These numbers roughly parallel CDC data, which reveal that as of September 2021 confirmed COVID-19 cases for Latinos were substantially higher than for whites, with rates for Black Americans in between Latinos and whites (and rates for Asian Americans lower than for whites).[28]

As we showed in figure 4.5 in chapter 4, in March 2020—when we first surveyed our respondents—there were very few differences in COVID-19–related health behaviors across racial groups. White respondents were slightly more likely to say they were seeking information about the diseases and avoiding contact with others than respondents from other races. Black and Latino respondents were more likely to say they were buying hand sanitizer. And starting with wave 2 (April 2020), we added a question about mask wearing to our survey. Overall, there are high levels of masking among all Americans, and while there are some differences in terms of levels across racial groups, these differences are not large enough to account for the vast differences in caseloads and deaths by racial group. These differences are much more likely caused by differences in the context of their behavior, that is, what percentage of people in the group were frontline works as well as whether they had access to testing, health care, and vaccines, which we discuss in more depth in chapter 11.

When we consider the racial dimensions of policy attitudes, emotions, and other factors, we can see even more clearly the pandemic's uneven effects. We do not find any evidence, for example, of racial differences in beliefs about testing availability, even though we found in chapter 6 that Democrats were far less likely to believe that tests were available. Whites were far more likely to blame Barack Obama for the COVID-19 pandemic and far less likely to blame Donald Trump than were Blacks. And as we found in chapter 7, Black and Latino/a respondents were more likely to have difficulty paying rent, more likely to have visited a food pantry, and more likely to have sought assistance from a charity for themselves and their family.

As this evidence shows, the pandemic was always going to be harder for minoritized communities. They experienced more precarity because of the pandemic, and they had stronger legacies of distrust toward and abuse by health care services, which would make government-led pandemic mitigation inherently difficult, hearkening back to inequality as an essential precondition (see chapter 1). And while we may have anticipated that minoritized groups would be scapegoated for the pandemic—the United States has a long history of blaming immigrants for pandemics[29]—as was the case for Asian American communities, we could not anticipate how fully the spotlight would turn to racial injustice in the summer of 2020, as it did following the murder of George Floyd.

Race and Protest

The pandemic spring of 2020 led into a summer of protests against racial injustice and police brutality following the killings of Black people by police in cities across the United States. On Memorial Day 2020 the United States was close to one hundred thousand deaths from coronavirus, cases were rising again, and many Americans were still working from home, going to school online, and social distancing.[30] On that day, George Floyd was murdered.

George Floyd was a forty-six-year-old Black man living in Minneapolis, Minnesota. On May 25, 2020, he was arrested on suspicion of having used a counterfeit $20 bill to purchase a pack of cigarettes at a local grocery store. After restraining and handcuffing him and placing him face down in the street, police officer Derek Chauvin knelt on Floyd's neck for nine minutes and twenty-nine seconds, surrounded by three other police officers and a crowd of onlookers who expressed horror and outrage as the event unfolded.[31] Bystanders recorded the encounter, where Chauvin pressed his body weight onto the neck of Floyd, who repeatedly said that he could not breathe. Mr. Floyd asphyxiated and died.

In the days following Floyd's murder, protesters filled the streets of Minneapolis. They were confronted with force by the police, who used tear gas and rubber bullets, and later by the National Guard. The protests that started in Minneapolis in late May 2020 spread across the country, with more than 4,700 demonstrations in more than 2,500 locations. In wave 3 of our survey, 115 out of 2104 respondents reported participating in the George Floyd protests: only four were Republicans; the rest were mostly Democrats. These protests—in small towns, suburbs, and cities alike in the United States and around the globe— were also prompted by the killing of other unarmed Black people such as Ahmaud Arbery in a subdivision near Brunswick, Georgia, and Breonna Taylor in her home in Louisville, Kentucky.[32] The protests continued all summer, with an estimated 20 million Americans taking part, making this one of the largest protest movements in American history. Our 115 George Floyd protestors included Americans of all races and incomes from thirty-four different states and the District of Columbia. To give a sense of the scale of these protests, only 15 of our survey respondents reported having participated in the much-discussed antilockdown/stay-at-home protests from the spring of 2020.

We will address some of the political consequences of these protests in chapter 9, where we discuss the implications of the pandemic on democracy. Here, we simply note that these protests were accelerated by the conditions of the COVID-19 pandemic that had so clearly revealed the racial inequalities in those who were sick and dying as well as heightened Americans' sensitivity to both the structural foundations and political choices that created and sustained these inequalities. Millions of people who would otherwise be at work or socializing or traveling were instead at home, more isolated and faced with the brutal reality that America's racial minorities were suffering. Police violence was not an uncommon occurrence, but it could be that a cross-section of Americans were paying attention because they were at home. Or, put another way, Americans were not as preoccupied by the many small distractions that happen in our day-to-day lives.

While we cannot conclude definitively that the COVID-19 pandemic created the conditions for the protests in the summer of 2020, it is clear that popular frustration was high enough to make an upsurge of mobilization unsurprising. Millions of people joined Black Lives Matter protests in their communities, despite stay-at-home orders and fears of community congregation. Pictures of protests and mass gatherings were distinct from those of contemporaneous Trump rallies and antilockdown protests because the vast majority of participants were wearing masks. While public officials such as CDC director Robert Redfield raised concerns that these protests might prove to be a "seeding event" for COVID,[33] one paper found "no evidence that urban protests reignited COVID-19 case growth during the more than three weeks following protest onset."[34] This, too, was unlike Trump rallies, many of which were held indoors and without masks or social distancing, and proved to be superspreader events.

Violence against Asian Americans

At the same time that George Floyd's murder focused global attention on Black lives in the United States, the COVID-19 pandemic was also revealing deep racism confronting Americans of Asian descent. The early links between the virus and China made by Trump, who tried repeatedly to brand COVID as the "China virus," among other pejoratives, would negatively affect Asian American and Pacific Islander (AAPI)–owned businesses and the lives of those in the community.[35] The earliest stages of the pandemic were characterized by stigmatization and prejudice toward people of perceived Asian ancestry in non-Asian countries.[36] And the United States saw unprecedent levels of hate crimes and violence perpetrated against AAPIs, from attacks on elderly Asian women on the streets of New York City to a homicidal rampage against Asian American workers in Atlanta.

Like other minority communities, many Asian American small businesses were negatively impacted by the shutdowns. But they also faced prejudice and fear sown by politicians about China and the virus. About half the Chinese restaurants in the United States closed in the spring of 2020, and Chinatowns across the country, once bustling immigrant communities, were left with many fewer restaurants and family-owned businesses by the time the economy started opening back up in late 2021.[37] Forty-four percent of Asian American women of working age (sixteen and above) reported being out of the workforce for more than six months, a result driven by their employment in the hard-hit leisure and travel industries as well as by their caregiving responsibilities.[38]

The Asian American community also suffered from increased levels of bigotry and violence. Asian Americans are often portrayed as perpetual foreigners in the United States, commonly stereotyped as a "yellow peril" in times of crisis.[39] The "yellow peril" myth is the idea that Asians are invaders, culturally inferior to whites, and the source of disease.[40] Such stereotypes were highlighted and repeated by Trump throughout his presidency and became especially explicit in the early months of the COVID-19 pandemic, when negative views of Asian Americans were associated with COVID concerns as well as xenophobic behavior.[41] As we described in chapter 7, this is sadly familiar, as people of Asian descent have long faced racist and xenophobic sentiments during pandemics in the United States and Canada.

Pandemics, public health, and disease scares lead to not only stigmatization of those groups who are associated with the source of the disease but also violence against them.[42] In a June 2020 report from the Pew Research Center, Asian Americans reported high levels of discrimination and fear. About four in ten Asian Americans said that people had acted uncomfortable around them since the coronavirus outbreak, 31 percent said that they had been the subject of slurs or jokes, and 26 percent expressed fear that someone would physically attack them because of their race.[43]

In the spring of 2020, federal law enforcement warned that the coronavirus would lead to an increase in hate crimes against Asian Americans based on the assumption that part of the public would associate COVID-19 with China and Asian Americans.[44] This warning proved prescient. According to the New York Police Department, hate crimes against Asian Americans rose 1,900 percent in New York City in 2020 over the previous year.[45] Stop AAPI Hate, an advocacy group for the AAPI community, set up an online reporting system for community members to report harassment. The system received more than 6,603 reports of hate incidents directed at AAPIs in the United States from March 2020 to March 2021, including verbal harassment, physical assaults, and spitting.[46] Firsthand accounts of these incidents reveal that in many, the assaults were related to people's fear and anger around the COVID-19 pandemic. One report from a sixty-seven-year-old man in San Francisco illuminates the negative effects of bigoted language on Asian Americans: "I was standing in an aisle at [a hardware store] when suddenly I was struck from behind. Video surveillance verified the incident in which a white male used his bent elbow to strike my upper back. Subsequent verbal attacks occurred with

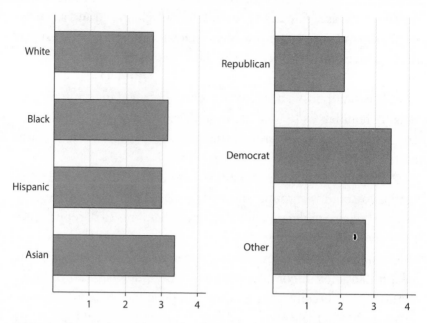

FIGURE 8.5. Concern about violence against the AAPI community, by race and partisanship

'Shut up, you Monkey!,' 'F**k you Chinaman,' 'Go back to China' and 'Stop bringing that Chinese virus over here.'"

In March 2021, we asked respondents about this violence against Asian Americans. This final wave of our survey—which selected large new samples of Black, Hispanic, and Asian Americans—went into the field a week after a white man killed eight people, six of them Asian women, in a shooting spree in metropolitan Atlanta at three local spas. On the survey, we asked respondents how serious they thought the problem of anti-Asian violence was during the pandemic on a four-point scale from 1 ("not at all") to 4 ("a serious problem"). Forty percent of respondents overall said that this violence was a very serious problem, and an additional 29 percent said that it was a somewhat serious problem. Figure 8.5 shows the average level of concern among respondents in the survey separately by the racial group and partisan affiliation of the respondent.

Among all groups, white respondents expressed the least amount of concern about violence against their Asian American neighbors. Latino, Black, and Asian respondents all saw the violence as significantly more serious than white respondents did, with Asian respondents expressing the most concern. Fifty-seven percent of Asian American respondents thought that the violence was very serious compared to 47 percent of Black respondents, 41 percent of Latino respondents, and 31 percent of white respondents. The high levels of concern among Black respondents reflect the empathy that marginalized groups express for one another.[47]

These concerns were well founded. In a study by Pew, by April 2021 almost half (45%) of Asian Americans report experiencing an incident tied to their racial or ethnic background since the start of the pandemic.[48] In this alarming environment, Biden signed an executive order in January 2021 to direct the federal government to advance equity and justice for underserved communities, including AAPI communities, as well as an executive order in May 2021 to establish a commission on Asian Americans, native Hawaiians, and Pacific Islanders to end anti-Asian bias and xenophobia and increase inclusion.[49]

As with so many other aspects of the COVID-19 pandemic, partisanship plays a central role in understanding Americans views on the anti-AAPI violence. Looking to figure 8.5, we find that Democrats expressed more concern about anti-AAPI violence than did Republicans, with independents/nonpartisans in the middle. We have noted how Trump used racially charged language to describe the COVID-19 pandemic, but other conservative and Republican leaders, such as Secretary of State Mike Pompeo, were also vocal in linking the coronavirus to China, calling it the "Wuhan virus" and the "China virus."[50] Republican senator Tom Cotton even implied that a Chinese lab developed the virus,[51] a stubborn rumor that persisted well into 2021.[52] Conservative media and social media, in turn, amplified the link between China and the disease, creating a connection between the illness and Asian Americans as a social group.[53]

These facts may help to explain the lower levels of white concern about anti-AAPI violence that we find in figure 8.5. People who accepted that the coronavirus pandemic can be blamed on China and who transfer that blame to Asian Americans in the United States should be less concerned about violence against a group that

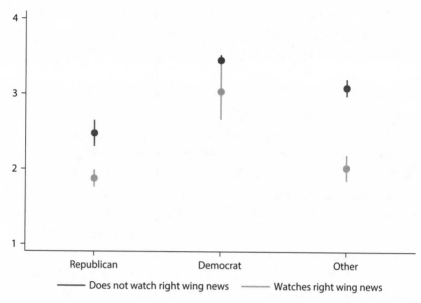

FIGURE 8.6. How serious is anti-Asian violence, by partisanship and news source

it blames for a deadly disease. Republicans should be the most likely to accept this connection made by Republican leaders and therefore be less concerned than Democrats about anti-Asian violence.

This should be especially true of people who watch and trust right-wing media. In previous chapters, we have found that consuming news from right-wing sources can heighten partisan differences in beliefs about, for example, the appropriate responses to the pandemic. To test if this is true for evaluation of the severity of anti-AAPI violence, figure 8.6 shows the average level of concern for anti-Asian violence among Republicans, Democrats, and Others, separating out respondents by whether they report watching right-wing news sources.[54] Each dot is a prediction calculated from a multiple regression model that adjusts for a range of demographic and geographical confounders, and the bars represent 95 percent confidence intervals around those predictions.

There are two main takeaways from this graph. First, Democrats are more concerned overall about anti-Asian violence than are Republicans and independents/nonpartisans. This helps to explain the higher levels of concern among respondents of color, who are more likely to identify as Democrats. Second, watching right-wing news dampens concern about violence against Asian Americans among all partisan groups. News sources do not explain away partisan differences in concern about anti-AAPI violence, though, as Democrats who watched right-wing news were more concerned about anti-AAPI violence than Republicans who did not. In that sense, our findings about right-wing news sources and concern about anti-AAPI violence mirror findings from previous chapters. Highly partisan news sources appear to exacerbate partisan differences in beliefs about anti-AAPI violence, but we cannot reduce differences in beliefs across parties to differences in where partisans get their news. In the end, partisanship is the fundamental divide in how Americans think about racial politics.

Conclusion

The COVID-19 pandemic both revealed and exacerbated the underlying racialized social and economic inequality in the United States. Communities of color in the United States have long suffered worse health outcomes than whites, and so too were communities of color hit especially hard by COVID-19. Blacks, Latinos, and Native Americans were more likely to get COVID-19, suffer worse complications, and die at higher rates compared to whites even when taking into account underlying health conditions.[55] Among Asian American communities, Pacific Islanders were more likely to die of COVID-19 than whites, while other Asian American groups fared similarly to whites. These unequal outcomes are the product of centuries-long health inequalities between white Americans and communities of color, sustained through structural and economic inequalities but fueled anew by the COVID-19 pandemic.

Racial inequality in health outcomes is not a product of partisanship itself, but as we have shown in this chapter, partisanship helps to explain how Americans interpret the racial politics of the COVID-19 pandemic. And of course, partisan politics has sustained the racialized inequalities in access to quality health care that explain the racial differences in health outcomes during the COVID-19 pandemic. In these dynamics, we can see not only how race matters for American politics but also how American politics has shaped the racial consequences of a pandemic that affects all Americans.

The racialized health inequalities brought to light by the COVID-19 pandemic are only part of the story, however. Amid the pandemic, long-simmering issues of police violence and anti-Black racism came to light during the summer of 2020. The pandemic also brought special hardship to the AAPI community in the United States because of unfounded fears. In chapter 9, we turn to consider how COVID-19 and racial justice interacted with the broader political environment and the 2020 presidential election.

9

Voting for Your Life

COVID-19 AND AMERICAN DEMOCRACY

> We were getting ready to win this election. Frankly we did win
> this election. So our goal now is to ensure the integrity, for the
> good of this nation—this is a very big moment, this is a major
> fraud on our nation—we want the law to be used in a proper
> manner. So we'll be going to the US Supreme Court. We want
> all voting to stop. We don't want them to find any ballots at
> 4 o'clock in the morning and add them to the list. It's a very
> sad moment."
>
> —PRESIDENT DONALD TRUMP, NOVEMBER 4, 2020

The presidential election on Tuesday, November 3, 2020, was unlike
any election in U.S. history. Presidential elections happen every four
years in the United States, and given the stakes for U.S. politics, they
are always moments of high political drama. But this one was different. The pandemic affected the election not just as the predomi-
nant issue of the election but also in determining *how* the election
would happen. Millions of Americans voted early for the first time,
such that "voting day" became a misnomer. By the time November 3
had come around, over one hundred million Americans had already

voted either in person or by mail.[1] This was unprecedented. According to an NBC poll, just over half of adults planned to vote early.[2] This would mean that more votes would be cast, so more votes needed to be counted.

Those who voted in person wore masks and socially distanced to protect themselves during the COVID-19 pandemic. Poll workers ensured not only the integrity of the election but also its safety, wiping down polling booths with disinfectant between voters. And the pandemic certainly affected campaigns leading up to November 3. The Democratic nominee, former vice president Joe Biden, had held no in-person events or mass rallies between March and November, whereas President Donald Trump found himself at the center of public controversy every time he held an in-person rally. And the round-the-clock vote counting—designed to satisfy hungry election-night cable news audiences—did not follow the same pattern across states. Many states were allowed to count the unprecedented surge of mail-in ballots ahead of time, while others, such as Pennsylvania, were not. Biden would not be formally acknowledged as the election winner until four days later, when his birth state of Pennsylvania put him over the electoral college threshold of 270 electoral votes. In the face of a contentious campaign of disinformation by the White House, which made baseless allegations of rampant voter fraud in every battleground state that Trump lost, the drama of the 2020 presidential election continued for months. Even years later, millions of Americans, most of them Republicans, believed that Trump actually won the election and that it was stolen from him.[3] Almost nothing was normal about the 2020 election season.

We have argued and illustrated throughout this book that partisan politics played a central role in the evolution of the COVID-19 pandemic in the United States. So far, we have focused on the role of partisanship in shaping health behaviors, attitudes, and policy debates. As important as these issues are, they cannot be separated from the fact that the COVID-19 pandemic erupted during an election year. This means that in addition to fighting a pandemic, the Trump administration was fighting for reelection in what was already set to be one of the most bitter partisan battles in American history.

This chapter examines how Americans' views of democracy evolved over the course of the pandemic. COVID-19 gave Americans a new context to think about old questions in American democracy, such as the proper role of government in a liberal democracy and citizens' duty to criticize their leaders in times of national crisis. These issues intersected with long-standing questions of race and racism in American democracy, which became a national conversation after the murder of George Floyd in May 2020. By the early summer of 2020, protests across the United States in defense of Black lives—and counterprotests by defenders of the police, white nationalists, and others—had begun a national conversation on race, police, and protest in American democracy.[4]

Beyond this upsurge in protest, COVID-19 also made salient an entirely new set of issues in American politics, such as making it possible for Americans to vote by mail and raising the prospect of actually postponing elections, that had never before received such national attention. Taken together with Trump's norm-shattering presidency, the COVID-19 pandemic upended presidential politics as usual. And it was not over after the election results came in: Trump's defeat by Biden occasioned an unprecedented assault on the legitimacy of the election by his Republican supporters in which Trump, his surrogates, and conservative media outlets used the occasion of record vote-by-mail numbers to suggest that ballots were stuffed, thousands voted illegally, and counting was corrupted. This conspiracy culminated in the January 6, 2021, insurrection at the U.S. Capitol.

It is fitting that a chapter on elections and American democracy focuses squarely on partisanship. Just as partisanship shaped the politics of the COVID-19 response, so too did Americans' partisan attachments govern their views about government criticism, executive authority, the legitimacy of elections, and even how individuals interpret their civic duty. Where the story in this chapter takes a novel turn is in wave 6, fielded after the inauguration of President Biden and Vice President Kamala Harris. We see here the "pure" effects of partisanship on Americans' political views, as Democrats' and Republicans' views on the same issues flip to reflect to what one of us (Goodman) has termed the "positional incentives" of their party in or out of power.[5] That is, Democrats who were worried about the state of democracy when Trump was president became more optimistic when Biden was elected; Republicans who supported executive authority under Trump became much more opposed once Biden took office.

In the conclusion to this chapter, we revisit this point to consider what it says about partisanship, policy attitudes, and their implications for the health of American democracy in the post-COVID world. Put baldly, partisanship now divides Americans so thoroughly that it is increasingly difficult to disentangle partisan disagreements about policy from partisan disagreements about the future of American politics and the nature of American democracy itself.

Power, Liberties, and Partisanship

We first began to track respondents' views about the role of government in wave 2 of our survey, in April 2020. Although questions about civil rights and executive authority in extraordinary times arose just as soon as the pandemic broke out, by April it was clear that a central area of conflict in the pandemic would be between those who sought a firm government response and those who held that government action was either unnecessary or counterproductive. We addressed a number of the specific policy prescriptions associated with the COVID-19 pandemic in chapter 5 (on pandemic policy) and chapter 6 (on the economy), finding that in general Republicans were skeptical of government encroachment but eager to jump-start the economy and ease the social and economic costs of recovery. Democrats, motivated by worry, also wanted to see a greater role played by government to curb the pandemic but, of course, were conflicted about investing new authority in a president with a proclivity for ignoring democratic norms who was recently impeached for a quid pro quo with an authoritarian regime to interfere in the 2020 presidential election.

But we also want to know about the state of American democracy more generally and Americans' general orientations toward political

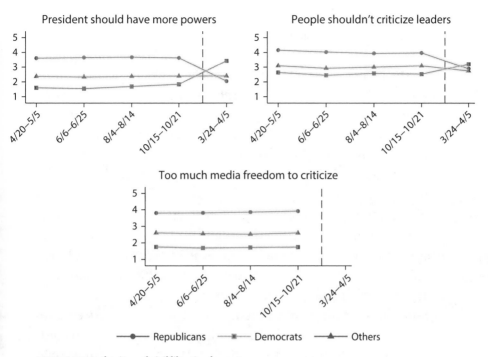

FIGURE 9.1. Authority and civil liberties, by party

authority, civil liberties, and media freedoms. The first of these was a key issue in our discussion of how the government would respond to the pandemic in chapter 5, but the latter two were increasingly salient as the Trump administration worked desperately to avoid losing the 2020 presidential election. So here, we look at views about presidential authority, bipartisan comity, and the media. Importantly, we asked the first two of these survey items under both the Trump and Biden presidencies, allowing us to see just how much Americans' views on rights and liberties depend on whether their own preferred candidate is in office. Figure 9.1 shows trends from waves 2–6 in our respondents' attitudes about presidential powers, whether or not people should come together in a crisis, and whether the media have too much freedom to criticize the government.

Beginning with the top left graph in figure 9.1, our data show that even though Republicans are, on the whole, much more opposed than Democrats and independents and nonpartisans to active policy responses that acknowledge the social and economic costs of the pandemic, we also find that they were much more favorable toward presidential authority under the Trump administration. The reverse is true for Democrats: as favorable as they were toward an active policy response, they strongly disagreed with the position that the president should be given more powers under the Trump administration. These positions, though, flip under the Biden administration. This finding is consistent with the expectation that you want your side to have more power when your side is in office.

These findings are bolstered by the results for two of the other survey items in figure 9.1, where we also find that the Republicans believe that we need to come together in a time of crisis and that criticizing the people in charge and questioning their decisions only divides us further. The partisan differences in the former, moreover, flip after the inauguration of Biden in January 2021. These trends in Americans' views of civil liberties and executive authority suggest a deep partisan cleavage in how Americans understand democracy: Republicans favor presidential powers and are skeptical of media criticism and social divisions only when their party holds the presidency, and the reverse is true among Democrats. These partisan differences were remarkably durable: they remained strong and quite statistically significant even when we accounted for respondents' race, age, education, and other demographic and geographic factors using a multiple regression approach. These results are worrying signs that under conditions of deep partisan polarization, it is difficult to separate "normal" politics about issues from deeper political conflict about the institutions of democracy.[6]

Stepping back, these findings about civil liberties and executive authority reveal the contradictions inherent in the partisan politics of the pandemic. Republicans during the Trump administration favored a presidency with wide powers to act but did not support most of the policies that the administration might have implemented, whereas Democrats wanted those policies but without granting the president unfettered authority to implement them. These two findings are not incompatible with one another; Democrats may suspect that the policies Trump would implement were not those that they support, while Republicans may believe that Trump would only implement the politics they favor. Still, these results suggest a much deeper challenge facing American democracy than simple disagreement over how to respond to the pandemic: Americans' support for democratic norms is contingent on positional advantage, that is, whether you support the incumbent or challenger party. This division strikes at the heart of American democracy. If citizens do not agree on basic democratic values, then we are having a disagreement not about politics but instead about the foundation of democracy itself.

To gain more insight into what this divide over democratic values means, in wave 4 of our survey (August 2020) we asked our respondents a number of questions about the qualities of a good citizen. What does it mean to be a good democratic citizen? What is expected of democratic citizens, and what do they expect of each other? Most of the questions we asked drew on a body of literature in political science that identifies the key attributes of citizenship in advanced democracies, focusing on liberal values such as tolerance and engaged citizenship behaviors such as protesting. Other items look to different values that Americans might hold about a good citizen: someone who obeys the law or someone who speaks English. Scholars of citizenship in American politics have argued that there are sizable partisan cleavages on what makes for a good citizen.[7]

To this collection of standard items, we add two additional questions: (1) "Is a good citizen someone who wears a mask?" and (2) "Is a good citizen someone who protests against unjust laws?" To understand why we added these two items, it helps to recall what was happening in American politics in the summer of 2020. The first wave of the pandemic had crested in the United States by the beginning of May, but the number of deaths was steadily rising again by August. The months of June and July had occasioned something of a return to normal among many Americans, which we observed as partisan divergence between Democrats and Republicans in behaviors such as avoiding gatherings and contact with others and wearing a mask (see chapter 3). At the same time, public health authorities warned that reduced adherence to pro–social health behaviors would lead to a subsequent rise in cases, a prediction that was borne out only several months later. In this context, as we have argued in previous chapters, mask wearing emerged as perhaps the single most important observable indicator of one's commitment to adhering to public health guidance.

The other major development in American politics at this time, though, was the dramatic upsurge in protest and mobilization in the wake of the murder of George Floyd. As we described in chapter 8, Floyd's murder sparked Black Lives Matter protests across the United States and around the world from Paris, France, to West Papua, Indonesia.[8]

In the United States, several competing media narratives about protesting emerged over the summer. One focused on the long history of police violence against Black men, from the shooting of Philando Castile to the death of Freddie Gray in Baltimore police custody and countless other examples. A competing set of narratives, however, characterized the protests as incidents of disorder and violence, invoking racialized tropes in portraying protestors of color as rioters run amok or alleging that protests had been overrun by leftist or anarchist groups such as those affiliated with the Antifa movement.[9] In the context of calls from many Black Lives Matter protestors to "defund the police," many seeking to defend Americans' police forces against criticism were attracted to this narrative. One of these individuals was Kyle Rittenhouse, a 17-year-old from Illinois, who traveled to Wisconsin, armed with his father's semi-automatic rifle, who fatally shot two individuals and wounding a third, during protests in response to the non-fatal shooting of Jacob Blake. Rittenhouse's lawyer argued his actions were in self-defense, and he was found not guilty after trial in November 2021. Throughout and after, Rittenhouse was lauded as a patriotic darling of the conservative right.

Beyond the obvious racial dimensions of these protests, together they raised the fundamental question of whether protest is an essential part of what it means to be a good American citizen.

With this context in mind, figure 9.2 shows how Americans in August 2020 conceived of what makes a good citizen. The bars show

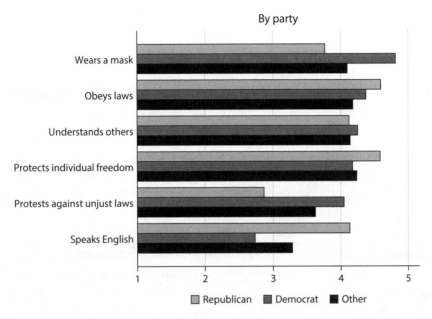

FIGURE 9.2. What makes a good citizen? By party

the average response of each group on a scale of 1 (strongly disagree) to 5 (strongly agree).

We see broad partisan agreement that a good citizen is tolerant (makes an effort to understand others). This is a key norm of liberal democracy, and it is reassuring to see bipartisan consensus on its value. But we observe striking divisions across party in several other responses. Look first to the item on mask wearing: although most Americans of all parties believed that wearing a mask is what a good citizen does, Democrats were nearly unanimous in strong support of this position, whereas Republican support is more muted. Instead, Republicans reserved their greatest enthusiasm for protecting individual freedoms, which—in the context of a contentious debate about mask wearing as a sign of excessive state control over individual choices—we interpret as a reflection of Republicans' reactions against policies such as mask mandates, restricting gatherings of people in public places, and shuttering businesses that reflect the tension between individual freedoms and public welfare in the context of the pandemic.

Turning now to items that are related to the Black Lives Matter protests of the summer of 2020, Democrats expressed strong support for the idea that a good citizen protests against unjust laws. Republicans were mixed on this, with the plurality of Republicans disagreeing with the position that a good citizen should protest against unjust laws (indeed, Republicans were strongly supportive of the position that a good citizen should obey laws, a view also held, albeit somewhat less intensely, by the majority of Democrats).

This Republican position on protesting is worth considering in a wider context. While the motivation of protests in June through August (when the survey was in the field) was racial justice, there were also mass protests back in April and early May in which citizens assembled outside of state capitals and at busy downtown intersections to protest state stay-at-home orders and mask mandates. Urged on by Trump, who was eager to reopen America's economy and get his approval ratings higher, protestors from Long Beach, California, to Augusta, Maine, carried signs ranging from "Stop the Shutdown!" to "All business is essential!" to the pithier "I need a haircut!" In famous images taken at a protest in Denver, Colorado, on April 20, "Operation Gridlock" protestors driving trucks and waving American flags were locked in a stand-off with nurses wearing scrubs and personal protective equipment. A Yahoo/YouGov poll in late April showed that while a plurality of Republicans opposed the antilockdown/antishutdown protestors (47%), 36 percent were in support.[10] This disjuncture is important to note. Republicans support the view that a good citizen protests against laws that they themselves think are unjust, in this case economic closure and stay-at-home orders, but they do not support policies ending police violence.

Taken together, these citizenship items from wave 4 and the analysis over time of executive authority and civil liberties paint a picture of an American populace divided over more than just policy issues and health behaviors. Rather, Americans' views about basic civic values and civil liberties reflected both their partisan affiliations and the positional incentives that followed from whether their party held the presidency or not. In the next section, we will see how these differences in partisan views also spilled over to affect how Americans grappled with concrete policy questions for the conduct of the 2020 elections.

The Partisan Politics of Election Administration

The 2020 presidential election was especially contentious because partisans debated not only the substance of the candidates but also the infrastructure of the election itself, that is, how the election was going to be conducted. With in-person voting during a pandemic a serious public health risk in the minds of many Americans, state governments sought alternatives. Two options were of particular import: expanding the availability of alternatives to in-person voting such as voting by mail, and delaying the election itself. Although the latter option seems extreme, it was actually implemented in sixteen states during the early months of the pandemic, which coincided with the latter half of the presidential primary season.[11] New York governor Andrew Cuomo even tried to cancel his state's 2020 presidential primary altogether, arguing that the primary results were already settled and that in-person voting was too risky from a public health perspective.

Both delaying elections and implementing vote by mail are fraught political decisions. Efforts to delay presidential primaries were met with some opposition: a federal judge rejected Governor Mike DeWine's plan to delay the March primary in Ohio, calling it "a terrible precedent."[12] The timing of an election is sacrosanct in the United States, where officeholders have fixed terms and presidential elections occur regularly every four years on the second Tuesday after the first Monday in November. (This is unlike parliamentary systems, where elections can be more unpredictable, called by the prime minister to strategically extend their tenure or provoked by a vote of "no confidence" by a majority of the parliament.) So, it is noteworthy that both Republicans such as DeWine and Democrats such as Cuomo sought to delay primary elections out of concern for public health. No serious calls for delaying the presidential election were heard from Republican party elites or prominent news sources when it came to the November 2020 general election, although Trump himself did float the idea in July, with no success.[13]

In contrast to delaying elections, voting by mail is a less dramatic step to protect public health during election season. Mail-in ballots are the norm for elections in states such as Washington, but in most U.S. states voting by mail is comparatively rare and requires that voters go through an administrative process to secure an absentee ballot. Absentee ballots are legal in all fifty states and under federal law must be made available to populations such as those serving in the military, but the specific provisions through which they are made available vary by state.

Trump's repeated assertions that the 2020 election would be stolen, which were echoed widely in conservative political circles and on conservative media, fed another narrative that voting by mail would increase the likelihood of voter fraud.[14] Although rarely articulated openly, the argument was simple. Voting by mail makes it harder for election officials to monitor who is actually filling out ballots, which suggests that a motivated fraudster could amass ballots of registered voters who did not intend to vote and fill them out with the candidate of their choice. Although voter fraud is illegal in every jurisdiction in the country and there is precious little evidence that voter fraud via mail actually occurs, by the spring of 2020 Trump's stance against voting by mail was clear.[15]

Holding aside Trump's baseless allegations about mail-in voter fraud, the partisan electoral consequences of increasing ballot access through voting by mail are ambiguous.[16] The most vulnerable populations to COVID-19 are the elderly, the immunocompromised, and those with preexisting medical conditions. Forcing such voters to vote in person would decrease their turnout. And yet among this population, the elderly in particular are more likely to vote Republican than are young people, and the immunocompromised and those with preexisting medical conditions do not neatly break down along partisan lines. What this means is that at least in principle, voting by mail might have increased rather than suppressed Republican turnout. At the same time, voting by mail also increases access to voters

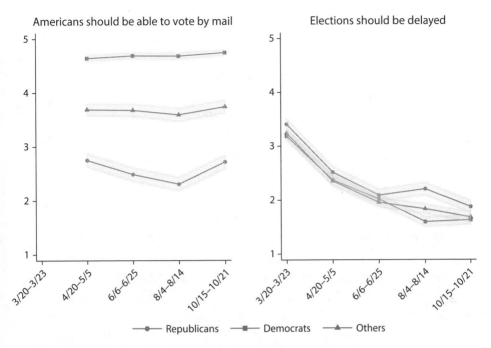

FIGURE 9.3. Voting by mail and delaying elections, by party

of lower socioeconomic status, including those for whom voting is difficult during normal working hours. Voting by mail may also increase turnout among those voters for whom long lines at crowded polling stations are unattractive. These groups are more likely to vote Democrat, and this is what may have driven Republicans' hostility to voting by mail.

As the pandemic broke out in the midst of primary season, we began asking Americans their opinions on delaying elections in wave 1 of our survey. Starting in wave 2 of our survey, we also asked respondents whether as a general matter it was important for Americans to have the opportunity to vote by mail. We repeated each of these questions each wave until wave 5, right before the 2020 election. In figure 9.3, we show trends in support for voting by mail and delaying elections across parties.

In the earliest wave of the pandemic, all Americans of all partisan affiliations expressed some willingness to delay elections. But support among all parties for delaying elections dropped precipitously as the pandemic wore on.[17] This is probably a consequence of the fact that in the early waves of our survey respondents understood "elections" to mean "primaries," but by the end they understood "elections" to be referring to the general election. Strikingly, though, we can see an emerging partisan divide on this question starting in the late summer of 2020: as Democratic support for delaying elections continued to plummet, the declining trend in Republican support stalled. It is not clear what explains this late-emerging partisan cleavage over whether or not to delay the November 2020 elections. But we also observe in figure 9.3 that this cleavage emerged just as Republican Party support for voting by mail was at its lowest. One interpretation is that a subset of Republicans came to think in the months approaching the election that Trump was unlikely to prevail, perhaps due to their erroneous belief that postal ballots would be subject to massive election fraud, and became willing to support delaying the November elections in his defense.

Turning to voting by mail, though, the partisan differences that we see in figure 9.3 are sharp and durable. Unsurprisingly, Democrats were nearly unanimous in strong support for allowing all Americans to vote by mail. Republicans were much more lukewarm on this question on average, as by late April the question of vote by mail was already politicized by the president. On April 7, Trump ranted about "corrupt" mail-in voting in front of the press: "There's a lot of dishonesty going on with mail-in voting, mail-in ballots."[18] On April 8 he tweeted, "Tremendous potential for voter fraud, and for whatever reason, doesn't work out well for Republicans." In other words, Trump had already cued his base to oppose voting by mail.

If we disaggregate these results by news source, an important pattern emerges, as shown in figure 9.4.

Republicans and Others who watch right-wing news sources were far less supportive of voting by mail than those who do not. This points to the essential role of conservative media in accelerating the partisan divide over postal voting in the 2020 election. We find no evidence in figure 9.4, however, that news sources affect beliefs about whether or not elections should be delayed.

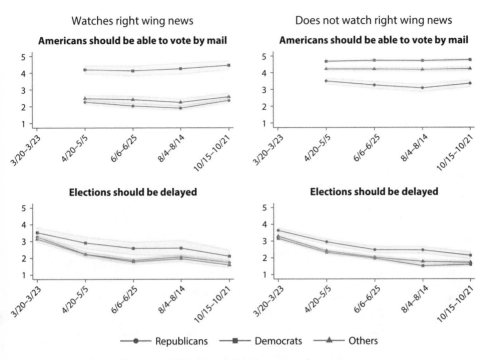

FIGURE 9.4. Voting by mail and delaying elections, by party and news source

The relatively lower average level of support for voting by mail may mask some intraparty divisions among Republicans on this question. To probe this possibility, we investigated whether elderly Republicans would be more supportive of voting by mail (to protect their own health). Our data show exactly the opposite pattern. We find that elderly Republicans were actually most opposed to voting by mail. Although surprising, this finding makes sense in the context of our earlier findings: if elderly Republicans are the least worried about COVID policy, which we showed in chapter 5, then it stands to reason that they would also not object to voting in person. But it is worth pausing to consider the implications of this finding. It comprises strong evidence of partisanship leading a subset of voters—elderly Republicans—to hold preferences that are demonstrably inconsistent with their interests, at least from a public health perspective.

We can delve even further into how Americans linked COVID-19 to elections in the context of a hotly contested presidential election

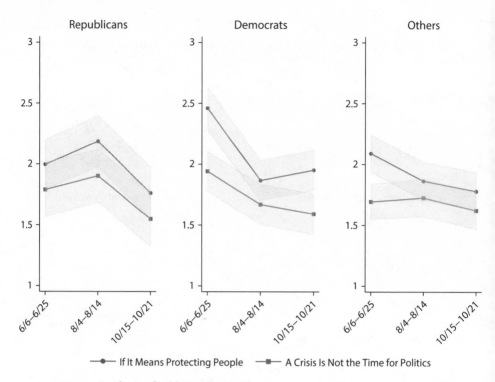

FIGURE 9.5. Justification for delaying elections, by party

season by analyzing the justifications available for delaying elections using a survey experimental approach, the logic of which is identical to those we presented in chapters 5 and 7. In waves 3–5 of our survey, we presented our respondents with two different justifications for why elections should be delayed. Roughly half of the respondents in each of these three waves were randomly assigned to read "We should delay elections if it means protecting people," whereas the others were assigned to read "We should delay elections because a crisis is not the time for politics." Because these two justifications were assigned randomly to each respondent, we can examine what drives respondents' support and opposition to delaying elections by comparing across responses to the two versions of the question.

We show the results of this exercise in figure 9.5. For each party, we trace out average levels of support for delaying elections depending on which prompt the respondent received, recognizing that these differences across prompts will themselves vary across the partisan identity of the respondent as well.

It turns out that voters of all sorts tend to be more responsive to the public health justification for delaying elections, although rarely is this difference statistically significant (it is only so in wave 3 and 5 among Democrats and in wave 3 among Others). This is a reassuring sign in a time of bitter partisan division of low support across all parties for delaying elections to suppress political opposition during a pandemic.

The Partisan Politics of Electoral Legitimacy

For more worrying signs of the heavy partisan politicization of the 2020 election, we turn to the question of the perceived legitimacy of the election itself. Recall that Trump had repeatedly raised suspicions about the conduct of the 2020 election, suggesting that mail-in voting would lead to fraud and implying (along with a host of right-wing media figures) that widespread illegal voting by ineligible or unregistered voters would hand the election to Democrats. Republican Party–led state governments in battleground states such as Pennsylvania, Michigan, and Georgia contributed to the uncertainty by passing regulations that restricted the counting of absentee or mail-in ballots until election day or right before it.[19] Both Republicans and Democrats preemptively set up legal teams in expectation of a bitter fight over the results. Unsurprisingly, election experts worried that a close election would lead to contested claims about the legitimacy of the results.[20] As we know with the benefit of hindsight, such worries were all too prescient.

In anticipation of such an outcome, in wave 5 of our survey—conducted just weeks before the general election itself—we implemented another survey experiment to probe how respondents would interpret the results of the presidential election. Specifically, we asked respondents "If [Trump/Biden] wins the election, we will know American elections are rigged" and randomly assigned respondents to read either "Trump" or "Biden" as the victor. We present the results of two analyses in figure 9.6, dividing respondents by

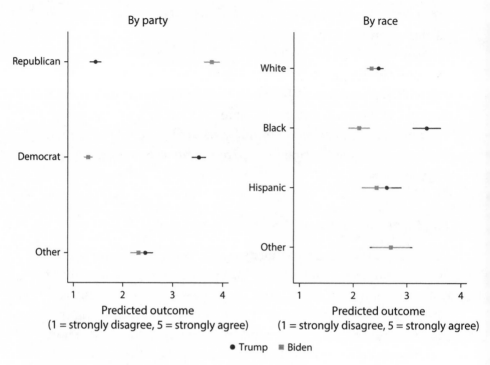

FIGURE 9.6. Perceptions of the legitimacy of the 2020 election

their partisan affiliation (left panel) and by race (right panel). Note that these are prospective evaluations: respondents did not yet know the outcome of the election but were simply projecting forward to what they would believe under these two different scenarios.

The partisan differences in perceived legitimacy of the results were simply enormous. Republicans, when asked about the legitimacy of a Trump victory, strongly disagreed almost unanimously that a Trump victory would signify that those elections were rigged. A Biden victory, by contrast, would be perceived as strong evidence that elections were rigged. Precisely the opposite pattern emerges among Democrats. Among those who are members of neither party, the identity of the victor had no relationship with the perceived legitimacy of the election.

These results are overwhelming evidence that citizens interpret the integrity and legitimacy of the election itself based on their preferred partisan outcome. The implications for American democracy are stark. Free, fair, and irreversible elections are the sine qua non of democracy: absent freedom of choice, fairness of the vote count, and a firm guarantee that the results will not be reversed upon an outcome that the government does not prefer, elections are not democratic.[21] What happens when citizens do not believe that elections are fair? And what happens when what citizens believe depends on what party they support? As one of us (Pepinsky) has recently argued, these conditions are no less than an existential threat to democracy itself.[22] Citizens cannot be expected to view the results of elections to be legitimate if they do not think that the elections were conducted freely and fairly.

Such differences in the perceived legitimacy of elections do not obtain when we break down our analysis by respondent race (we do adjust our results here to account for different patterns in partisan affiliation by race and ethnic group). The exception is Black respondents, among whom a Trump victory would have been much more likely to be interpreted as evidence that the elections were rigged than a Biden victory. This suspicion is well founded: restrictive voting laws passed by Republican-led state legislatures, limited access to polling stations in predominantly Black neighborhoods, and long waits at polling places keep Black voters (as well as wage workers, who don't get time off from work) from participating in and trusting the democratic process. But we emphasize again that our results are not driven by the fact that most Black Americans tend to be Democrats. Instead, our results reflect the very real understanding among Black Americans of just how fragile electoral democracy is in the United States. It was only during the civil rights era that full participatory rights were secured for Black Americans, and the practices of electoral administration in majority-Black districts across the country to this day are a painful reminder of just how unequal American elections are—a fact that resonates with our discussion in chapter 8 of the myriad other ways in which America's racial inequalities are with us today.

Another important finding emerges when we disaggregate respondents by their main source of news, as shown in figure 9.7. Republicans who watch right-wing news were especially likely to believe that the election was rigged if Biden won, and Democrats

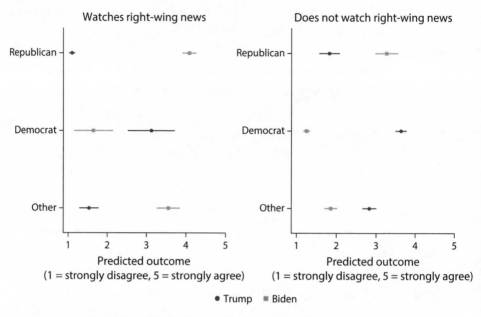

FIGURE 9.7. Perceptions of the legitimacy of the 2020 election, by news source

who do not watch right-wing news were especially likely to believe that the election was rigged if Trump won. But look at those labeled "Others," who hold no partisan attachment or affiliate with a third party. Those who watch right-wing news were more likely to believe the election was rigged if Biden won, whereas those who do not were more likely to believe that the election was rigged if Trump won. Here, in sum, we see clear evidence that the partisan media environment of 2020 shaped the views of nonpartisans too.

But broadly speaking, our analysis reveals that American partisanship by the fall of 2020 had come to drive perceptions about not only which presidential candidate was the right choice for America but also whether elections were fair and free from interference. We emphasize that the public's belief that elections are secure and that their votes are counted as intended are the key to the legitimacy of elections. Perceptions that elections are rigged can undercut beliefs in the whole enterprise of a democratic mandate in an electoral transition. To see the implications of such motivated reasoning about the legitimacy of elections, we can look to other countries around the world facing bitterly contested elections in which each side rejects any result that goes against it. In these situations, citizens may boycott or otherwise refuse to participate in elections that they believe are unfair. Governments may suspend elections on the suspicion that they will not return the outcome that they desire. Citizens on both sides may mobilize, sometimes peacefully and sometimes not, to demand recalls, recounts, and do-overs. All of this bodes ill for the health of American democracy.

In the end, Biden handily defeated Trump in the 2020 elections. And just as anticipated, Trump decried the results as fraudulent, launching a sustained legal battle to try to stop the certification of the results.[23] And sadly, our worries about the consequences of partisan disagreement about the legitimacy of the 2020 election—which we predicted publicly weeks before the election took place[24]—proved prescient. Unable to present any evidence whatsoever of electoral fraud in any of the battleground states where the slow counting of the election results had prompted his challenge, Trump's legal team was ultimately defeated in the courts more than forty times.[25] One hundred forty-seven Republican Party members of Congress nevertheless voted against certification of the election results when asked to do so in early January. This vote came the same day, January 6, 2021, that Trump loyalists stormed the Capitol building in an insurrection hoping to somehow stop Vice President Mike Pence from certifying the electoral college vote, thereby reversing Trump's defeat by force.

It is hard to imagine a more direct public assault on the institutions of American democracy than the events of January 6. They followed from Trump's continued assault on America's political institutions, his demonization of the Democratic Party, and his refusal to tolerate any form of news that called into question his authority or popularity—each a symptom of the preexisting conditions we laid out in chapter 1. Although we cannot know whether such an outcome would have taken place without the extra stress on American society and politics produced by the COVID-19 pandemic, we believe that the frustrations felt by millions of Americans

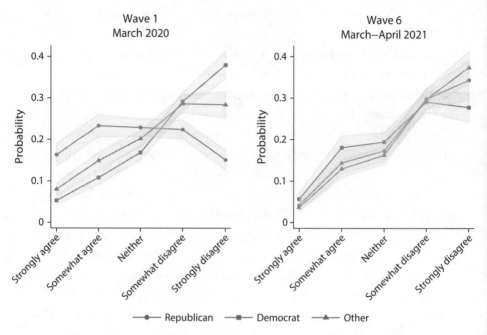

FIGURE 9.8. American democracy is healthy, by party

were channeled by this particular segment of the American public into violent antigovernment action.

The January 6 insurrection shocked Americans of all partisan affiliations, although in the subsequent months many Trump supporters sought to reinterpret the events as less shocking than they had been portrayed[26] or even as a natural and legitimate form of protest. Even though the insurrection was wholly unsuccessful in reversing Trump's electoral defeat, it laid bare just how deeply divided Americans are. Analysts from across the political spectrum concluded that American democracy was in a dangerous state, a view that we also find among our survey respondents. In figure 9.8 we compare our respondents' views about the health of American democracy in wave 1 (March 2020) and wave 6 (April 2021). In both waves, we asked respondents to what extent they agreed with a simple statement: "American democracy is healthy." The lines trace out the probability that respondents gave one of the five possible responses to this question, divided up by their partisan affiliation and controlling for a range of demographic and geographic differences across respondents.

Unsurprisingly, in March 2021 Democrats were very likely to strongly disagree with the view that American democracy is healthy. Such sentiments were shared as well by those without a partisan identification in the "Others" category. Only Republicans expressed some agreement with this view, with most reporting that they either somewhat agreed, somewhat disagreed, or neither agreed nor disagreed with the statement. This moderation among Republican Party respondents disappeared by April 2021. Following the events of 2020 and early 2021, Republicans joined Democrats and Others in expressing strong disagreement with the position that American democracy is healthy. The view from April 2021 is clear that almost no Americans strongly agree with the statement that American democracy is healthy, regardless of their partisan affiliation.

One might have expected Democrats to become more favorable toward American democracy by wave 6. This would match the findings we reported in figure 9.1, where Democrats expressed great opposition to executive authority and people coming together just until Biden was inaugurated and then immediately became more supportive of executive authority. In this case, however, Biden's victory did nothing to erase Democrats' anxieties about the health of American democracy. Tragically, one of the few political positions about which Americans of all partisan affiliations can agree is that American democracy is not healthy.

Conclusion

The COVID-19 pandemic made an already tenuous democratic situation even more precarious. America had been experiencing for years what political scientists have termed "democratic backsliding," accelerated by Trump's personalistic ruling style and patrimonial practices and the failure of the Republican Party to uphold "institutional guardrails" that protect democracy from authoritarian power grabs.[27] The pandemic made the United States even more vulnerable. National health emergencies require leadership and coordination, and that is often manifest in a consolidation of power. Sometimes states pass national security laws so they can act fast, as the United States did with the Patriot Act after 9/11. But security laws can be used by authoritarian leaders for undemocratic ends, such as Brazil's president Jair Bolsonaro's violent crackdown on critics of his COVID-19 response. Consolidating power in a crisis can be a precarious exercise for democracies, so keeping an eye on democratic norms is a vital exercise.

What are we to make of partisanship and the 2020 election? On one hand, the implications are plain: Americans are sharply divided according to their partisan identity in ways that are increasingly associated with broad indictments of the condition of American democracy rather than simply their satisfaction with the government in office. It is one thing for Democrats to express their opposition to Trump during his time in office and Republicans their opposition to Biden after he had succeeded Trump. It is quite another for America's partisans to hold such sharply divergent views about holding elections and granting powers to the president. If democracy is to be a viable system for managing the inevitable political conflicts that will emerge in a country as large and heterogeneous as the United States, Americans must not externalize their partisan frustrations to the system itself. By the spring of 2021, though, one of the only areas of true bipartisan popular consensus was that American democracy is not healthy.

Some of our findings in this chapter might be, at first glance, reassuring. Although it is generally worrisome that so many partisans favor granting greater power to the presidency in times of crisis, it is good that these positions change when the party occupying the presidency changes. Opposition parties are a check against government excess; this is one major benefit of democracy, that a loyal opposition exists to make sure that the party in power does not exceed its authority. And yet we see still additional cause for worry in the finding that partisan positions flip depending on the party in office. In our view, this finding reinforces our conclusions that partisanship explains not just voters' policy preferences but also their views about democracy itself. This worrying conclusion, of course, also resonates with our findings throughout this book about how partisanship has thoroughly pervaded the American experience with COVID-19.

10

Shots in Arms

THE PARTISAN POLITICS
OF VACCINATION

> I'm perplexed by the reluctance of some to get vaccinated,
> totally perplexed.
>
> —SENATOR MITCH MCCONNELL (R-KY)

A pandemic can end in several ways. One is to find a cure. Another
is to wait for herd immunity, a process that may take years with millions of otherwise preventable deaths along the way. Still another is
to end social life as we know it until the virus abates, which would
require totalitarian control over the world's population. But the most
desirable way to end a pandemic—the way that saves the most lives—
is to develop a vaccine. Vaccination teaches our immune systems
how to respond to a new disease by producing antibodies to fight
it off. For many, including President Donald Trump, early development of a vaccine was a priority, and mass vaccination would usher
the end of the pandemic, or, at least, a manageable plateau of caseloads as COVID became endemic.

The timeline of the COVID-19 vaccine was almost miracu-
lous. The World Health Organization was first notified of a unique

cluster of cases, first thought to be pneumonia of unknown cause, in the city of Wuhan, China, on December 31, 2019, though it is believed that human-to-human transmission was occurring as early as mid-October, circulating undetected for months.[1] The virus was later determined to be a novel coronavirus, SARS-CoV-2, and by midsummer both Moderna and Pfizer established themselves as leaders in the mRNA vaccine development. Moderna was the first to publish phase I clinical trials on July 14 (Pfizer published its results on August 12),[2] and by December 11 the U.S. Food and Drug Administration issued emergency use authorization, allowing the Pfizer-BioNTech COVID-19 vaccine to be distributed in the United States. The Moderna vaccine received emergency use authorization on December 18, and the one-shot Janssen (Johnson & Johnson) received emergency use authorization on February 27, 2021. That's less than a year from discovery to distribution. By comparison, the mumps vaccine took four years to develop, and many vaccines take much longer than that.

In addition to the three vaccines available in the United States, more than a dozen others have been approved for use in at least one country around the world, ranging from the widely available Oxford-AstraZeneca vaccine to Russia's Sputnik V and China's Sinopharm and Sinovac, among others. Most of these vaccines (and all three authorized for use in the United States) are highly effective against the coronavirus: they reduce contagion, ease COVID-19 symptoms among those who do test positive, and essentially eliminate the risk of dying from COVID-19. The side effects for nearly everyone are moderate, amounting to a day or two of fever-like symptoms. More serious side effects, such as the heart problems associated with the Johnson & Johnson vaccine, are vanishingly rare. And vaccines authorized for usage in the United States also proved to be effective against subsequent variants, including delta (peaking in November 2021) and omicron (first spreading in December 2021).

But developing a vaccine is only half of the job. To end a pandemic, you need to convince people to take it. And you need to vaccinate the *global* population, not just *your* population. Of course, not everyone is eligible for a vaccine. Individuals with severe allergies or with underlying health conditions may not be able to be vaccinated. But if enough of the population gets vaccinated, these people can still be protected, as the virus is unable to spread further (this is herd immunity, achieved via vaccinations rather than through mass infections). No vaccine is 100 percent effective, but vaccines protect individuals and the communities they live in. Vaccines are a miracle of modern medicine and have essentially eradicated diseases such as polio and smallpox that once plagued the world. But the human costs required to end the pandemic through mass isolation or herd immunity are enormous, meaning that the only serious public health response to COVID-19 was to develop a vaccine and distribute it widely.

The Trump administration's Operation Warp Speed oversaw the development of a suite of COVID-19 vaccines that could be authorized for emergency use just over a year after the virus was first discovered, something few observers would have thought possible. Yet the project faced criticism for ignoring the logistics of distributing the vaccines[3]—a vaccine does no good if it cannot be distributed promptly to those who need it—and key figures such as project leader Moncef Slaoui faced charges from Democrats of self-dealing and profiteering.[4] Trump himself received a vaccine in January, but unlike every other world leader and most members of Congress, he did not do so publicly, thus missing a key opportunity to endorse uptake from his base. He also accused Pfizer, without evidence, of deliberately waiting until after election day to release its trial results, speculating on Twitter that Democrats and even the Food and Drug Administration "didn't want to have me get a Vaccine WIN, prior to the election."

Here we see how politics can either hasten the end of a pandemic or draw it out longer than necessary. Bipartisan endorsement of vaccines—where political, religious, and community leaders model good behavior by publicly getting a vaccine themselves—have been a mainstay of American public health campaigns for nearly a century. For instance, the effort to eradicate polio was thoroughly bipartisan.[5] And beloved Sesame Street character Big Bird got a measles vaccine on television in the 1970s to encourage kids to do the same. But when an (ageless) Big Bird got a COVID-19 vaccine in November 2021, Senator Ted Cruz referred to it as "government propaganda," and conservative media elites went so far as to label Big Bird a communist.[6] Prominent Republicans also adopted a habit of not reporting whether they received a vaccine, with vaccine denial becoming a point of pride among many.[7] And after months of opposing vaccine mandates and perpetuating vaccine skepticism, the most visible conservative voices have asserted that President Joe Biden was to blame for low vaccination rates, with Fox News host and former Trump press secretary Kayleigh McEnany audaciously referring to the Biden administration as the nation's "biggest contributor to vaccine hesitancy."[8] And by December 2021 when eight hundred thousand Americans had died from COVID-19, a staggering two hundred thousand had been lost after vaccines were available. This magnitude of preventable death is hard to fathom.

Like nearly every other aspect of the pandemic, partisan differences in health behavior emerged in the context of vaccinations, echoing the long precedent in American politics of vaccines being perceived as more safe by members of the president's political party than those who are not.[9] For example, during the 2009 H1N1 flu pandemic, conservative media figures such as Glenn Beck and Rush Limbaugh publicly denounced the vaccine rollout by the Obama administration, with the result that Republicans proved less amenable to vaccination than Democrats.[10] And true to form, Fox News would sow seeds of skepticism in vaccination on air while privately over 90 percent of company employees were vaccinated, with strict daily testing for those who were not.[11] As we will see, even though Trump's leadership jump-started the rapid development of safe and highly effective COVID-19 vaccines, the mass rollout under the Biden administration was hamstrung by politicized vaccine hesitancy, in particular among Republicans.

Vaccine Intent and Vaccine Hesitancy

We first asked our respondents about COVID-19 vaccines in wave 2, at the end of April. By this time the dangers of COVID-19 were plain to see, as were the social, economic, and personal costs of lockdowns and physical distancing. We asked respondents how likely they would be to get a COVID-19 vaccine if one were available, with an answer on a four-point scale ranging from "definitely not" to "certainly yes." We expected high levels of excitement at the possibility of a vaccine, but what we found was surprising. Only 51 percent of respondents reported that they would certainly get the vaccine, a bare majority. Substantial proportions of respondents indicated some degree of hesitation and even outright opposition to getting the vaccine.

Our survey data also allowed us to look more closely at whether levels of vaccine hesitancy varied by party, race, income, or education. The simple conclusion is that partisanship matters more than any other variable we have measured. Democrats were substantially more likely to report a strong interest in a vaccine in late April 2020 than were Republicans and Others. And although a plurality (but not a majority) of Republicans and Others expressed strong interest in a vaccine, each was substantially more likely to express some degree of vaccine hesitancy than were Democrats. Once again, the partisan politics of COVID-19 had set in early, this time shaping Americans' approach to the one public health measure that could bring the pandemic to a close.

Consistent with the troubled history of public health initiatives in the United States, our data also show that Black respondents expressed higher levels of vaccine hesitancy (controlling again for income, education, partisanship, and other factors) than white Americans. But rather unexpectedly, we find no relationship between education, income, and vaccine hesitancy in April 2020 once we account for race and partisanship. We had expected to find, for example, that more highly educated Americans would be more likely to report a willingness to get vaccinated or that Americans living in rural areas would report less willingness to get vaccinated. But it turns out that once we know respondents' race and partisan affiliation, there are no further differences in vaccine hesitancy that we might attribute to education or geography (or income or any number of other factors that we considered). The central challenge facing America's public health authorities would be to combat the racial and political divisions in American society.

We conducted nearly the same analysis just about a year later for wave 6 of our survey (April 2021). America's political and public health landscapes had changed dramatically in the intervening twelve months, with Biden having succeeded Trump and the death toll having surpassed half a million Americans. But more importantly, vaccines were no longer hypothetical: they were available by this time to all Americans over the age of sixty-five, and many frontline workers and others had managed to obtain a vaccine as well. So, we were able to run basically the same analysis to see if our respondents' views had changed in any way after a year of pandemic politics and with a new president and vaccines that were increasingly available.

Once again, we find a dramatic difference in vaccine hesitancy among the partisans (this only includes those who had not been vaccinated yet). Sixty percent of Democrats who had not yet been vaccinated said they were extremely likely to get vaccinated; this was twice as likely as Republicans and one and a half times as likely as independents/Others. Racial differences matter as well, although they are more muted in wave 6. The only novel finding is that by wave 6, education seems to matter as well: those respondents with a postgraduate degree were significantly less hesitant than those without postgraduate education. Even with a free, safe, extremely effective, and readily available vaccine, not all Americans wanted to get it, and the reluctance was systematically related to politics rather than health risk. The message remains the same: vaccine hesitancy was a partisan public health issue in April 2021, just as a hypothetical analysis predicted a year previously.

While vaccine hesitance and acceptance are heavily tied to partisanship, the way party identification operates here is by serving as a catch-all for other social identities. For instance, the Republican Party does not formally maintain an antivaccine platform, but an individual who votes Republican may hold a "science skeptical" worldview. A Kaiser Family Foundation study asked individuals, in their own words, why they didn't get vaccinated, and answers varied dramatically from "This event seems more and more just like the flu. Everyone is exposed and has the same chance of getting it.

I never got a flu vaccine either" to "My daughter has had covid. . . . My thought is I am either immune or I have antibodies" and "I really don't want to be sick from a vaccination so I kind of lost interest."[12] Although none of these responses actually referenced a political party, partisanship is a good indicator of whether or not an individual holds these sorts of skeptical views toward vaccination.

Of course, vaccine hesitancy was expressed by Democrats and Republicans, but mixed or inconsistent messaging on the Right directly undermined Republican Party efforts to endorse the vaccine among its more vaccine-skeptical supporters. While some Republicans, such as Governor Spencer Cox of Utah, were eager to promote vaccination and get his state to Biden's 70 percent goal by the Fourth of July, others such as Florida governor Ron DeSantis sent mixed signals. While he himself was vaccinated with the single-shot Johnson & Johnson vaccine, he did not do so publicly like other governors.[13] Moreover, his politics have buoyed antivaxxers efforts by preserving the "vaccination as personal choice" stance; he signed an executive order prohibiting vaccine passports, most notably threatening to fine cruise ships that require passengers to be vaccinated. We see a consistent theme in these efforts to frame vaccination mandates as an effort to undermine individual liberty, mirroring our discussion of civil liberties and government authority in chapter 5.

In a second example, the Tennessee Department of Health halted vaccine outreach to kids—not just COVID-19 vaccines but also vaccines for all diseases, including deadly ones such as whooping cough and rotavirus—amid pressure from the Republican Party. This is the Republican Party at the state level explicitly siding against vaccines and against science.[14] And the major source of vaccine skepticism for conservatives is Fox News. As the delta variant surged across undervaccinated southern U.S. states in July 2021, hosts Tucker Carlson and Laura Ingraham mused on air that vaccines could be dangerous, with Carlson going so far as to describe Biden's vaccination push as "the greatest scandal in my lifetime, by far."[15] So, while McConnell—a polio survivor—mused about the mystery of vaccine hesitancy, his very party was conveying messages that undercut a push toward herd immunity.

The Racial Politics of the COVID-19 Vaccine Rollout

On May 4, 2021, Biden set an ambitious goal of having 70 percent of American adults partially vaccinated by Independence Day. Some parts of the United States far surpassed this mark but the country ultimately fell short of his July 4 goal.[16] Across many parts of the country, from rural western Colorado to southern Missouri to the Northern Tier of Pennsylvania and most of the rural South, vaccination rates were far below Biden's target. In the end, thirty-two states did not meet Biden's goal. States at the bottom of the list include Mississippi, Louisiana, and Wyoming, all below 50 percent. This loss was a major contrast to Biden's earliest vaccine win. The Biden White House came into office in January 2021 with the ambitious goal to deploy one hundred million shots in the first one hundred days, a goal he hit by day fifty-eight. Of course, uptake in the early days was limited only by supply. After that, the challenge became convincing individuals and expanding access to underserved populations.

Biden made racial equity in vaccination an explicit goal.[17] In framing vaccine access as about equity in addition to simply availability, the Biden administration acknowledged that many communities of color already suspected that health authorities would not be responsive to their community's needs. In wave 6—after the vaccine rollout had begun—we asked three closely related questions about the racial dimension of vaccine access, specifically whether respondents believed that vaccine distribution plans were taking into account the needs of Black, Hispanic, and Asian American communities. We show the results for the first of these questions, broken down by race, in figure 10.1.[18]

Not surprisingly, Black Americans were less confident that vaccine distribution plans would meet the needs of Black communities than were white Americans. But also note that most Americans of any race were only somewhat confident in plans to get vaccines to Black communities. In a sad commentary on the racialized politics of health equity in the United States, Americans of all races largely agree that access is a problem for Black Americans.

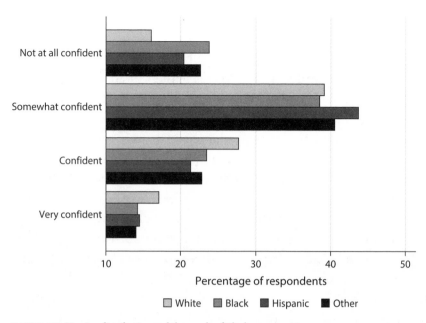

FIGURE 10.1. Vaccine distribution and the needs of Black communities

These views are borne out by the data on vaccination. By late April 2021, 44 percent of the adult population in the United States was fully vaccinated,[19] but there were significant disparities in vaccination by race and ethnicity. The percentage of white Americans who received at least one COVID-19 vaccine dose was 1.6 times higher than for Black Americans and 1.5 times higher than for Latinos, with Asian Americans having similar rates of vaccination as whites.[20] Despite barriers to accessing health care and high levels of being uninsured, Native Americans and Alaska Natives were more likely than other groups to be vaccinated by the spring of 2021. These high rates of vaccination were due in part to the early and robust supply of vaccines to the Indian Health Service, high levels of trust in tribe leaders, and long-standing strategies developed to reach rural and isolated communities.[21]

For explanations for persistently low levels of vaccinations across certain portions of the United States, we can look to any number of factors, from logistical issues and the challenges of distribution to the distance that many rural citizens have to drive to get to vaccination sites. But we and others have noticed that partisanship and race might explain these patterns as well.[22] For example, reading Trump's antivaccination tweets increased vaccination concern among Trump voters.[23] Ethnic and racial minorities in the United States, particularly Black Americans and Latinos, express more hesitancy about the COVID-19 vaccines.[24] These differences in intention among Black and Latino individuals are a product of mistrust in the medical profession,[25] experiences of bias from health care professionals, marginalization, poorer care, and a historical legacy of research abuse.[26]

We used two strategies to investigate the role of race and partisanship in shaping the vaccine rollout. First, we looked at the total uptake of vaccines across states according to how supportive a state was of Trump in the 2020 presidential election. The data in figure 10.2 run from early January until December 1, 2021.

There is plainly a divergence in the period between March and July 2021 in states that voted for and against Trump. This is the critical moment for the U.S. vaccine effort in which vaccines were available to any healthy adult, and yet we see vaccination rates lagging significantly in the most pro-Trump states. This is particularly striking when compared to the earliest months of 2021, when vaccines were mostly available only to essential workers and the elderly and during which there were no differences in vaccine uptake across states. The mid-2021 divergence—arriving just as Biden was hoping to ramp up vaccination rates—is a powerful reminder of how thoroughly partisan the COVID-19 pandemic had become.[27]

Another way to look at this result is to examine the correlation between 2020 vote share and vaccines administered by the states over time. In figure 10.3, we use the same data as in figure 10.2 to calculate the correlation—controlling for state population—between the 2020 vote share for Trump in each state and the number of vaccines administered per one hundred residents. We do this for every day starting in early January and ending on December 1, 2021. Each point in figure 10.3, then, describes the relationship between Trump support and vaccination rates across the states, with negative numbers indicating that on that particular day states with higher Trump support in 2020 were administering fewer vaccines.

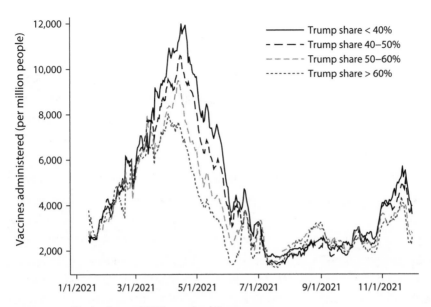

FIGURE 10.2. Vaccinations and 2020 state-level Trump support

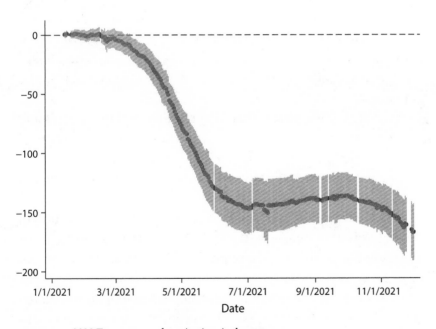

FIGURE 10.3. 2020 Trump vote and vaccinations in the states

In the first two months that vaccines were available, the points are close to zero, which means that there was no relationship between partisanship and vaccination rates. But we can see clearly that after the first tranche of vaccines were administered to essential workers and the elderly and once supply increased, partisanship took hold. Every single day beginning in April 2021 and persisting through today, there are more vaccines being administered as a share of state population in Biden-supporting states than in Trump-supporting states.

The results in figure 10.2 and figure 10.3, though, are aggregated up to the state level, and we know that even those states that were most strongly in support of Trump in 2020 have substantial numbers of Trump opponents. So to look more carefully at the partisan politics of vaccination, in figure 10.4 we use data from the Centers for Disease Control and Prevention (CDC) to compare across counties around the country, looking to see the correlation between county-level vote share for Trump in 2020 and the percentage of adults eighteen years of age or older in that county who are fully vaccinated by the middle of June 2021.[28] We look specifically at six very different states—California, Florida, Idaho, Kentucky, North Carolina, and Wisconsin—in order to capture differences between blue and red states across regions of the country (all states are available in the appendix).

In each of these states, there is a striking negative correlation between Trump's vote share in 2020 (expressed as a share of the total votes for Trump and Biden) and vaccination, a pattern that is equally evident in red states such as Idaho, blue states such as California, and swing states such as North Carolina and Wisconsin.

When we run the same analysis to compare the proportion of a county's Black population to vaccination rates in the same states (all states are available in the appendix),[29] a very different pattern emerges as indicated in figure 10.5.

In most states, there is no relationship whatsoever between the share of the county's Black population and vaccination rates. This is true both in states with large Black populations such as North Carolina and Florida and in those with small Black populations such as Idaho.

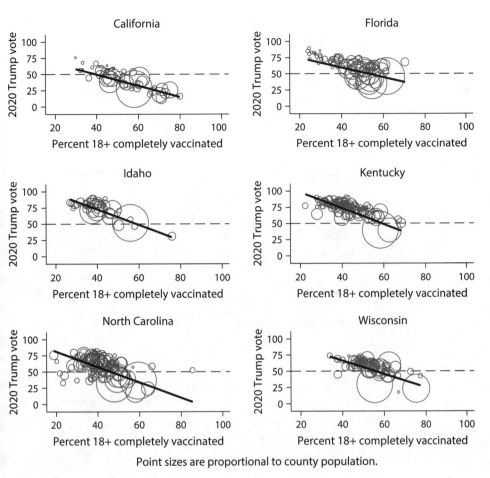

Point sizes are proportional to county population.

FIGURE 10.4. 2020 Trump support and vaccination rates, June 15, 2021

These findings only apply to a single snapshot in time, June 15, 2021. But they have important implications for how we should understand the partisan and racial politics of the COVID-19 vaccination rollout. We showed above that Republicans and Black Americans expressed higher levels of vaccine hesitancy than Democrats and white Americans, but it is only partisanship that seems to predict lower levels of vaccination rates across American counties. Overall vaccination rates among Black Americans were lower as of June 15, but we interpret this as a consequence of the health inequities and racialized differences in public health delivery that we discussed in

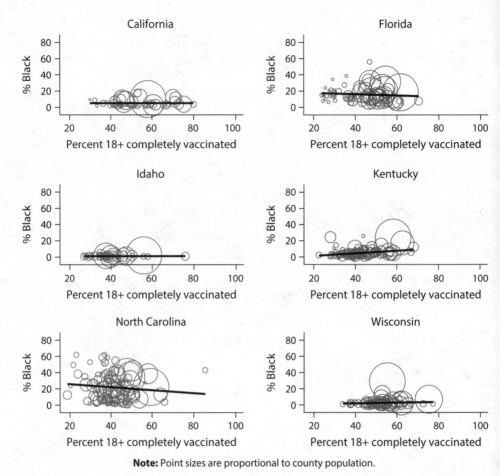

Note: Point sizes are proportional to county population.

FIGURE 10.5. Black population and vaccination rates, June 15, 2021

chapter 1 that could be overcome with more access and targeted campaigns. When it comes to partisanship, though, the findings are more consistent with a different interpretation: vaccine skepticism and support for Trump go hand in hand.

Conclusion

The politics of COVID-19 vaccines are much bigger than partisan considerations within the United States. Key political questions include the fairness, equity, and ethics of efforts by the Trump administration and the Boris Johnson government in the United Kingdom to secure first-use vaccine supplies at the expense of billions of other people around the world.[30] Others include vaccine diplomacy especially by Russia and China, which developed a number of COVID-19 vaccines that have not been approved for emergency use in the United States but have been widely distributed elsewhere.[31] Vaccine donations is also a critical political question, with pressure being placed on Biden in May 2021 to distribute eighty million doses to surging hotspot countries such as India, South Korea, and Taiwan. Still other political questions include the role of authoritarian governments in pushing out vaccines, given emerging reports of their limited effectiveness.[32]

These considerations remind us that the COVID-19 pandemic will only truly come to an end when vaccines have been distributed throughout the world and with sufficient uptake in all countries. Only mass vaccination has the chance of stopping the spread of the virus and ensuring that it does not evolve into new, more dangerous forms. After a catastrophic year of health policy mismanagement and bitter partisan division over every aspect of the COVID-19 pandemic, Americans find themselves in the enviable position of being at the front of the line for access to vaccines. As COVID-19 spikes anew in India, Peru, and Uganda, Americans can visit the nearest local drug store, mall, or elementary school to obtain a safe, free, and remarkably effective vaccine. To put it crudely, the United States lost the battle against COVID-19, but Americans could win the race to the vaccine.

But even with an ample supply of vaccines, there was still a stubborn segment of the U.S. population who would not take the vaccine and would not inoculate their kids. By Thanksgiving 2021, 58.9 percent of the U.S. population was vaccinated. This number varies widely by state, with Vermont (72.51%) and New York (68.07%) at the top of the chart and Idaho (44.95%) and West Virginia (41.5%) at the bottom.[33] Vaccine mandates at major companies across the country, such as Walmart and United Airlines, certainly aided the push, but holdouts prevent communities from reaching critical mass to end the pandemic. And individuals go out of their way to avoid vaccine mandates. One Florida couple was arrested and fined $8,000 after traveling to Hawaii with fake COVID vaccination cards, including cards for their children who were too young for vaccination at the time, that could cost hundreds of dollars on the black market.[34] Six Seattle police officers were let go for not complying with a statewide vaccine mandate.[35] And some people even seek out extreme "detox" measures and disinformation to "undo the vaccine," such as Borax baths.[36]

The pandemic did not end when vaccines became available. The partisan divisions that have characterized every aspect of the pandemic stood in the way of a complete and effective vaccination campaign. When we started the research on this book, we thought that COVID-19 would further divide an already divided American electorate. When we finished it, we realized that the reverse is also true: we need to heal American politics if we are to ever bring the pandemic to an end.

Conclusion

In August 2021 Daniel Wilkinson, a forty-six-year-old U.S. Army veteran who served two tours of duty in Afghanistan, had abdominal pain so severe that his mother took him to a hospital in Belleville, Texas, an hour outside of Houston.[1] An emergency room physician diagnosed him with gallstone pancreatitis, a serious condition but rarely fatal. Wilkinson needed a procedure to treat the pancreatitis and a bed in an intensive care unit. But owing to the steep rise of COVID-19 cases in the area, there were no beds available at the local hospital. Doctors called hospitals in Texas, Oklahoma, Arkansas, Kansas, and Colorado for seven hours and finally found him a spot at the Houston Veterans Administration hospital. But by the time he made it to Houston his organs were failing, and doctors could not perform the routine surgery that would have saved his life. Daniel Wilkinson died from this treatable illness on August 21; he did not die from COVID-19, but instead because of COVID-19.

That same month, three conservative talk radio personalities died from COVID-19.[2] Marc Bernier, age sixty-five, from Daytona Beach, Florida, had publicly rejected COVID-19 vaccines and compared Florida's public health commissioner to the Nazis for urging the public to get vaccinated. Dick Farrell, from West Palm Beach,

Florida, had condemned the vaccine and Anthony Fauci on his social media page and in appearances on the right-wing television channel Newsmax. Despite these public statements, after he was hospitalized Farrell privately expressed regret about his opposition to vaccination and urged his friends to get the vaccine.[3] In Nashville, Phil Valentine had publicly criticized vaccine mandates for taking away freedom of choice and recorded a song mocking the vaccine.[4] After being hospitalized for pneumonia caused by COVID-19, he put out a press release regretting that he had not been more "provaccine."

Bernier, Farrell, and Valentine had each rejected the vaccine and encouraged their listeners to do the same. All three of them died from COVID-19 at a time in which the most powerful nation in the world had made three fully safe and remarkably effective vaccines available at no cost to any adult. Their deaths are tragic because they were preventable, and their lives reflect the sad truth about the continuing partisan politics of COVID-19.

The summer of 2021 was meant to be the turning point, when all Americans could return to something close to normal. The Biden administration had set a goal to get 70 percent of eligible Americans vaccinated by July 4.[5] The Centers for Disease Control and Prevention (CDC) was encouraging Americans to take off their masks if they were fully vaccinated.[6] Through collective efforts, Americans were promised a "summer of freedom," when the nation would emerge "from one of the darkest years in our nation's history into a summer of hope and joy."[7]

But that's not what happened. Fueled by the deadlier and more transmissible delta variant and with tens of millions of Americans still unvaccinated, the summer and fall of 2021 proved to be some of the deadliest months of the pandemic. Breakthrough cases of COVID-19 in fully vaccinated individuals were increasingly common as vaccines gradually and inevitably lost their effectiveness over time, but the risk of death for the unvaccinated was far higher. The CDC reported that in September 2021, the risk of dying from COVID-19 was fourteen times higher for unvaccinated Americans than for fully vaccinated Americans.[8]

What the Biden administration's optimistic messaging missed was that partisan politics is very difficult to dislodge. All of the structural conditions that made responding to the pandemic so difficult in the early days of 2020 still persisted in late 2021, only to be aggravated by the more contagious delta variant and continued vaccine skepticism among millions of Americans. The health care system was still overburdened, and the economic fallout from the pandemic had led to furloughs and forced retirements of health care workers, further hobbling understaffed hospitals. High rates of community transmission (primarily among the unvaccinated) drove high levels of hospital admissions, producing overworked emergency departments and long wait times—such as the wait that killed Daniel Wilkinson. Inequality across the United States remained high; if anything, the disproportionate harms suffered by communities of color further deepened racial and wealth disparities.

These factors do not fully explain the American predicament, however. The partisan conflict over the COVID-19 pandemic, which emerged in the early months of 2020 before anyone could have imagined that eight hundred thousand Americans would die, never abated. Donald Trump left office, and the Republicans lost control of the Senate, but partisan politics remained at the core of the COVID-19 pandemic in the United States.

Perhaps conservative radio talk show hosts such as Bernier, Farrell, and Valentine knew they would lose their audiences if they advocated the same policies as the Biden administration. Much like masking was so emblematic of the partisan politics of the pandemic in the summer of 2020, vaccination became a thoroughly partisan matter in 2021. In the same way that many Republican politicians resisted mask mandates, many of these politicians—from Florida to Texas—also resisted vaccine mandates. These antimasking and antivaccine messages sustain a feedback loop that reinforces the link between Republican identity and resistance to public health measures.

Partisan polarization has thus fed the continued divisions among the American mass public. And these divisions have hardened in ways that prevent even stalwart Republican Party politicians and conservative media elites from reaching out to their supporters and viewers with public health recommendations that can save lives. For example, in October 2021 Fox News anchor Neil Cavuto—a cancer survivor who also has multiple sclerosis—encouraged his audience to get vaccinated for their own safety after getting a breakthrough COVID case. In response, he received death threats.[9] Crowds at a rally in Alabama in August 2021 booed Trump himself when he recommended that people get the vaccine.[10] Like the conservative radio hosts, Trump was both an instigator of the polarization of public health and ultimately one of its targets.

So, when delta tore through the American population in the late summer of 2021, the partisan gap in vaccinations that we identified in chapter 11 had only grown. A Pew Research Center poll in August found that 86 percent of Democrats had received at least one shot, compared to 60 percent of Republicans.[11] While racial and ethnic gaps in vaccine uptake narrowed over time, a Kaiser Family Foundation survey found strong and enduring differences by partisanship such that "self-identifying as a Republican or leaning Republican is one of the strongest identification predictors of remaining unvaccinated."[12] This created a uniquely morbid outcome: a growing partisan gap in death. By October 2021, the gap in COVID-19 death tolls between red and blue Americans was growing faster than any point in the pandemic.[13] That is, there were more COVID-19 deaths in counties that voted for Trump throughout 2021 than in counties that voted for Biden.

In 2020 in the absence of widely available and effective vaccines, there was no partisan pattern in COVID-19; by 2021, death itself had become partisan.

As we have emphasized through this book, no country was spared from the pandemic. Countries with strong starts fell victim to new variants or lax stay-at-home orders. Countries that faced early disasters, such as Italy and Brazil, learned from the past and came to excel in vaccination policies.[14] What made American COVID so unique and so tragic was that a bad start seemed impossible to rectify. Trump's partisan approach to managing the COVID-19 pandemic outlived his presidency. Partisan polarization continued to hamper the ability of the United States to bring the virus to an end, prolonging the suffering and killing hundreds of thousands of Americans even when effective vaccines are widely available to anyone who wants them.

Could It Have Been Any Other Way?

We have traced the ways that the partisan politics of the pandemic in the United States has led to more cases and deaths in America than in other countries with similar levels of polarization, high levels of material prosperity, and even conservative leaders. What might have altered the trajectory of the partisan pandemic in the United States?

LEADERSHIP

Most obviously, a different president in the White House would almost certainly have handled the pandemic differently. Trump was particularly unsuited to managing a large, complex crisis due to his brand of politics, the timing of the crisis during an election year, general disdain toward the oftentimes unglamorous and unpopular work of governance, and deliberate practice of undermining the federal bureaucracy. Moreover, Trump's practice of charismatic populism portrayed him as uniquely knowledgeable, with a particular authority that other politicians and health leaders lacked.[15] Public health crises require the input and knowledge of medical and scientific experts in both setting policy and communicating with the public. But Trump's leadership style was to not defer to other actors, and he demanded the media spotlight. It is shocking to realize just how much of the American public discourse about the COVID-19 pandemic was focused on Trump.

Trump was not only vain; he was also stubborn. Rather than learning from the pandemic as it unfolded and we gained a better understanding of its epidemiology, Trump considered new information from the perspective of image management. To him, correcting mistakes and updating expectations would signal weakness. He therefore preferred to sideline, ignore, and criticize experts when they suggested that he might be wrong. During the infamous press briefing in which Trump suggested, without any medical evidence, that ultraviolet light or even injecting disinfectant could "knock out" coronavirus,[16] White House coronavirus response coordinator Dr. Deborah Birx—an HIV/AIDS immunologist—sat quietly in frame, nodding along. She never corrected him in public. She would later admit that moment haunted her: "I still think about it every day."[17]

Small government is part of the Republican Party philosophy; another Republican president might have gutted the federal bureaucracy. States' rights is also part of that philosophy; another Republican might have limited the role of the federal government in managing the COVID-19 pandemic, empowering the states instead. As for support for individual liberty and the free market, another Republican may have rejected costly and invasive policies such as contact tracing or prioritized economic opening over prolonged stay-at-home orders. But rejecting health science is not a Republican Party platform. Trump's decisions made the pandemic worse.

Moreover, Trump's choices were puzzlingly short-sighted. The opportunity was there to frame COVID as a war, which would buoy support in an election year. As a wartime president, Trump could have led a bipartisan effort as commander in chief to mitigate the virus. He even built a narrative for thinking about COVID as an "invisible enemy." But there was no follow-through. Instead of developing a "plan of attack," he pivoted to reopening the American economy. He chose the enemy to be economic malaise or political opponents, not the virus. And once this course was set, he would not deviate.

DIFFERENT MESSENGERS

In a health crisis people want to hear from their leaders, but they also want to hear from medical professionals and health experts. And they want assurance that the information they are hearing is truthful; they want information to make sense of what is happening, and they want guidelines for how to navigate in a situation of uncertainty. Around the world, heads of state coupled their own messages of reassurance and leadership with those from public health authorities such as France's minister of solidarity and health Olivier Véran and Taiwan's minister of health and welfare Chen Shih-Chung. It is hard to imagine any other 2016 presidential candidate such as Hillary Clinton or Jeb Bush publicly contradicting infectious disease specialists the way Trump did. By publicly undercutting experts on live television, Trump left Americans uncertain about what to think, making them susceptible to misinformation and other politically self-serving influences. At the state level, Republican governors such as Mike DeWine in Ohio and Larry Hogan in Maryland successfully led their states' early responses, working in lockstep with their states' public health professionals. Political elites needed to make the connections between the values they hold, the party they identify with, and what behaviors come with that identity.

As we argued in chapter 1, partisanship is more enduring than values and shapes how people apply those values to new issues. This means that partisan leaders are not completely constrained by a single vision of what party membership means.[18] Elites can actively connect different values and beliefs to partisan identity depending on context and incentives. We can imagine many ways that a committed Republican administration might have approached the pandemic differently. For example, we know that people who identify as politically conservative are, on average, more sensitive to pathogens and concerned about contagions such as viruses.[19] Using moral language about the responsibility to protect others, Republican and conservative leaders might have attached conservative values to preserving life, strengthening communities, and cooperation.[20] But because leaders on the American political right have spent years telling their followers not to trust institutions, media, and political elites, convincing more conservative citizens to mask up, stay home, or vaccinate was harder than for those on political left, whose ideology is more supportive of an active and robust government response. Alternatively, Republicans could have pulled on the thread of Trumpian authoritarianism to compel obedience and discipline, in which loyal party members follow a strong president's dictates on combating COVID-19.

In fact, COVID did present the Republican Party with moments of achievement. Most significantly, Republicans could have claimed vaccines as a signature Republican victory in the fight against COVID-19. Operation Warp Speed might have been portrayed as an early Trump achievement that directed billions of dollars toward supporting American innovation. Vaccines could have been touted as the Republican key to unlocking economic recovery. And that the United States received among the world's first doses could have been touted as a savvy bit of negotiating by America's entrepreneur in chief. Imagine if Trump had gone on television in February 2021 to urge Americans to get the "Trump Vaccine, available at no cost to you, but only while supplies last."

Sadly, the Trump administration chose a different path. Even though Trump was vaccinated back in January 2021, he chose not to do it publicly. He instead politicized vaccines early on, publicly raising baseless accusations against Pfizer, which he suggested delayed positive vaccine trial results until after election day.[21] He chose personal, petty grievances over what was best for not just Americans' health but also his own party. Perhaps the Republican Party could have kept the Senate—maybe kept Trump in the presidency—on the backbone of public health achievements. The COVID States Project estimates that Republican governors lost an average of 22 points on their approval ratings from 2020 to 2021 due to their handling of the pandemic, whereas Democratic governors lost an average of 14 points.[22] Rather than focusing on the actual accomplishments of his pandemic management, Trump spent most of 2020 complaining that the media does not give him enough credit and undermining public health officials.

ELECTION TIMING AND GEOGRAPHY

We can imagine alternative scenarios to what happened in the first months of 2020. For instance, what if the pandemic had arrived in the United States through Jacksonville or Cincinnati rather than Seattle and New York? What if it hadn't been an election year? These may not have changed how COVID-19 spread, but they would certainly have altered the president's incentives to respond. Had 2020 not been an election year, Trump may not have been so eager to see the Dow Jones rebound or so quick to reopen businesses to signal confidence to struggling American workers. In previous disasters such as hurricanes, there is evidence that districts that are key to the reelection of a sitting president were more likely to get federal dollars to help with recovery.[23] Trump—as a transactional businessman par excellence—would not expend precious resources on states that could not give him something in return. Had the pandemic emerged in red states rather than blue states, perhaps he would have been quicker to find an effective response.

Trump's reelection pitch in 2020 was to "Keep America Great," appealing to his base of Republican voters. Had the first cases been in safe-Republican or competitive states, perhaps the White House would have acted with more urgency and coordinated with states to roll out testing, personal protective equipment, and hospital equipment rather than leaving states to compete with one another over medical supplies.[24] The fact that the pandemic hit blue states first—states that would not be part of his reelection strategy—probably explains why Trump was so uninterested in developing a national testing plan in coordination with the federal government that could have allowed a safer reopening of the economy.[25] And combining the early politicization of the pandemic with Trump's preoccupation with image management in an election year, this strategy did not allow for adjustment as red states began to get hit hard by the realities of the ever-spreading novel coronavirus. A perverse epilogue to this strategy is that Trump has never been penalized by this voter base, not even for ignoring and abandoning his fellow Republicans.

FUNCTIONING BUREAUCRACY WITH NO INTERFERENCE

Last, we can imagine that a fully functioning and well-prepared federal agency would have been sufficient to make progress against COVID-19 in the early days of the pandemic. Most countries found themselves short on personal protective equipment, but the dearth of supply, coupled with a lack of central coordination and the Trump administration's obstreperous rejection of Barack Obama–era best practices, unnecessarily bound the U.S. government's hands in regard to the pandemic response from the outset. By early 2020, much of the federal bureaucracy in the United States was understaffed and underresourced. Many agencies did not have a Senate-confirmed permanent director and lacked the ability to respond effectively to the complex needs of the pandemic. Trump was actively hostile to certain federal agencies, referring to civil servants as members of a "deep state" intent on harming his presidency.[26] Investigations from the House Select Subcommittee on the Coronavirus Crisis later revealed that not only were federal agencies unprepared for a quick response to the pandemic due to their internal issues such as staffing and morale, but there was also political interference in addition to pressure from the White House on issues of science and health.

Scientific agencies such as the CDC are supposed to function independently from the partisan branches of government. Yet interviews with agency leaders and reviews of memos, emails, and documents have shown that political appointees tried to change or affect the CDC's guidance and weekly scientific reports about the prevalence of COVID-19 and mitigation policies.[27] Dr. Christine Casey, editor of the CDC's *Morbidity and Mortality Weekly Report*, describes an email that she received from an adviser to the Department of Health and Human Services and a Trump political appointee that she interpreted as a request to stop a scientific report because it harmed the president. She was later instructed to delete the email. A fully functioning health bureaucracy that operated without pressure from the White House could not have avoided the pandemic altogether. But it could have led a more coordinated response from the beginning.

As the nursery rhyme goes, "If wishes were horses, beggars would ride." As of December 2021, the pandemic had taken more than eight hundred thousand American lives. This is more than any other country in the world. The United States is the richest and most powerful country on Earth, with all the science and technology and best minds at our disposal. The U.S. government put billions of dollars into research and development to fast-track a vaccine, and what did we do with it? You can fund the best science in the world, but if you can't convince a critical mass of the community to wear a mask, to take a vaccine, or to endure small sacrifices for their fellow community members, then the best science will not defeat COVID-19.

Looking Ahead

The death toll from COVID-19 has exceeded that of the average flu season twenty-six times over. COVID-19 has killed more Americans than, as singular events, the 1918 influenza pandemic, the American Civil War, World War I, the Japanese attack on Pearl Harbor, World War II, and the 9/11 attacks. In fact, more Americans died from COVID-19 the week before Thanksgiving 2021 than on 9/11 and Pearl Harbor combined. In this book we have traced out the many ways that the United States failed to respond to the COVID-19 pandemic, setting in motion partisan patterns that made the pandemic worse than it had to be. What does this failure portend for difficult issues such as climate change, natural disasters, or yet another pandemic? Have we Americans proven that we cannot work together to solve crises? How does the country recover and move forward?

We have documented so many points of deficiency—from the government's response to citizen behavior—that it is easy to be pessimistic about America's future. But there are important bright spots, aspects of the pandemic that speak to the resilience and fortitude of the American public. Hundreds of millions of Americans upended their lives, learning how to worship and run religious services, teach and attend school, argue matters in court, treat patients, and more, all virtually. Hundreds of millions of Americans—a vast majority— wore face masks in supermarkets, on buses, and in schools and places of work without incident. Through a partnership between the federal government and private industry, pharmaceutical companies developed and tested lifesaving COVID-19 vaccines and brought them to market within a year. A divided Congress and a Republican president came together to help pass economic relief for the unemployed, renters' relief, business loans, money for hospitals, and direct tax credits for families, among many other provisions to support Americans. Prompted by continued economic fallout from the pandemic and experiences with the long, slow climb back from the Great Recession of 2007–2009, the Biden administration passed a set of policies that broadened the reach of the federal government in ways not seen since President Lyndon Johnson's Great Society. Some of these policies—such as direct payments to families with young children, funding for broadband, expanding mass vaccination, and support for rural hospitals—are a direct response to the pandemic. They mark a fundamental shift in how the federal government interacts with the American public.

Americans also accomplished a lot on their own without the federal government. Americans organized to support one another through mutual aid societies and working through civic organizations such as food banks. When the pandemic exposed the fissures in society such as racial inequality in health care and racialized police violence, millions took to the street in response. The Black Lives Matter marches in the summer of 2020 in the wake of George Floyd's death were the largest protest movement in American history.[28] The pandemic also demonstrated the importance and salience of politics to Americans' everyday lives; voter turnout in 2020 election was the highest since 1900.[29]

Our findings show that self-interest does not always overwhelm partisanship in shaping health behaviors, emotions, or what types of policies people want in a crisis. People want to stay consistent with their identities and derive self-esteem from those identities, and they bristle at being required to change their behavior even if doing so will help them avoid falling ill to a deadly virus. People will pursue surprising behaviors to be able to stay true to their party label, such as taking ivermectin instead of a vaccine. They will even construct fantastical beliefs, such as that the whole pandemic is not real or that it is a political conspiracy (i.e., a "plandemic"). This makes partisanship a really powerful tool, one that can smooth a stone or sharpen a dagger.

But partisan identities are malleable, and partisan divisions can be overcome. We know, for example, that people who age into

Medicare or get access to health insurance through the Affordable Care Act become more supportive of those programs, even among Republicans who were traditionally less supportive of government-run programs than their Democratic counterparts.[30] People more at risk for effects of the disease are more likely to get vaccinated regardless of their partisanship: as of December 2021, 99 percent of people aged sixty-five and above had at least one dose of a COVID vaccine. The challenge is to find ways to overcome partisan politics for the rest of us before it is too late.

Lessons Going Forward

With this point in mind, we close this book by outlining a series of lessons that we hope Americans and their political leaders can learn from the COVID-19 pandemic. Politics made the pandemic worse than it had to be, but we cannot ask for a world without politics. Instead, we must grapple with how our politics might serve Americans better and how we as engaged citizens can support one another for the common good.

Most obviously, America's preexisting conditions explain—in part—why the pandemic was so devastating in the United States. Partisanship divides Americans, and Trump was uniquely unqualified to manage this pandemic, but we draw our attention here to the social and economic inequalities that characterize the United States today. American health care is too unequal and our system of health care delivery is too wobbly and ineffective to be able to withstand a public health emergency such as COVID-19. Health care reform has been an ongoing political challenge since the 1930s, and there are few issues that captivate Americans' attention as have Medicare, the Affordable Care Act, and the out-of-pocket costs associated with health coverage. The COVID-19 pandemic confirms what many have long argued: that the United States needs a better, more inclusive, and more equitable health care system. The United States is too big, too diverse, and too unequal to withstand a shock such as COVID-19 without thoroughgoing reform to the way that health care is purchased, subsidized, and delivered.

Beyond these preexisting conditions, however, one lesson to draw from America's COVID-19 tragedy is about the importance of public health communication in supporting the work of our public health authorities. As social scientists, we think it is essential to remember that public health—like science more generally—is a social phenomenon. Science does not speak for itself, and findings and recommendations are often messy, contested, and hard to communicate. And ordinary people—the three of us included—have their own beliefs, biases, and values that affect how they receive the information provided to them. With these facts in mind, government panels on public health and climate science should include social scientists who can help other scientists understand the importance of identity in shaping changes in attitudes and behaviors. Vaccines are only effective if people are willing to have them put in their arms. When science needs to change minds and get people to act, social scientists can help craft messages that resonate with different groups. To the extent that partisanship is a social identity in the United States—one of our motivating premises in this book—it follows that public health communication strategies must take partisanship into account.

Even with a better understanding of the social dimensions of public health communications, though, the United States suffers from low levels of trust in government and widespread skepticism of public authority, especially at the federal level. Low trust in institutions also begets low social trust, which is a huge impediment for collective problem solving. Low trust in government means that elected officials struggle to establish authority in hard times. Low trust in each other means that community-based solutions are not intuitively valuable, leading some to default to more individualized responses instead. These are long-standing issues in American public life, but we nevertheless believe that American citizenship needs sturdier foundations.

This means investing in at least two separate dimensions of American citizenship. One is practical and immediate: we need positive campaigns touting the benefits of public health interventions such as vaccines outside of times of crisis in order to build reservoirs of active support for public health measures that can protect us all. These reservoirs of support should foster the development of prosocial norms that are less likely to be undermined by politicians, media figures, and celebrities with nonmainstream views. Most Americans had never thought to question the public health benefits of vaccination prior to the COVID-19 pandemic, not least because vaccinations are so remarkably effective at eliminating disease that the vast majority of Americans never have to consider the consequences of diseases such as whooping cough and scarlet fever. But this very fact makes it easy for Americans to forget that vaccinations are a miracle of our modern world.[31] We need Americans to actively and positively associate public health achievements such as vaccination with civic obligation toward the common good.

The second investment in American citizenship is more difficult to achieve. One common argument about why some (mostly small and homogenous) countries have avoided the worst of the pandemic is that these are societies that are characterized by high levels of political trust. For example, social scientists have held out Denmark as an example where public health communications are particularly effective owing to Danes' trust in government and institutions.[32] Similar arguments have been made about countries such as South Korea and Taiwan. We acknowledge that trust in government and trust in fellow citizens makes pandemic management easier. But we cannot simply legislate trust. Social trust and trust in government are not policy choices that governments can switch on or off. Even a competently executed pandemic management strategy would founder in the United States. Building social trust takes time, but it is just as essential to achieving the common good as is having a President who trusts his advisers and focuses on science rather than partisan division.[33]

One explanation for why Americans have such low trust in government is that the government has not earned the public's trust in recent years. Viewed this way, we can see how trust in government might be fortified by reinforcing the importance of well-functioning, professional, and impartial federal and state institutions for making government work.[34] This is an area in which American politicians can act right now if they so desire. Congress has the authority to implement legislative safeguards to preserve the independence of key federal agencies such as the CDC and the Food and Drug Administration as well as all other federal bureaucracies that are tasked with implementing the policies that Congress produces. Likewise, Congress can demand that all executive-appointed offices are staffed in an orderly and timely fashion with administrators who bring subject matter expertise to the job. Of course, America's partisans will disagree on the details of administrative appointments. But if there is one thing that the COVID-19 pandemic has taught us it is that we need competent authorities making decisions, not politicians seeking to exploit the news cycle for personal political gain.

Politics is the act of working collectively even when we disagree. We still have the capacity to do politics, to work together in times of crisis. But we must learn the right lessons from the COVID-19 pandemic. We cannot guarantee that partisan polarization and America's other preexisting conditions will look any better when the next crisis arrives in the United States. But we can shore up the load-bearing walls that support our political institutions. If we buttress our institutions with social science, good citizenship and accountable and prepared institutions, and reflect soberly on the deadly price we paid for these lessons, perhaps the next crisis won't produce such tragic outcomes. The pandemic is not yet over, but the lessons that we are still learning from COVID-19 should guide policy makers toward a better response to future crises.

Epilogue

We finished writing *Pandemic Politics* in December 2021, just as the highly infectious omicron variant emerged. Omicron spread faster than the original Wuhan variant and ripped across America in a matter of weeks. Given its high transmissibility, omicron sent Americans to the hospital at rates that surpassed even those at our most virulent peak of December 2020. And like all its predecessors, omicron proved fatal. By late January 2022, over fifteen thousand people were dying per week from COVID. These were the same rates as March 2020. Despite nearly two years of the COVID-19 pandemic, it seemed as though nothing had changed and that we had learned nothing. Hospitals were once again overflowing. We still had a president who was slow to react, despite a change in government. And at-home tests were once again in short supply.

And the political divisions were also unchanged. Democrats supported government mitigation efforts, mask mandates, vaccine mandates, and pro–social health measures. Republicans supported individual choice, economic openness, and "returning to normal" while virulently (no pun intended) opposing vaccine mandates. If anything, with omicron the political fault lines that formed in the earliest days of the pandemic metastasized. The partisan differences we observed in March 2020 in the United States only strengthened over time. Antivacccine movements had consolidated in message in the United States and around the world and were exhibiting stubborn resilience in places such as Germany and Canada. Given what we have learned of the divisive partisan politics of COVID-19, the politics of omicron were utterly predictable.

Omicron did not alter what we already learned in writing this book. If anything, it strengthened our conclusion. Partisanship still drove attitudes about mask wearing, safe reopening, and vaccines. In one study from January 2022, Pew reported an almost 40-point gap between Democrats who favored showing proof of COVID-19 vaccination to shop inside stores (58%) compared to Republicans (19%). That gap became wider for eating inside restaurants, going to a sporting event or concert, and travel by airplane, where 80 percent of Democrats support a vaccine requirement compared to 31 percent of Republicans.[1]

Omicron was remarkable not just because of how widespread it was but also because it was the apogee of pandemic politics. We were seeing death tolls that matched the earliest days of the pandemic despite a widely available free vaccine. Even with strong evidence that the best protection against omicron was vaccination, entrenched political opposition to vaccination and vaccine mandates remained. The politics of vaccination had become self-destructive. By the close of January 2022, 75 percent of Americans were vaccinated with at least one dose (64% fully vaccinated). But even though this was sufficient to protect many against serious infection and hospitalization, it was not enough to establish herd immunity to protect the unvaccinated. The vast majority of the deaths wrought by omicron were avoidable.

It was also too late to do anything politically. Since the delta variant wave (July 2021), President Joe Biden had been referring to the COVID-19 pandemic as the "pandemic of the unvaccinated." With every week, the correlation between COVID-related deaths and Trump support increased. In October 2022, the Kaiser Family Foundation found that 60 percent of unvaccinated people identified as Republican (compared to 17% Democrats).[2] Donald Trump himself was booed again by a Republican audience in Dallas, Texas, in December 2021 for endorsing the COVID booster shot. The message had overtaken the messenger. The pandemic became the politics.

As we write in late February 2022, the United States has surpassed nine hundred thousand deaths. We will likely reach a million Americans dead from COVID-19 by the end of March. Partisanship did not kill everyone; health access, racial inequality, and comorbidities were lethal in this once-in-a-century pandemic. But so was partisanship. It killed more Americans than died in the American Civil War. The pandemic was a new kind of civil war, American versus American waged through distrust, enmity, and misinformation. And it was a cold war. We didn't have to brandish firearms. Our weapon was politics, and the battlefield is the air we breathe.

APPENDIX

Here we provide further information on survey details as well additional analyses for the interested reader.

Survey Details

Our sample was collected by YouGov, a high-quality survey firm. YouGov recruits and maintains an online respondent pool using a procedure called active sampling, in which restrictions are put into place to ensure that only people contacted are allowed to participate, to form a pool of registered users. YouGov panels are populated by a host of recruitment strategies, including standard advertising and strategic partnerships with a broad range of websites. YouGov employs internal rules for determining eligibility and exclusion criteria, and researchers play no role in selecting the participants. Participants in YouGov panels are fairly compensated with points, which may be redeemed for rewards including cash and gift cards (e.g., Amazon, Best Buy, Target). Researchers play no role in assigning point value.

This research was approved by the Institutional Review Board for Human Participant Research at Cornell University (Protocol 2003009479), the Institutional Review Board at the Office of Research Integrity and Protections at Syracuse University (Protocol 20-099), and the University of California, Irvine (through a procedure of self-exemption with confirmation from the Office of Research, March 6, 2020). In obtaining a representative sample, the pool of participants was nationally diverse and random within the sampling frame. The research does not differentially affect vulnerable populations, nor does it differentially benefit or harm particular groups. Participants had to click "yes" to affirm informed consent and, if confirmed, were directed to the start of the survey.

YouGov samples were matched to a sampling frame derived from the full 2016 American Community Survey one-year sample on age, gender, race, and education. Matched cases were weighted to the sampling frame using propensity scores, with a propensity function that includes age, gender, race/ethnicity, years of education, and census region. The weights were then poststratified on 2016 presidential vote choice and a four-way stratification of gender, age (four categories), race (four categories), and education (four categories) to produce the final weight. We employ sampling weights in all of the statistical analyses that we describe in the sections below, but when simply tabulating respondents we use raw unweighted (data).

Here, we describe our respondents' demographic characteristics in wave 1 by tabulating age, gender, race, income, education, marital status, employment status, urban-rural status, state of residence, and partisan identity.

TABLE A.1: Wave 1 Respondents, by Age

	Frequency	Percent
18-	424	14.1
30-	840	28.0
45-	1,068	35.6
65-	668	22.3

TABLE A.2: Wave 1 Respondents, by Gender

	Frequency	Percent
Male	1,404	46.8
Female	1,596	53.2

TABLE A.3: Wave 1 Respondents, by Race

	Frequency	Percent
White	2,171	72.4
Black	308	10.3
Hispanic	322	10.7
Other	199	6.6

TABLE A.4: Wave 1 Respondents, by Income

	Frequency	Percent
Less than $30K/yr	1,335	44.5
$30–70K/yr	651	21.7
$70–120K/yr	625	20.8
More than $120K/yr	389	13.0

TABLE A.5: Wave 1 Respondents, by Education

	Frequency	Percent
High school or less	989	33.0
Some college	1,042	34.7
College grad	606	20.2
Postgrad	363	12.1

TABLE A.6: Wave 1 Respondents, by Marital Status

	Frequency	Percent
Married	1,443	48.1
Separated	48	1.6
Divorced	331	11.0
Widowed	183	6.1
Never married	846	28.2
Domestic/civil partnership	149	5.0

TABLE A.7: Wave 1 Respondents, by Employment Status

	Frequency	Percent
Employed, student, or retired	2,805	93.5
Unemployed	195	6.5

TABLE A.8: Wave 1 Respondents, by Urban-Rural Status

Rural Code	Frequency	Percent
Metro (1m-)	1,534	51.4
Metro (250k-1m)	703	23.6
Metro (-250k)	308	10.3
Nonmetro (20k-, Metro adj.)	131	4.4
Nonmetro (20k-, Nonmetro adj.)	57	1.9
Nonmetro (-20k, Metro adj.)	133	4.5
Nonmetro (-20k, Nonmetro adj.)	72	2.4
Rural (Metro adj.)	18	0.6
Rural (Nonmet. adj.	26	0.9

TABLE A.9: Wave 1 Respondents, by State of Residence

	Frequency	Percent
Alabama	39	1.3
Alaska	7	0.2
Arizona	81	2.7
Arkansas	44	1.5
California	260	8.7
Colorado	44	1.5
Connecticut	31	1.0
Delaware	14	0.5
District of Columbia	8	0.3
Florida	224	7.5
Georgia	101	3.4
Hawaii	12	0.4
Idaho	20	0.7
Illinois	116	3.9
Indiana	62	2.1
Iowa	29	1.0
Kansas	16	0.5
Kentucky	43	1.4
Louisiana	41	1.4
Maine	14	0.5
Maryland	44	1.5
Massachusetts	57	1.9

	Frequency	Percent
Michigan	111	3.7
Minnesota	45	1.5
Mississippi	28	0.9
Missouri	67	2.2
Montana	15	0.5
Nebraska	13	0.4
Nevada	45	1.5
New Hampshire	24	0.8
New Jersey	67	2.2
New Mexico	30	1.0
New York	175	5.8
North Carolina	89	3.0
North Dakota	8	0.3
Ohio	111	3.7
Oklahoma	27	0.9
Oregon	59	2.0
Pennsylvania	178	5.9
Rhode Island	8	0.3
South Carolina	47	1.6
South Dakota	10	0.3
Tennessee	52	1.7
Texas	185	6.2
Utah	29	1.0
Vermont	10	0.3
Virginia	99	3.3
Washington	72	2.4
West Virginia	26	0.9
Wisconsin	60	2.0
Wyoming	3	0.1

TABLE A.10: Wave 1 Respondents, by Partisanship

	Frequency	Percent
Republican	775	25.8
Democrat	1,176	39.2
Other	1,049	35.0

Note: We repeated our survey for a total of six waves. The dates of each wave and the sample sizes in each appear in table A.11.

TABLE A.11: Wave Dates and Samples Sizes

Wave Number	Date	Sample Size
1	March 20–23, 2020	3,000
2	April 20–May 4, 2020	2,401
3	June 6–25, 2020	2,104
4	August 4–14, 2020	1,949
5	October 15–21, 2020	1,871
6	March 24–April 5, 2021	3,000

Additional Details for Chapter 4

In chapter 4, we showed there to be substantial differences in health behavior among Democrats, Republicans, and others. But periodically, we also encountered a question: are those differences the product of partisanship or something else—such as income, education, or race—that also happens to be related to partisanship? Take the example of income. If higher-income people are more likely to identify as Republicans and if higher-income people have different kinds of health behaviors than lower-income people, then the fact that Democrats and Republicans differ might be explained by income rather than partisanship.

To address this question, we relied on a standard statistical technique known as multiple regression. Taking the running example of income and partisanship, the basic idea is this. First, look to see how much of a relationship there is between income and behavior. Then, accounting for that difference associated with income, see if there is any remaining difference between Democrats and Republicans. In the language of statistics, we change our focus from *the correlation between partisanship and behavior* to the *partial correlation between partisanship and behavior, conditional on income*. Variables such as income in this example are known as "confounding variables" or "confounders," and when we account for them we write that we have "adjusted" or "controlled" for these confounders.

Multiple regression does not allow us to answer all questions that we might want to ask using our data. It is a statistical procedure, not a magic mirror: the aphorism that "correlation does not imply causation" applies equally to multiple regression analyses. However, multiple regression does give us powerful tools to isolate partisanship from other factors that might explain the patterns in our health behavior data. We will never conclude based on multiple regression analyses that partisanship causes anything—we cannot prove cause-and-effect using data such as this—but we will conclude that partisan differences cannot be explained by a whole host of other economic, demographic, or geographical factors.

To check whether wave 1 differences by party are explained by something other than partisanship, look to figure A.1. To read it, look first to the points. Each is associated with a different health behavior (the titles of the subplots) and a party (which appears on the y-axis on the left-hand side of each subplot). Arrayed across the bottom of each plot along its x-axis is a scale from 0 to 1. We can read the predicted proportion of respondents from each political party who report each COVID-19 behavior by looking to the y-axis of each subplot for the party and to the x-axis to the predicted proportion. As part of this exercise, we can also calculate the uncertainty in our predictions, which we represent with the bars that go through each point. When these error bars overlap, we cannot conclude that respondents differ by partisanship. When they do not overlap, we are more confident that whatever partisan differences we uncover are not simply due to chance (hereafter we will use the term "confidence intervals").

In a similar fashion, we investigate the enduring partisan differences that we identified across the six survey waves using a multiple regression approach. In this case, we can follow our respondents' employment status over the course of the pandemic as well as other measures of how Americans were interacting with the crisis—such as whether they were praying more frequently or looking at the news more frequently—that might also explain these partisan trends. We can also account for state-level policy differences as well as local-level COVID-19 caseloads and death tolls over time, each of which

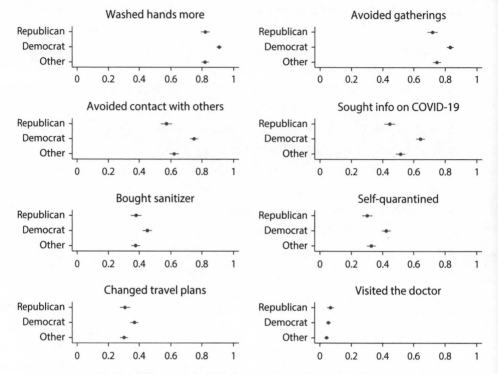

FIGURE A.1. Partisan differences in health behavior, adjusting for confounders

might explain the partisan differences that we have identified above. The results of our statistical analysis appear in figure A.2.

Strikingly, the partisan trends in health behaviors over time depicted in figure A.2 are nearly identical to what we identified in figure 3.8, which did not account for other socioeconomic and geographic differences across respondents. Even in this more sophisticated statistical analysis, we find that over the course of 2020 Americans' COVID-19 health behavior became ever more divided as the pandemic progressed.

To see just how powerful these tools can be, consider the statistical analysis that produced figure A.2. This was generated through an extended version of multiple regression analysis known as a multilevel regression model,[1] which makes adjustments to the differences among Democrats, Republicans, and others. The multilevel regression model

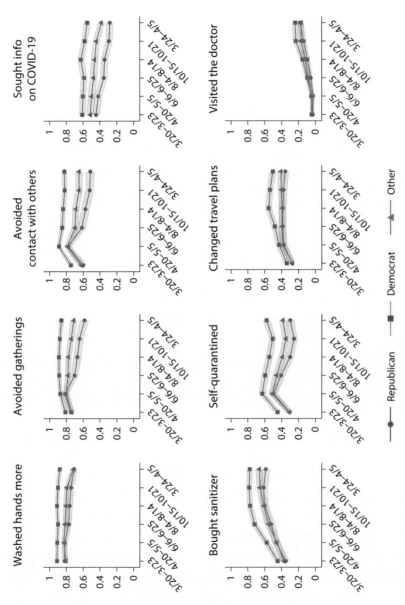

FIGURE A.2. Health behaviors across six waves, adjusting for confounders

Republican   Democrat   Other

> Adjusts for important factors such as race, income, education, unemployment status, frequency of prayer, and interest in reading the news that might differentiate Democrats, Republicans, and others;
>
> Adjusts for local-level COVID-19 caseloads and death tolls at each wave of our survey, which might also matter if Democrats and Republicans live in different kinds of localities that differ in the severity of the pandemic at various points in time (think Seattle versus Tulsa in wave 1 and so forth);
>
> Allows for differences in health behaviors across states;
>
> Allows for there to be a unique correlation between partisanship and health behavior that differs across each wave of the survey (i.e., perhaps differences between Democrats and Republicans are different in wave 1 than wave 2); and
>
> Allows there to be factors that are unique to *each individual in the survey* that might explain differences in health behavior across waves, assuming only that they can be described as following a specified statistical distribution.

As this discussion makes clear, this is a very flexible way to think about what might divide Democrats, Republicans, and others, acknowledging that there are likely to be differences over the course of the pandemic, across states, and across individuals. That we still find partisan differences to be so consistently visible is a testament to the utility of these complex statistical models for revealing the role of partisanship in health behavior.

Our lasso regression approach also tells us that partisanship matters more than any other variable that we have measured. Loosely speaking, if partisanship "matters," then this procedure should select partisan variables as good predictors of health behaviors; if partisanship is "more important" than other variables in predicting health behaviors, partisan variables ought to be selected more frequently than other variables. We implemented this lasso procedure forty-eight separate times, once per each of the six waves for each health behavior. The results are unambiguous. Partisanship is not only a very good predictor of nearly every health behavior (the exception is visiting a doctor, which our results above also showed are not very closely tied to partisanship) but is also selected more frequently in total than any other variable that we have measured. We can conclude from this exercise that more than just being correlated with health behaviors, partisanship is actually the best predictor of health behaviors that we have in our data.

Additional Details for Chapter 6

Here, we describe in more detail the survey experiment whose results appear in figure 5.12. The idea behind a survey experiment is simple: we randomly assign respondents to several groups, then respondents are asked a question that differs across groups on one important detail. We then compare responses across groups of respondents to ascertain how much that detail matters. Randomization gives us a key advantage: we can assume that on average there is no difference among groups who got each treatment and the control group. Comparing responses across groups thereby allows us to estimate the effect of the treatment. If there are no differences in support for a policy across groups, despite the groups having been asked about different levels of government (federal vs. state), we can be confident that the level of government in question does not matter.

The results in figure 5.12 plot the predicted level of support for each policy, alongside 95 percent confidence intervals, based on specified level of government ("we," "the federal government," or "the state government") and separated out by partisanship. When confidence intervals overlap, we conclude that there is no effect of the experiment—in other words, that the level of government does not affect support for the policy.

Additional Details for Chapter 11

In Chapter 11 we presented two figures—figure 10.4 and figure 10.5—that showed county-level correlations between partisanship, race, and vaccination for six important states. The figures below depict variation in all fifty states.

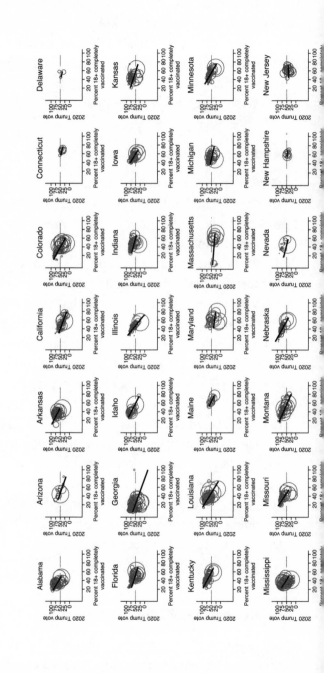

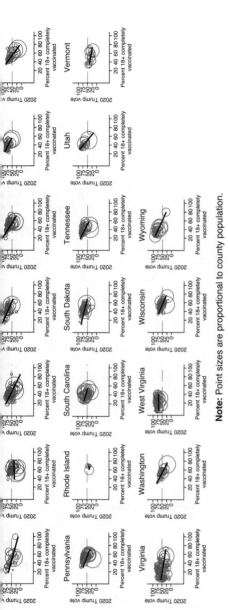

FIGURE A.3. 2020 Trump support and vaccination rates, June 15, 2021 (all states)

Note: Point sizes are proportional to county population.

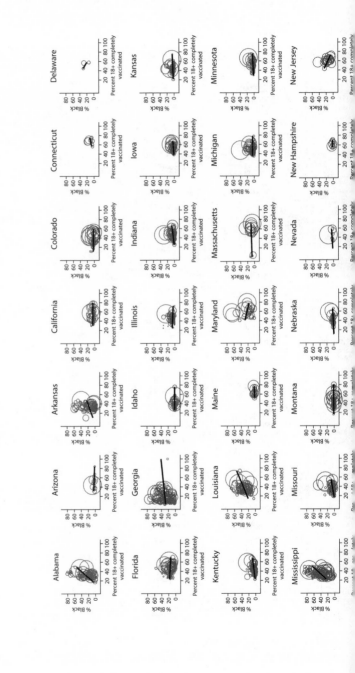

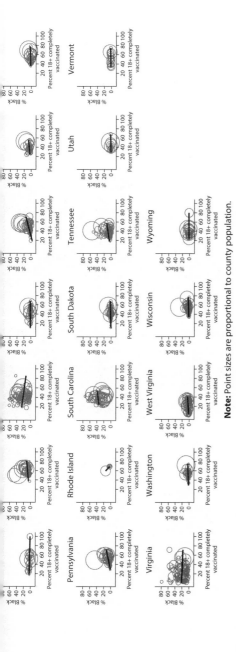

Note: Point sizes are proportional to county population.

FIGURE A.4. Black population and vaccination rates, June 15, 2021 (all states)

NOTES

Introduction

1. Taylor Lorenz, Kellen Browning, and Sheera Frenkel, "TikTok Teens and K-Pop Stans Say They Sank Trump Rally," *New York Times*, June 21, 2020.

2. Bryan Anderson, Gary D. Robertson, and Jill Colvin, "Trump Says GOP Is Pulling Convention from North Carolina," Associated Press, June 2, 2020.

3. Jamilah King, "Eight Trump Campaign Staffers Test Positive for Coronavirus after Tulsa Rally," *Mother Jones*, June 27, 2020.

4. Sean Murphy, "Health Official: Trump Rally 'Likely' Source of Virus Surge," Associated Press, July 8, 2020.

5. Bert Douglas Bernheim, Nina Buchmann, Zach Freitas-Groff, and Sebastián Otero, "The Effects of Large Group Meetings on the Spread of COVID-19: The Case of Trump Rallies," Stanford Institute for Economic Policy Research Working Paper No. 20-043, 2020.

6. Ashley Parker and Josh Dawsey, "Seven Days: Following Trump's Coronavirus Trail," *Washington Post,* December 5, 2021.

7. Stephanie Soucheray, "Coroner: First US COVID-19 Death Occurred in Early February," Center for Infectious Disease Research and Policy, April 22, 2020, https://www.cidrap.umn.edu/news-perspective/2020/04/coroner-first-us-covid-19-death-occurred-early-february.

8. For flu rates, see "Disease Burden of Flu," Centers for Disease Control and Prevention, January 7, 2022, https://www.cdc.gov/flu/about/burden/index.html.

9. Daniel Carpenter, "Is Health Politics Different?," *Annual Review of Political Science* 15, no. 2012 (2012): 287–311.

10. Olivia Waxman, "The Inspiring Depression-Era Story of How the 'March of Dimes' Got Its Name," *Time*, January 3, 2018.

11. Bethany Albertson and Shana Kushner Gadarian, *Anxious Politics: Democratic Citizenship in a Threatening World* (New York: Cambridge University Press, 2015).

12. John E. Mueller, "Presidential Popularity from Truman to Johnson," *American Political Science Review* 64, no. 1 (1970): 18–34; William D. Baker and John R. Oneal, "Patriotism or Opinion Leadership? The Nature and Origins of the 'Rally 'Round the Flag' Effect," *Journal of Conflict Resolution* 45, no. 5 (2001): 661–87.

13. Richard C. Eichenberg, Richard J. Stoll, and Matthew Lebo, "War President: The Approval Ratings of George W. Bush," *Journal of Conflict Resolution* 50, no. 6 (2006): 783–808.

14. Morris P. Fiorina and Samuel J. Abrams, "Political Polarization in the American Public," *Annual Review of Political Science* 11 (2008): 563–88.

15. Jennifer McCoy and Murat Somer, "Toward a Theory of Pernicious Polarization and How It Harms Democracies: Comparative Evidence and Possible Remedies," *Annals of the American Academy of Political and Social Science* 681, no. 1 (2019): 235.

16. Marc J. Hetherington, "Resurgent Mass Partisanship: The Role of Elite Polarization," *American Political Science Review* 95, no. 3 (2001): 619–31.

17. Ezra Klein, *Why We're Polarized* (New York: Simon & Schuster, 2020).

18. Erin C. Cassese, "Straying from the Flock? A Look at How Americans' Gender and Religious Identities Cross-Pressure Partisanship," *Political Research Quarterly* 73, no. 1 (2019): 169–83.

19. Kathy J. Cramer, *The Politics of Resentment: Rural Consciousness in Wisconsin and the Rise of Scott Walker* (Chicago: University of Chicago Press, 2016).

20. Lilliana Mason, *Uncivil Agreement: How Politics Became Our Identity* (Chicago: University of Chicago Press, 2018), 14.

21. Gabriel S. Lenz, *Follow the Leader? How Voters Respond to Politicians' Policies and Performance* (Chicago: University of Chicago Press, 2013).

22. Julia Azari. "Weak Parties and Strong Partisanship Are a Bad Combination," Vox, November 3, 2016.

23. Samara Klar, and Yanna Krupnikov, *Independent Politics: How American Disdain for Parties Leads to Political Inaction* (New York: Cambridge University Press, 2016).

24. Matthew Levendusky, *The Partisan Sort: How Liberals Became Democrats and Conservatives Became Republicans* (Chicago: University of Chicago Press, 2009); Lilliana Mason, "A Cross-cutting Calm: How Social Sorting Drives Affective Polarization," *Public Opinion Quarterly* 80, no. S1 (2016): 351–77.

25. Bernard Berelson, Paul Lazarsfeld, and William McPhee, *Voting: A Study of Opinion Formation in a Presidential Campaign* (Chicago: University of Chicago Press, 1954).

26. "Writer Michael Anton Makes the Case for Why Trump Should Be Reelected," National Public Radio, October 20, 2020.

27. Noam Gidron, James Adams, and Will Horne, *American Affective Polarization in Comparative Perspective* (Cambridge: Cambridge University Press, 2020).

28. Michael Dimock and Richard Wike, "America Is Exceptional in the Nature of Its Political Divide," Pew Research Center, November 13, 2020, https://www.pewresearch.org/fact-tank/2020/11/13/america-is-exceptional-in-the-nature-of-its-political-divide/.

29. Albertson and Gadarian, *Anxious Politics*.

30. Leonardo Bursztyn, Aakaash Rao, Christopher Roth, and David Yanagizawa-Drott, "Misinformation during a Pandemic," NBER Working Paper No. 27417,

2020; Jim Tankersly, Maggie Haberman, and Roni Caryn Rabin, "Trump Considers Reopening Economy, over Health Experts' Objections," *New York Times*, March 23, 2020.

31. Matthew Hartfield and Samuel Alizon, "Introducing the Outbreak Threshold in Epidemiology," *PLOS Pathogens* 9, no. 6 (2013): e1003277–e77.

32. Kim Yi Dionne and Fulya Felicity Turkmen, "The Politics of Pandemic Othering: Putting COVID-19 in Global and Historical Context," *International Organization* 74, no. S1 (2020): E213–E30.

33. Lena H. Sun and Joel Achenbach, "Unvaccinated People Were 11 Times More Likely to Die of Covid-19, CDC Report Finds," *Washington Post*, September 10, 2021.

Chapter 1

1. Shanto Iyengar, Yphtach Lelkes, Matthew Levendusky, Neil Malhotra, and Sean J. Westwood, "The Origins and Consequences of Affective Polarization in the United States," *Annual Review of Political Science* 22 (2019): 130.

2. Arthur Lupia, *Uninformed: Why People Know So Little about Politics and What We Can Do about It* (New York: Oxford University Press, 2016); Christopher H. Achen and Larry M. Bartels, *Democracy for Realists: Why Elections Do Not Produce Responsive Government* (Princeton, NJ: Princeton University Press, 2017); Bernard Berelson, Paul Lazarsfeld, and William McPhee, *Voting: A Study of Opinion Formation in a Presidential Campaign* (Chicago: University of Chicago Press, 1954); Michael X. Delli Carpini and Scott Keeter, *What Americans Know about Politics and Why It Matters* (New Haven, CT: Yale University Press, 1996).

3. Richard R. Lau and David P. Redlawsk, *How Voters Decide: Information Processing in Election Campaigns* (New York: Cambridge University Press, 2006).

4. Milton Lodge and Charles S. Taber, *The Rationalizing Voter* (New York: Cambridge University Press, 2013).

5. Larry Bartels, "Beyond the Running Tally: Partisan Bias in Political Perceptions," *Political Behavior* 24, no. 2 (2002): 117–50.

6. Lilliana Mason, *Uncivil Agreement: How Politics Became Our Identity* (Chicago: University of Chicago Press, 2018).

7. Henri Tajfel, *The Social Psychology of Minorities*, Vol. 38 (London: Minority Rights Group, 1978).

8. Angus Campbell, Philip Converse, Warren E. Miller, and Donald Stokes, *The American Voter* (Chicago: University of Chicago Press, 1960).

9. John Zaller, *The Nature and Origin of Public Opinion* (New York: Cambridge University Press, 1992).

10. Donald P. Green, Bradley Palmquist, and Eric Schickler, *Partisan Hearts and Minds: Political Parties and the Social Identities of Voters* (New Haven, CT: Yale University Press, 2004); Thomas E. Nelson and Donald R. Kinder, "Issue Frames and Group-Centrism in American Public Opinion," *Journal of Politics* 58, no. 4 (1996): 1055–78.

11. Henri Tajfel and John C. Turner, "The Social Identity Theory of Intergroup Behavior," in *Political Psychology: Key Readings*, ed. J. T. Jost and J. Sidanius, 276–3 (New York: Psychology Press, 2004).

12. Eli J. Finkel, Christopher A. Bail, Mina Cikara, Peter H. Ditto, Shanto Iyengar, Samara Klar, Lilliana Mason, et al., "Political Sectarianism in America," *Science* 370, no. 6516 (2020): 533–36; Shanto Iyengar, Gaurav Sood, and Yphtach Lelkes, "Affect, Not Ideology: A Social Identity Perspective on Polarization," *Public Opinion Quarterly* 76, no. 3 (2012): 405–31.

13. Alan I. Abramowitz and Steven Webster, "The Rise of Negative Partisanship and the Nationalization of US Elections in the 21st Century," *Electoral Studies* 41 (2016): 12–22.

14. Diana Mutz, "Effects of 'In-Your-Face' Television Discourse on Perceptions of a Legitimate Opposition," *American Political Science Review* 101, no. 4 (2007): 621–35.

15. Shanto Iyengar and Masha Krupenkin, "Partisanship as Social Identity: Implications for the Study of Party Polarization," Paper presented at The Forum, 2018.

16. Bill Bishop, *The Big Sort: Why the Clustering of Like-Minded America Is Tearing Us Apart* (Boston: Houghton Mifflin Harcourt, 2009).

17. Dhrumil Mehta, "The Media Really Has Neglected Puerto Rico," FiveThirtyEight, September 28, 2017.

18. James N. Druckman, Jordan Fein, and Thomas J. Leeper, "A Source of Bias in Public Opinion Stability," *American Political Science Review* (2012): 430–54.

19. Lodge and Taber, *The Rationalizing Voter*.

20. Ezra Klein, *Why We're Polarized* (New York: Simon & Schuster, 2020), 48.

21. George C. Edwards and B. Dan Wood, "Who Influences Whom? The President, Congress, and the Media," *American Political Science Review* 93, no. 2 (1999): 327–44.

22. Gabriel S. Lenz, *Follow the Leader? How Voters Respond to Politicians' Policies and Performance* (Chicago: University of Chicago Press, 2013).

23. Adam Berinsky, "Assuming the Costs of War: Events, Elites, and American Public Support for Military Conflict," *Journal of Politics* 69, no. 4 (2007): 975–97.

24. John Zaller, "Information, Values, and Opinion," *American Political Science Review* 85, no. 4 (1991): 1215–37.

25. Voteview: Congressional Roll-Call Votes Database, https://voteview.com/.

26. Eric Bradner and Phil Mattingly, "McCain, Graham Lead in GOP Criticism of Trump Ban, Many Others Stay Mum," CNN, January 29, 2017.

27. Jeff Stein, "Top Republicans Denounced Trump's Muslim Ban on the Trail. Now They Support His Executive Order," Vox, January 28, 2017.

28. Charlotte Alter, "How the Anti-Trump Resistance Is Organizing Its Outrage," *Time*, October 18, 2018.

29. Kevin Roose, "What Is QAnon, the Viral Pro-Trump Conspiracy Theory?," *New York Times*, September 3, 2021.

30. Robert S. Erikson and Laura Stoker, "Caught in the Draft: The Effects of Vietnam Draft Lottery Status on Political Attitudes," *American Political Science*

Review (2011): 221–37; Vesla M. Weaver and Amy E. Lerman, "Political Consequences of the Carceral State," *American Political Science Review* (2010): 817–33.

31. Ted Brader, *Campaigning for Hearts and Minds: How Emotional Appeals in Political Ads Work* (Chicago: University of Chicago Press, 2006); Cigdem V. Sirin, Nicholas A. Valentino, and José D. Villalobos, "The Social Causes and Political Consequences of Group Empathy," *Political Psychology* 38, no. 3 (2017): 427–48.

32. Dennis Chong, Jack Citrin, and Patricia Conley, "When Self-Interest Matters," *Political Psychology* 22, no. 3 (2001): 541–70.

33. Nolan McCarty, Keith T. Poole, and Howard Rosenthal, *Polarized America: The Dance of Ideology and Unequal Riches* (Cambridge, MA: MIT Press, 2016); Alan I. Abramowitz, "Peak Polarization? The Rise of Partisan-Ideological Consistency and Its Consequences," in *State of the Parties Conference* (Akron: University of Akron, 2021).

34. "Majority Support Trump Impeachment," Monmouth University Polling Institute, January 25, 2021, https://www.monmouth.edu/polling-institute/reports/monmouthpoll_US_012521/.

35. Jeffrey M. Jones, "Trump Job Approval at Personal Best 49%," *Gallup*, February 4, 2020.

36. Samara Klar and Yanna Krupnikov, *Independent Politics: How American Disdain for Parties Leads to Political Inaction* (New York: Cambridge University Press, 2016).

37. Shanto Iyengar et al., "The Origins and Consequences of Affective Polarization in the United States," *Annual Review of Political Science* 22 (2019): 129–46.

38. Max Weber, *Economy and Society: An Outline of Interpretive Sociology*, Vol. 1 (Berkeley: University of California Press, 1978.)

39. Jennifer L. Merolla and Elizabeth J. Zechmeister, *Democracy at Risk: How Terrorist Threats Affect the Public* (Chicago: University of Chicago Press, 2009).

40. Donald J. Trump, "Donald Trump's Speech at the Republican Convention, as Prepared for Delivery," CNN, July 16, 2016, https://www.cnn.com/2016/07/22/politics/donald-trump-rnc-speech-text/index.html.

41. Angelo Panebianco, *Political Parties: Organization and Power* (New York: Cambridge University Press, 1988).

42. Herbert Kitschelt, "Formation of Party Cleavages in Post-Communist Democracies: Theoretical Propositions," *Party Politics* 1, no. 4 (1995): 447–72.

43. To understand how clientelism differs from programmatic policy making, see Herbert Kitschelt, "Linkages between Citizens and Politicians in Democratic Polities," *Comparative Political Studies* 33, no. 6–7 (2000): 845–79.

44. "The Replacements: Why and How "Acting" Officials Are Making Senate Confirmation Obsolete," The Brookings Institution, September 23, 2020, https://ourpublicservice.org/publications/the-replacements/.

45. Marisa Taylor, "Exclusive: U.S. Axed CDC Expert Job in China Months before Virus Outbreak," Reuters, March 22, 2020.

46. Michael Tesler, *Post-Racial or Most-Racial? Race and Politics in the Obama Era* (Chicago: University of Chicago Press, 2016).

47. Andrea Schneiker, "Populist Leadership: The Superhero Donald Trump as Savior in Times of Crisis," *Political Studies* 68, no. 4 (2020): 857–74.

48. Jan Teorell, Aksel Sundström, Sören Holmberg, Bo Rothstein, Natalia Alvarado Pachon, and Cem Mert Dalli, "The Quality of Government Standard Dataset, Version Jan21," University of Gothenburg: The Quality of Government Institute, 2021, http://www.qog.pol.gu.se doi:10.18157/qogstdjan21.

49. Kenneth J. Arrow, "Uncertainty and the Welfare Economics of Medical Care," *American Economic Review* 53, no. 5 (1963): 941–73.

50. Nicole Huberfeld, Sarah H. Gordon, and David K. Jones, "Federalism Complicates the Response to the COVID-19 Health and Economic Crisis: What Can Be Done?," *Journal of Health Politics, Policy and Law* 45 (6) (2020): 951–65.

51. One such ranking is "Health Care Rankings: Measuring How Well States Are Meeting Citizens' Health Care Needs," *US News and World Report*, https://www.usnews.com/news/best-states/rankings/health-care.

52. Radha Chitale, "The Best and Worst States for Heart Attack," ABC News, July 9, 2009.

53. Scott L. Greer and Peter D. Jacobson, "Health Care Reform and Federalism," *Journal of Health Politics, Policy and Law* 35, no. 2 (2010): 203–26.

54. Jamila Michener, *Fragmented Democracy: Medicaid, Federalism, and Unequal Politics* (New York: Cambridge University Press, 2018).

55. Alan Blinder, "In Rural Alabama, a Longtime Mistrust of Medicine Fuels a Tuberculosis Outbreak," *New York Times*, January 17, 2016.

56. Scott L. Greer and Phillip M. Singer, "The United States Confronts Ebola: Suasion, Executive Action and Fragmentation," *Health Economics Policy and Law* 12, no. 1 (2017): 81–104.

57. "Cost to Treat Ebola: $1 Million For Two Patients," NBC News, November 18, 2014.

58. Richard Pérez-Peña, "Nurse Who Contracted Ebola in the U.S. Sues Her Hospital Employer," *New York Times*, March 2, 2015.

59. Alex Ura, "Dallas Hospital Apologizes for 'Mistakes' in Ebola Care," *Texas Tribune*, October 16, 2014.

60. Avidit Acharya, Matthew Blackwell, and Maya Sen, *Deep Roots: How Slavery Still Shapes Southern Politics* (Princeton, NJ: Princeton University Press, 2018).

61. "Labor Force Statistics from the Current Population Survey," Bureau of Labor Statistics, https://www.bls.gov/web/empsit/cpsee_e16.htm.

62. "Figure 1. Real Median Household Income by Race and Hispanic Origin: 1967 to 2017," U.S. Census Bureau, https://www.census.gov/content/dam/Census/library/visualizations/2018/demo/p60-263/figure1.pdf.

63. "Quarterly Residential Vacancies and Homeownership, Third Quarter 2021," U.S. Census Bureau, November 2, 2021, https://www.census.gov/housing/hvs/files/currenthvspress.pdf.

64. Marc Morjé Howard, *Unusually Cruel: Prisons, Punishment, and the Real American Exceptionalism* (Oxford: Oxford University Press, 2017).

65. John Gramlich, "The Gap between the Number of Blacks and Whites in Prison Is Shrinking," Pew Research Center, April 30, 2019.

66. Frank Edwards, Hedwig Lee, and Michael Esposito, "Risk of Being Killed by Police Use of Force in the United States by Age, Race-Ethnicity, and Sex," *Proceedings of the National Academy of Sciences* 116, no. 34 (2019): 16793–98.

67. "Racial Inequalities in Homelessness, by the Numbers," National Alliance to End Homelessness, June 1, 2020, https://endhomelessness.org/resource/racial-inequalities-homelessness-numbers/.

68. "Nonwhite School Districts Get $23 Billion Less Than White Districts Despite Serving the Same Number of Students," EdBuild, https://edbuild.org/content/23-billion.

69. "Who Votes in America?," Population Reference Bureau, October 1, 2000, https://www.prb.org/resources/who-votes-in-america/.

70. Allana T. Forde, Danielle M. Crookes, Shakira F Suglia, and Ryan T. Demmer, "The Weathering Hypothesis as an Explanation for Racial Disparities in Health: A Systematic Review," *Annals of Epidemiology* 33 (2019).

71. Michael Tesler, "The Spillover of Racialization into Health Care: How President Obama Polarized Public Opinion by Racial Attitudes and Race," *American Journal of Political Science* 56, no. 3 (2012): 690–704.

72. Tesler, *Post-Racial or Most-Racial?*

73. Marissa Melton, "Is 'Make America Great Again' Racist?," VOA, August 31, 2017.

74. Michael Tesler, "Trump Voters Think African Americans Are Much Less Deserving Than 'Average Americans',", Huffington Post, December 19, 2016.

75. Jennifer Karas Montez et al., "US State Policies, Politics, and Life Expectancy," *Milbank Quarterly* 98, no. 3 (2020): 668–99.

76. Jamila Michener, "Race, Politics, and the Affordable Care Act," *Journal of Health Politics, Policy and Law* 45, no. 4 (2020): 547–66.

77. Christopher Adolph, Kenya Amano, Bree Bang-Jensen, Nancy Fullman, and John Wilkerson, "Pandemic Politics: Timing State-Level Social Distancing Responses to COVID-19," *Journal of Health Politics, Policy and Law 46*, no. 2 (2021): 211–33.

78. "List of Ethnic Groups in the United States by Household Income," Wikipedia, https://bit.ly/3cq6qUS.

Chapter 2

1. Carey Goldberg, "Got Extra Masks or Goggles? Mass. Hospitals Already Running Short, Ask for Donations." *WBUR News*, March 17, 2020.

2. Liz Adlerman, "As Coronavirus Spreads, Face Mask Makers Go into Overdrive." *New York Times*, February 6, 2020.

3. Beth Healy, "Miscommunication, Missing Supplies Strain COVID-19 Coordination between Mass. And FEMA," WBUR News, April 12, 2020.

4. "A 'War' for Medical Supplies: States Say FEMA Wins by Poaching Orders," National Public Radio, April 15, 2020.

5. Noam M. Levey, "Hospitals Say Feds Are Seizing Masks and Other Coronavirus Supplies without a Word," *Los Angeles Times*, April 7, 2020.

6. Kristen Holmes, Carma Hassan, and David Williams, "New England Patriots Team Plane with 1.2 Million N95 Masks Arrives from China to Help Ease Shortages," CNN, April 3, 2020.

7. "A 'War' for Medical Supplies."

8. Bethany Albertson and Shana Kushner Gadarian, *Anxious Politics: Democratic Citizenship in a Threatening World* (New York: Cambridge University Press, 2015).

9. Maggie Haberman, "Trade Adviser Warned White House in January of Risks of a Pandemic," *New York Times*, April 6, 2020.

10. Eric Lipton, "The 'Red Dawn' Emails: 8 Key Exchanges on the Faltering Response to the Coronavirus," *New York Times*, April 11, 2020.

11. This was revealed in a U.S. Office of Special Counsel Complaint & Disclosure Form, available at Katz, Marshall & Banks, https://bit.ly/3qPHG0v.

12. Centers for Disease Control and Prevention, "Public Health Screening to Begin at 3 U.S. Airports for 2019 Novel Coronavirus ('2019-nCoV')," January 17, 2020, https://www.cdc.gov/media/releases/2020/p0117-coronavirus-screening.html.

13. "Interview: Bret Baier and Martha MacCallum Host a Town Hall with Donald Trump," YouTube, March 5, 2020, https://www.youtube.com/watch?v=cukyV5UGuEE.

14. Aki Peritz, "The Intelligence Community Got the Pandemic Right. Then Politicians Botched It," *Washington Post*, September 11, 2020.

15. Eric Lipton, David E. Sanger, Maggie Haberman, Michael D. Shear, Mark Mazzetti, and Julian E. Barnes, "He Could Have Seen What Was Coming: Behind Trump's Failure on the Virus," *New York Times*, April 11, 2020.

16. Haberman, "Trade Adviser Warned White House in January of Risks of a Pandemic."

17. Greg Miller and Ellen Nakashima, "President's Intelligence Briefing Book Repeatedly Cited Virus Threat," *Washington Post*, April 27, 2020.

18. June-Ho Kim, Julia Ah-Reum An, SeungJu Jackie Oh, Juhwan Oh, and Jong-Koo Lee, "Emerging COVID-19 Success Story: South Korea Learned the Lessons of MERS," Our World in Data, March 5, 2021, https://ourworldindata.org/covid-exemplar-south-korea.

19. Max Fisher and Choe Sang-Hun, "How South Korea Flattened the Curve," *New York Times*, April 10, 2020.

20. Lothar H. Wieler, Ute Rexroth, and René Gottschalk, "Emerging COVID-19 Success Story: Germany's Push to Maintain Progress," Our World in Data, March 20, 2021, https://ourworldindata.org/covid-exemplar-germany.

21. Christina Farr, "Germany's Coronavirus Response is a Master Class in Science Communication," CNBC, July 21, 2020.

22. Ned Stafford, "Covid-19: Why Germany's Case Fatality Rate Seems So Low," *BMJ* 369 (2020).

23. "22 Days of Dither and Delay on Coronavirus That Cost Thousands of British Lives," *The Times*, May 23, 2020.

24. Swapnil Mishra, James A. Scott, Daniel J. Laydon, Seth Flaxman, Axel Gandy, Thomas A. Mellan, H. Juliette T. Unwin, et al., "Comparing the Responses

of the UK, Sweden and Denmark to COVID-19 Using Counterfactual Modelling," *Scientific Reports* 11, no. 1 (2021).

25. Joe Biden, "FLASHBACK by Joe Biden: Trump is Worst Possible Leader to Deal with Coronavirus Outbreak," *USA Today*, January 27, 2020.

26. "Trump Tells Woodward He Deliberately Downplayed Coronavirus Threat," National Public Radio, September 10, 2020.

27. Morgan Phillips, "Trump Lashes Out at Woodward Book as a 'Political Hit Job' as McEnany Defends President over Coronavirus Comments," Fox News, September 9, 2020.

28. "Scientist Tapped to Lead CDC Does Not Inspire Confidence," *Star Tribune*, March 22, 2020.

29. Helen Branswell, "Coronavirus Concerns Trigger Global Run on Supplies for Health Workers, Causing Shortages," Statnews, February 7, 2020.

30. U.S. Department of State, "The United States Announces Assistance to Combat the Novel Coronavirus," February 7, 2020, https://www.usaid.gov/coronavirus/updates/state/mar-20-2020-united-states-announces-assistance-combat-novel-coronavirus.

31. Vivian Salama, "Not a 'Good Look': White House Fight over Masks Signaled Covid-19 Plans Running Awry," CNN, October 2, 2020.

32. Eric Lipton et al., "He Could Have Seen What Was Coming."

33. Jonathan Chait, "Trump: I Was Right, Coronavirus Cases 'Will Go Down to Zero, Ultimately,'" *New York Magazine*, April 28, 2020.

34. "First on CNBC: CNBC Transcript: National Economic Council Director Larry Kudlow Speaks CNBC's Kelly Evans on CNBC's 'The Exchange' Today," CNBC, September 22, 2020.

35. World Health Organization, "Diagnostic Detection of 2019-nCoV by Real-Time RT-PCR," January 17, 2020, https://www.who.int/docs/default-source/coronaviruse/protocol-v2-1.pdf?sfvrsn=a9ef618c_2.

36. Shawn Boburg, Robert O'Harrow Jr., Neena Satija, and Amy Goldstein, "Inside the Coronavirus Testing Failure: Alarm and Dismay among the Scientists Who Sought to Help," *Washington Post*, April 3, 2020.

37. Dan Vergano, "The Government Asked Us Not to Release Records from the CDC's First Failed COVID Test. Here They Are," Buzzfeed News, December 8, 2021.

38. Ibid.

39. Joanne Kenen, "How Testing Failures Allowed Coronavirus to Sweep the U.S.," Politico, March 8, 2020.

40. Reuters, "Only Three U.S. States Can Test for Coronavirus—Public Lab Group," Thomson Reuters Foundation News, February 21, 2020.

41. Centers for Disease Control and Prevention, "CDC Confirms Possible Instance of Community Spread of COVID-19 in U.S," February 26, 2020, https://www.cdc.gov/media/releases/2020/s0226-Covid-19-spread.html.

42. Michael D. Shear, Abby Goodnough, Sheila Kaplan, Sheri Fink, Katie Thomas, and Noah Weiland, "The Lost Month: How a Failure to Test Blinded the U.S. to Covid-19," *New York Times*, March 28, 2020.

43. Steve Eder, Henry Fountain, Michael H. Keller, Muyi Xiao, and Alexandra Stevenson, "430,000 People Have Traveled from China to U.S. since Coronavirus Surfaced," *New York Times*, April 4, 2020.

44. Pew Research Center, "COVID-19 Discussion Increasingly Popular in Twitter Posts Sent by Members of Congress," April 2, 2020, https://www.pewresearch.org/fact-tank/2020/04/02/tweets-by-members-of-congress-tell-the-story-of-an-escalating-covid-19-crisis/ft_2020-04-02_congressionaltweets_01/.

45. Nancy Cook and Matthew Choi, "Trump Rallies His Base to Treat Coronavirus as a 'Hoax,'" Politico, February 28, 2020.

46. David Frum, "This Is Trump's Fault," *The Atlantic*, April 7, 2020.

47. Jeremy W. Peters and Michael M. Grynbaum. "How Right-Wing Pundits Are Covering Coronavirus," *New York Times*, March 11, 2020.

48. Heidi Tworek, "Lessons Learned from Taiwan and South Korea's Tech-Enabled COVID-19 Communications," Brookings Institution, October 6, 2020.

49. Centers for Disease Control and Prevention, "Transcript for the CDC Telebriefing Update on COVID-19," February 26, 2020, https://www.cdc.gov/media/releases/2020/t0225-cdc-telebriefing-covid-19.html.

50. Grace Panetta, "Trump Reportedly Threatened to Fire a Top Doctor at the CDC for Sounding the Alarm about the Coronavirus in February," Business Insider, April 22, 2020.

51. Nathaniel Meyersohn, "CVS and Walgreens Warn There Could Be a Shortage of Hand Sanitizer," CNN, February 28, 2020.

52. Dan Diamond, "Trump Advisers Privately Warned of 'Critical Mistakes' as Pandemic Loomed," *Washington Post*, September 14, 2021.

53. Frum, "This Is Trump's Fault."

54. Harry Enten, "Flu Shots Uptake Is Now Partisan. It Didn't Use to Be," CNN, November 14, 2021.

55. Brad Heath, "Americans Divided on Party Lines over Risk from Coronavirus: Reuters/Ipsos Poll," Reuters, March 6.

56. Naeun Lauren Kim and Hyunjoo Im, "Do Liberals Want Curbside Pickup More Than Conservatives? Contactless Shopping as Protectionary Action against the COVID-19 Pandemic," *International Journal of Consumer Studies*, May 7, 2021.

57. Guy Grossman, Soojong Kim, Jonah M. Rexer, and Harsha Thirumurthy, "Political Partisanship Influences Behavioral Responses to Governors' Recommendations for COVID-19 Prevention in the United States," *Proceedings of the National Academy of Sciences* 117, no. 39 (2020): 24144–53.

58. Maria Sobolewska and Robert Ford, *Brexitland: Identity, Diversity and the Reshaping of British Politics* (Cambridge: Cambridge University Press, 2020).

59. YouGov, "Do You Think the Coronavirus Outbreak Has Brought the UK Together, or Pulled It Further Apart?," March 30, 2020, https://yougov.co.uk/topics/politics/survey-results/daily/2020/03/30/e959b/2.

60. Guy Falconbridge and Kate Holton, "Healthy Again, British PM Says Too Risky to Relax Lockdown Yet," Reuters, April 26, 2020.

61. YouGov, "Do You Think People Do, or Do Not, Have a Civic Duty to Self-Isolate for 14 Days If They Have Been in Contact with Somebody Who Has

Been Diagnosed with Coronavirus?," June 12, 2020, https://yougov.co.uk/topics/politics/survey-results/daily/2020/06/12/81a5a/1.

62. Quint Forgey, "Trump Floats His Own Coronavirus Hunches on 'Hannity,'" Politico, March 5, 2020.

63. COVID Tracking Project, "US Daily Reported Tests, Mar 1–Mar 7," Covidtracking.com.

64. Corinne Reichert, "Amazon Plans to Prosecute Sellers for Price Gouging during Coronavirus Outbreak," CNET, March 6, 2020.

65. Kevin Bohn, "US Surgeon General Says He Thinks Coronavirus Is Contained in Certain Areas of the Country," CNN, March 8, 2020.

66. Alexander Bolton, "GOP Senators Tell Trump to Make Fauci Face of Government's Coronavirus Response," The Hill, March 10, 2020.

67. Anita Kumar, "Trump Fears Emergency Declaration Would Contradict Coronavirus Message," Politico, March 11, 2020.

68. Ariadne Labs, "Global Learnings from South Korea: Protecting Health Care Workers from COVID-19," March 12, 2020, https://covid19.ariadnelabs.org/global-learnings-south-korea/.

69. "Coronavirus: Northern Italy Quarantines 16 Million People," BBC News, March 8, 2020.

70. Mark Jurkowitz and Amy Mitchell, "Cable TV and COVID-19: How Americans Perceive the Outbreak and View Media Coverage Differ by Main News Source," Pew Research Center for Journalism and Media, April 1, 2020, https://www.journalism.org/2020/04/01/cable-tv-and-covid-19-how-americans-perceive-the-outbreak-and-view-media-coverage-differ-by-main-news-source/.

71. David Leonhardt, "A Complete List of Trump's Attempts to Play Down Coronavirus," New York Times, March 15, 2020.

72. Yascha Mounk, "Cancel Everything," The Atlantic, March 10, 2020.

73. White House Coronavirus Task Force Briefing, April 3, 2020.

74. Trip Gabriel, "Ohio's G.O.P. Governor Splits from Trump, and Rises in Popularity," New York Times, April 28, 2020.

75. Jeff Zeleny, "Why These 8 Republican Governors Are Holding Out on Statewide Stay-at-Home Orders," CNN, April 4, 2020.

76. Ibid.

77. Samuel Bazzi, Martin Fiszbein, and Mesay Gebresilasse, "'Rugged Individualism' and Collective (In)Action during the COVID-19 Pandemic," Journal of Public Economics 195 (2021): 104357.

78. Jon Green, Jared Edgerton, Daniel Naftel, Kelsey Shoub, and Skyler J. Cranmer, "Elusive Consensus: Polarization in Elite Communication on the COVID-19 Pandemic," Science Advances 6, no. 28 (2020): eabc2717.

79. Joel B. Pollak, "Democrats Pushed Impeachment While Coronavirus Spread," Breitbart, March 13, 2020.

80. Lis Power and Rob Savillo. "Fox News Has Promoted Hydroxychloroquine Nearly 300 Times in a Two-Week Period," Media Matters for America, April 7, 2020.

81. OANN, "The Daily Ledger," April 7, 2020.

82. Maxim Ananyev, Michael Poyker, and Yuan Tian, "The Safest Time to Fly: Pandemic Response in the Era of Fox News," *Journal of Population Economics* 34, no. 3 (2021): 775–802.

83. **{AU: Please provide the complete source here..}{Simonov, 2020 #5588}**

84. Elliott Ash, Sergio Galletta, Dominik Hangartner, Yotam Margalit, and Matteo Pinna, "The Effect of Fox News on Health Behavior during COVID-19," *SSRN* 3636762, June 28, 2020.

85. Fox News, *Hannity*, April 7, 2020.

86. Amrita Narlikar, "In Brief: The Coronavrius and Germany," German Institute for Global and Area Studies, March 12, 2020.

87. David E. Lewis, "Is the Failed Pandemic Response a Symptom of a Diseased Administrative State?," *Daedalus* 150, no. 3 (2021): 68–88.

88. Andrew Restuccia and Rebecca Ballhaus, "Trump Shuns Use of Law Allowing Control over Manufacturers," *Wall Street Journal*, March 22, 2020.

89. Marielle Segarra, "How Did We End Up in a Ventilator Bidding War?," Marketplace, April 1, 2020.

90. Allison Quinn, "California Gov Was Reportedly Told He'd Have to Do the White House a Favor to Get Help with Testing Swabs," Daily Beast, July 18, 2020.

91. Orion Rummler, "Hogan Says National Guard Is Protecting Coronavirus Tests Sent from South Korea," Axios, April 23, 2020.

92. James Crump, "'It Was a Government of Chaos': Kushner's Coronavirus Task Force Whistleblower Says He Was Pressured to 'Fudge' Death Data Model," *The Independent*, September 23, 2020.

93. Aaron Blake, "The Trump Administration Just Changed Its Description of the National Stockpile to Jibe with Jared Kushner's Controversial Claim," *Washington Post*, April 3, 2020.

94. Katherine Eban, "'That's Their Problem': How Jared Kushner Let the Markets Decide America's COVID-19 Fate," *Vanity Fair*, September 17, 2020.

95. Ibid.

96. Christopher Adolph, Kenya Amano, Bree Bang-Jensen, Nancy Fullman, and John Wilkerson, "Pandemic Politics: Timing State-Level Social Distancing Responses to COVID-19," *Journal of Health Politics, Policy and Law* 46, no. 2 (2021): 211–33.

97. Amanda Moreland, Christine Herlihy, Michael A. Tynan, Gregory Sunshine, Russell F. McCord, Charity Hilton, Jason Poovey, et al., "Timing of State and Territorial COVID-19 Stay-at-Home Orders and Changes in Population Movement—United States, March 1–May 31, 2020." *Morbidity and Mortality Weekly Report* 69, no. 35 (2020): 1198.

98. Robert Anderton, Vasco Botelho, Agostino Consolo, António Dias da Silva, Claudia Foroni, Matthias Mohr, and Lara Vivian, "The Impact of the COVID-19 Pandemic on the Euro Area Labour Market," *ECB Economic Bulletin* 8 (2020).

99. Patricia Cohen, "'Still Catching Up': Jobless Numbers May Not Tell Full Story," *New York Times*, May 28, 2020.

100. Kim Parker, Rachel Minkin, and Jesse Bennett, "Economic Fallout from COVID-19 Continues to Hit Lower-Income Americans the Hardest," Pew Research

Center, September 25, 2020, https://www.pewresearch.org/social-trends /2020/09/24/economic-fallout-from-covid-19-continues-to-hit-lower-income -americans-the-hardest/.

101. Tiana N. Rogers, Charles R. Rogers, Elizabeth VanSant-Webb, Lily Y. Gu, Bin Yan, and Fares Qeadan, "Racial Disparities in COVID-19 Mortality among Essential Workers in the United States," *World Medical & Health Policy* 12, no. 3 (2020): 311–27.

102. Julie Satow, "Turning a Second Home into a Primary Home," *New York Times*, July 24, 2020.

103. Melinda Wenner Moyer, "Pods, Microschools and Tutors: Can Parents Solve the Education Crisis on Their Own?," *New York Times*, July 22, 2020.

104. Brett Samuels and Jessie Hellman, "Trump Says Testing May Be 'Frankly Overrated,'" The Hill, May 14, 2020.

105. Hannah Miao, "White House Abandoned Plan to Send 650 Million Face Masks across the U.S. in April, Report Says," CNBC, September 17, 2020.

106. Filipe Matoso and Mateus Rodrigues, "Coronavírus: Bolsonaro diz na TV que não há razão para pânico ainda que problema se agrave," G1, June 3, 2020.

107. "Coronavirus: Bolsonaro Downplays Threat of Pandemic to Brazil," BBC, March 25, 2020.

108. Katy Watson, "Coronavirus: Brazil's Bolsonaro in Denial and Out on a Limb," BBC, March 29, 2020.

109. Fábio Amato, "Coronavírus: MP concentra no governo federal poder para restringir circulação de pessoas," G1, March 21, 2020.

110. "Ministério da Saúde pressiona Manaus e diz ser 'inadmissível' não usar cloroquina contra Covid-19," *Folha de S.Paulo*, January 1, 2021.

111. Pedro C. Hallal, "SOS Brazil: Science under Attack," *The Lancet* 397, no. 10272 (2021): 373–74.

112. Rodrigo Pedroso, "Brazil's Bolsonaro Says He Will Not Be Vaccinated against Covid-19," CNN, October 13, 2021. Incidentally, his wife was vaccinated when the couple visited New York for the United Nations General Assembly meeting in September 2021.

113. Tamires D. A. Serdan, Laureane N. Masi, Renata Gorjao, Tania C. Pithon-Curi, Rui Curi, and Sandro M. Hirabara, "COVID-19 in Brazil: Historical Cases, Disease Milestones, and Estimated Outbreak Peak," *Travel Medicine and Infectious Disease* 38 (2020): 101733.

114. Aidan Connaughton, "Those on Ideological Right Favor Fewer COVID-19 Restrictions in Most Advanced Economies," Pew Research Center, July 30, 2021, https://www.pewresearch.org/fact-tank/2021/07/30/those-on-ideological-right -favor-fewer-covid-19-restrictions-in-most-advanced-economies/.

115. Yasmeen Abutaleb, Ashley Parker, Josh Dawsey, and Philip Rucker, "The Inside Story of How Trump's Denial, Mismanagement and Magical Thinking Led to the Pandemic's Dark Winter," *Washington Post*, December 19, 2020.

116. Brian Neelon, Fedelis Mutiso, Noel T. Mueller, John L. Pearce, and Sara E. Benjamin-Neelon, "Associations between Governor Political Affiliation and COVID-19 Cases, Deaths, and Testing in the US," *American Journal of Preventive Medicine* 61, no. 1 (2021): P115–19.

Chapter 3

1. Madeline Merinuk, "Songs to Sing While Washing Hands: Coronavirus Hand-Washing Songs," *Today.* March 11, 2020, https://www.today.com/health /songs-sing-while-washing-hands-coronavirus-hand-washing-songs-t175755.

2. Andrea Wurzburger, "Dwayne Johnson, Jimmy Fallon, Gloria Gaynor and More Share Their Coronavirus Hand-Washing Songs." *People,* March 24, 2020, https://people.com/health/coronavirus-hand-washing-songs-celebrities/.

3. Michelle Roberts, "Study Reveals Why Some People Get Covid Toe Condition," BBC News, October 6, 2020.

4. Niloufar Haidari, "Kim Kardashian Is Having a Luxurious Lockdown. Why Are People So Surprised?," *The Guardian*, October 29, 2020.

5. Bill Melugin and Shelly Insheiwat. "Fox 11 Obtains Exclusive Photos of Gov. Newsom at French Restaurant Allegedly Not Following COVID-19 Protocols." Fox 11 LA, November 17, 2020, https://www.foxla.com/news/fox-11-obtains -exclusive-photos-of-gov-newsom-at-french-restaurant-allegedly-not-following -covid-19-protocols.

6. Centers for Disease Control and Prevention, *CDC Health Disparities and Inequalities Report—United States, 2013*, https://www.cdc.gov/mmwr/pdf/other /su6203.pdf.

7. Shannon Guzman, "Multigenerational Housing on the Rise, Fueled by Economic and Social Changes," AARP, June 17, 2019, https://www.aarp.org/ppi/info -2019/multigenerational-housing.html.

8. Jennifer Kates et al., "Comparing Trump and Biden on COVID-19." Kaiser Family Foundation, September 11, 2020, https://www.kff.org/coronavirus-covid -19/issue-brief/comparing-trump-and-biden-on-covid-19/?utm_campaign=KFF -2020-Coronavirus&utm_med.

9. Jon Green, Jared Edgerton, Daniel Naftel, Kelsey Shoub, and Skyler J. Cranmer, "Elusive Consensus: Polarization in Elite Communication on the COVID-19 Pandemic," *Science Advances* 6, no. 28 (2020): eabc2717.

10. Only four states did not issue stay-at-home orders: Arkansas, Iowa, Nebraska, and North Dakota. South Dakota, Utah, and Wyoming had regional orders.

11. Deborah Netburn, "A Timeline of the CDC's Advice on Face Masks." *Los Angeles Times*, July 27, 2021, https://www.latimes.com/science/story/2021-07-27 /timeline-cdc-mask-guidance-during-covid-19-pandemic.

12. Gallup, "Coronavirus Pandemic," https://news.gallup.com/poll/308222 /coronavirus-pandemic.aspx.

13. In fact, there was such an acute scarcity of sanitizer that local distilleries and multinational companies alike—including Anheuser-Busch and Pernod Ricard SA (the company behind Absolut vodka and Jameson Irish whiskey)—started redirecting factories to meet demand.

14. A statistical test of the association between education and income reveals that in our sample these two demographic variables are quite closely related: the more education our respondents have, the higher their income.

15. Tyler T. Reny, "Masculine Norms and Infectious Disease: The Case of Covid-19," *Politics & Gender* 16, no. 4 (2020): 1028–35.

16. In fact, the opposite is true. Statistical tests of the relationship between gender and education and between gender and income find that women report lower education and income levels than men.

17. Vincenzo Galasso, Vincent Pons, Paola Profeta, Michael Becher, Sylvain Brouard, and Martial Foucault, "Gender Differences in COVID-19 Attitudes and Behavior: Panel Evidence from Eight Countries," *Proceedings of the National Academy of Sciences* 117, no. 44 (2020): 27285–91.

18. Irmak Olcaysoy Okten, Anton Gollwitzer, and Gabriele Oettingen, "Gender Differences in Preventing the Spread of Coronavirus," *Behavioral Science & Policy* 6, no. 2 (2020): 109–22.

19. Lisa S. Moussaoui, Nana D. Ofosu, and Olivier Desrichard, "Social Psychological Correlates of Protective Behaviours in the COVID-19 Outbreak: Evidence and Recommendations from a Nationally Representative Sample," *Applied Psychology: Health and Well-Being* 12, no. 4 (2020): 1183–204.

20. Christopher T. Rentsch, Farah Kidwai-Khan, Janet P. Tate, Lesley S. Park, Joseph T. King Jr., Melissa Skanderson, Ronald G. Hauser, et al., "Patterns of COVID-19 Testing and Mortality by Race and Ethnicity among United States Veterans: A Nationwide Cohort Study," *PLOS Medicine* 17, no. 9 (2020): e1003379.

21. Marcella Alsan, Stefanie Stantcheva, David Yang, and David Cutler, "Disparities in Coronavirus 2019 Reported Incidence, Knowledge, and Behavior among US Adults," *JAMA Network Open* 3, no. 6 (2020): e2012403.

22. The COVID-19 Tracking Project, https://covidtracking.com. The website ceased collecting new data as of March 7, 2021.

23. Matthew Levendusky, *The Partisan Sort: How Liberals Became Democrats and Conservatives Became Republicans* (Chicago: University of Chicago Press, 2009).

24. Juliane Corman and David Levin, "Support for Government Provision of Health Care and the Patient Protection and Affordable Care Act," *Public Opinion Quarterly* 80, no. 1 (2016): 114–79; Julianna Pacheco, Jake Haselswerdt, and Jamila Michener, "The Affordable Care Act and Polarization in the United States," *RSF: The Russell Sage Foundation Journal of the Social Sciences* 6, no. 2 (2020): 114–30.

25. Tom W. Smith, Michael Davern, Jeremy Freese, and Stephen Morgan, "General Social Surveys, 1972–2018," NORC at the University of Chicago, data accessed from the GSS Data Explorer, gssdataexplorer.norc.org. See also Harry Enten, "Flu Shots Uptake Is Now Partisan. It Didn't Use to Be," CNN, November 14, 2021, https://www.cnn.com/2021/11/14/politics/flu-partisan-divide-analysis/index.html.

26. Matthew A. Baum, "Red State, Blue State, Flu State: Media Self-Selection and Partisan Gaps in Swine Flu Vaccinations," *Journal of Health Politics, Policy and Law* 36, no. 6 (2011): 1021–59.

27. J. Eric Oliver and Taeku Lee, "Public Opinion and the Politics of Obesity in America," *Journal of Health Politics, Policy and Law* 30, no. 5 (2005): 923–54;

Cindy D. Kam, "'And Why Is That a Partisan Issue?' Source Cues, Persuasion, and School Lunches," *Journal of Politics* 82, no. 1 (2020): 361–66.

28. Mya Guarnieri Jaradat, "Stop Saying 'We're All in This Together.' You Have Money. It's Not the Same," *Washington Post*, April 18, 2020.

29. Ashley Kirzinger, Liz Hamel, Cailey Muñana, Audrey Kearney, and Mollyann Brodie, "KFF Health Tracking Poll—Late April 2020: Coronavirus, Social Distancing, and Contact Tracing," Kaiser Family Foundation, April 24, 2020, https://www.kff.org/global-health-policy/issue-brief/kff-health-tracking-poll-late-april-2020/.

30. Philip Ewing and Barbara Sprunt, "Trump Sets Easter Goal for Reopening American Economy," National Public Radio, March 24, 2020.

31. Gallup, "Coronavirus Pandemic."

32. Green et al., "Elusive Consensus."

33. Ian Millhiser, "A Republican Lawsuit Could Force Wisconsin to Reopen Immediately," Vox, May 5, 2020.

34. William H. Frey, "COVID-19 Continues Spreading into Counties with Strong Trump Support," Brooking Institution, May 20, 2020.

35. Guy Grossman, Soojong Kim, Jonah M. Rexer, and Harsha Thirumurthy, "Political Partisanship Influences Behavioral Responses to Governors' Recommendations for COVID-19 Prevention in the United States," *Proceedings of the National Academy of Sciences* 117, no. 39 (2020): 24144–53.

36. Ceren Budak, Ashley Muddiman, and Natalie (Talia) Stroud, "How Did U.S. Television News Networks Cover the Pandemic? Here's a Scorecard," *Washington Post's Monkey Cage*, February 3, 2021.

37. Ibid.

38. Jacob Kastrenakes, "Etsy Sales Doubled in April Thanks to Homemade Masks," The Verge, May 6, 2020.

39. Philip Bump, "The Partisan Revolt against Efforts to Fight the Virus Isn't as Big as You Might Think," *Washington Post*, May 13, 2020.

40. AJMC, "A Timeline of COVID-19 Developments in 2020," January 1, 2021, https://www.ajmc.com/view/a-timeline-of-covid19-developments-in-2020.

41. AJMC Staff, "What We're Reading: Pharma Companies Fund Antibiotic Start-ups; COVID-19 Can Be Airborne; WHO Launches Pandemic Review," July 10, 2020, https://www.ajmc.com/view/what-were-reading-pharma-companies-fund-antibiotic-startups-covid19-can-be-airborne-who-launches-pandemic-review.

42. Christina Morales, "Ted Cruz Was Seen on a Flight without a Mask. His Office Says He Followed Airline Policy," *New York Times*, July 13, 2020.

43. Kasra Zarei and John Duchneskie, "Coronavirus Cases Rise in States with Relaxed Face Mask Policies," *Philadelphia Inquirer*, June 24, 2020.

44. Fenit Nirappil and Julie Zauzmer Weil, "Trump Attended a Fundraiser without a Mask. The City Sent an Investigator to Inspect his Hotel," *Washington Post,* July 22, 2020.

45. Ashley Parker, Josh Dawsey, and Philip Rucker, "White House Implements Stringent Mask Policy—but Not for Trump," *Washington Post*, May 11, 2020.

46. The White House, "Executive Order on Protecting the Federal Workforce and Requiring Mask-Wearing," January 20, 2021, https://www.whitehouse.gov /briefing-room/presidential-actions/2021/01/20/executive-order-protecting-the -federal-workforce-and-requiring-mask-wearing/.

47. Derek K. Chu, Elie A. Akl, Stephanie Duda, Karla Solo, Sally Yaacoub, Holger J. Schünemann, Amena El-harakeh, et al., "Physical Distancing, Face Masks, and Eye Protection to Prevent Person-to-Person Transmission of SARS-CoV-2 and COVID-19: A Systematic Review and Meta-analysis," *The Lancet* 395, no. 10242 (2020): 1973–7.

48. Zarei, "Coronavirus Cases Rise in States with Relaxed Face Mask Policies."

49. "Poll: 82 Percent of Voters Support a National Face Mask Mandate," The Hill, August 3, 2020.

50. YouGov, "The Economist/YouGov Poll: January 16–19, 2021—1500 U.S. Adult Citizens," https://docs.cdn.yougov.com/4k61xul7y7/econTabReport.pdf.

51. Bill Chappell, "3rd Member of Congress Tests Positive for Coronavirus, Blames Capitol Attack Lockdown." National Public Radio, January 12, 2021.

52. Jesus Jimenez, "Airline Bars Alaska State Senator over Mask Policy Violation," *New York Times*, April 26, 2021.

53. Samuel Bazzi, Martin Fiszbein, and Mesay Gebresilasse, "'Rugged Individualism' and Collective (in)Action during the COVID-19 Pandemic," *Journal of Public Economics* 195 (2021): 104357.

54. Carl L. Palmer and Rolfe D. Peterson, "Toxic Mask-ulinity: The Link between Masculine Toughness and Affective Reactions to Mask Wearing in the COVID-19 Era," *Politics & Gender* 16, no. 4 (2020): 1044–51; Dan Cassino and Yasemin Besen-Cassino, "Of Masks and Men? Gender, Sex, and Protective Measures during COVID-19," *Politics & Gender* 16, no. 4 (2020): 1052–62.

55. "Face-off over Face-Masks: Europe's Latest North-South Split," *The Economist*, July 8, 2020.

56. "COVID-19 Behaviour Tracker," Institute of Global Health Innovation, Imperial College London, http://www.coviddatahub.com/.

57. Vincent Chi-Chung Cheng, Shuk-Ching Wong, Vivien Wai-Man Chuang, Simon Yung-Chun So, Jonathan Hon-Kwan Chen, Siddharth Sridhar, Kelvin Kai-Wang To, et al., "The Role of Community-wide Wearing of Face Mask for Control of Coronavirus Disease 2019 (COVID-19) Epidemic Due to SARS-CoV-2," *Journal of Infection* 81, no. 1 (2020): 107–14.

58. Helier Cheung, "Coronavirus: Why Attitudes to Masks Have Changed around the World," BBC News, July 14, 2020.

59. Anwar Mohammed, Regan M. Johnston, and Clifton van der Linden, "Public Responses to Policy Reversals: The Case of Mask Usage in Canada during COVID-19," *Canadian Public Policy 46*, no. S2 (2020): S119–S26.

60. YouGov, "YouGov—Coronavirus Tracker UK," https://docs.cdn.yougov .com/w13gbqyhqq/YouGov%20-%20Coronavirus%20tracker%20UK%207-8%20 Sep%202020.pdf.

Chapter 4

1. Joe Hernandez, "The FAA Has Seen A 'Significantly Higher' Number of Unruly Passenger Reports in 2021," National Public Radio, May 28, 2021.

2. Alicia Victoria Lozano, "Southwest Airlines Employee Hospitalized after Passenger Punched Her, Police Say," NBC News, November 13, 2021.

3. Francesca Street, "Dread at 30,000 Feet: Inside the Increasingly Violent World of US Flight Attendants," CNN, September 6, 2021.

4. Craig A. Smith and Phoebe C. Ellsworth, "Patterns of Cognitive Appraisal in Emotion," *Journal of Personality and Social Psychology* 48, no. 4 (1985): 813–38.

5. Richard S. Lazarus, "Cognition and Motivation in Emotion," *American Psychologist* 46, no. 4 (1991): 352–67; James Gross and Ross Thompson, "Emotion Regulation: Conceptual Foundations," In *Handbook of Emotion Regulation*, ed. James Gross, 3–26 (New York: Guilford, 2009).

6. W. Russell Neuman, George Marcus, Ann N. Crigler, and Michael MacKuen, eds., *The Affect Effect: Dynamics of Emotion in Political Thinking and Behavior* (Chicago: University of Chicago Press, 2007); Ted Brader and Nicholas A. Valentino, "Identities, Interests, and Emotions: Symbolic versus Material Wellsprings of Fear, Anger, and Enthusiasm," in *The Affect Effect: Dynamics of Emotion in Political Thinking and Behavior*, ed. W. Russell Neuman, George E. Marcus, Ann N. Crigler, and Michael MacKuen, 180–201 (Chicago: University of Chicago Press, 2007); Eric Groenendyk, Ted Brader, and Nicholas Valentino, "Appraising Political Emotions: Appraisals, Emotions, and Behavior in Response to Threatening News," ResearchGate, January 2011; Pavlos Vasilopoulos, "Terrorist Events, Emotional Reactions, and Political Participation: The 2015 Paris Attacks," *West European Politics* 41, no. 1 (2018): 102–27; Lene Aarøe, Michael Bang Petersen, and Kevin Arceneaux, "The Behavioral Immune System Shapes Political Intuitions: Why and How Individual Differences in Disgust Sensitivity Underlie Opposition to Immigration," *American Political Science Review* 111, no. 2 (2017): 277–94.

7. Shana Kushner Gadarian, "Scary Pictures: How Terrorism Imagery Affects Voter Evaluations," *Political Communication* 31, no. 2 (2014): 282–302; Arthur Lupia and Jesse Menning, "Politics and the Equilibrium of Fear: Can Strategies and Emotions Interact?," in *The Affect Effect: Dynamics of Emotion in Political Thinking and Behavior*, ed. George E. Marcus, W. Russell Neuman, and Michael MacKuen, 337–56 (Chicago: University of Chicago Press, 2008).

8. Davin L. Phoenix, *The Anger Gap: How Race Shapes Emotion in Politics* (New York: Cambridge University Press, 2019); Eric Groenendyk, "Current Emotion Research in Political Science: How Emotions Help Democracy Overcome Its Collective Action Problem." *Emotion Review* 3, no. 4 (2011): 455–63.

9. Jon Green, Jared Edgerton, Daniel Naftel, Kelsey Shoub, and Skyler J. Cranmer, "Elusive Consensus: Polarization in Elite Communication on the COVID-19 Pandemic," *Science Advances* 6, no. 28 (2020): eabc2717.

10. Susan Folkman and Richard S. Lazarus, "Coping as a Mediator of Emotion," *Journal of Personality and Social Psychology* 54, no. 3 (1988): 466.

11. George Marcus, W. Russell Neuman, and Michael MacKuen, *Affective Intelligence and Political Judgment* (Chicago: University of Chicago Press, 2000).

12. Bethany Albertson and Shana Kushner Gadarian, *Anxious Politics: Democratic Citizenship in a Threatening World* (New York: Cambridge University Press, 2015).

13. Steven W. Webster, *American Rage: How Anger Shapes Our Politics* (Cambridge: Cambridge University Press, 2020).

14. Ira Roseman, Martin Spindel, and Paul Jose, "Appraisals of Emotion-Eliciting Events: Testing a Theory of Discrete Emotions," *Journal of Personality and Social Psychology* 59, no. 5 (1990): 899–915.

15. Ken Alltucker and Grace Hauck, "Trump Addressed the Nation on Coronavirus. We Checked the Facts," *USA Today*, February 26, 2020.

16. Gross and Thompson, "Emotion Regulation"; Christina L. Jones, Jakob D. Jensen, Courtney L. Scherr, Natasha R. Brown, Katheryn Christy, and Jeremy Weaver, "The Health Belief Model as an Explanatory Framework in Communication Research: Exploring Parallel, Serial, and Moderated Mediation," *Health Communication* 30, no. 6 (2015): 566–76.

17. Robert F. Schoeni, Emily E. Wiemers, Judith A. Seltzer, and Kenneth M. Langa, "Association between Risk Factors for Complications from COVID-19, Perceived Chances of Infection and Complications, and Protective Behavior in the US," *JAMA Network Open* 4, no. 3 (2021): e213984.

18. Sarah E. Gollust, Rebekah H. Nagler, and Erika Franklin Fowler, "The Emergence of COVID-19 in the US: A Public Health and Political Communication Crisis," *Journal of Health Politics, Policy and Law* 45, no. 6 (2020): 967–81; Mark Pickup, Dominik Stecula, and Clifton Van Der Linden, "Novel Coronavirus, Old Partisanship: COVID-19 Attitudes and Behaviours in the United States and Canada," *Canadian Journal of Political Science/Revue canadienne de science politique* 53, no. 2 (2020): 357–64.

19. Emily Stewart, "Anti-Maskers Explain Themselves," Vox, August 7, 2020; Bill Hutchinson, "'Incomprehensible': Confrontations over Masks Erupt amid COVID-19 Crisis," ABC News, May 7, 2020.

20. Morris Fiorina, *Retrospective Voting in American National Elections* (New Have, CT: Yale University Press, 1981).

21. Christopher H. Achen and Larry M. Bartels, *Democracy for Realists: Why Elections Do Not Produce Responsive Government* (Princeton, NJ: Princeton University Press, 2017).

22. Donald M. Taylor and Janet R. Doria, "Self-Serving and Group-Serving Bias in Attribution," *Journal of Social Psychology* 113, no. 2 (1981): 201–11.

23. Thomas J. Rudolph, "Who's Responsible for the Economy? The Formation and Consequences of Responsibility Attributions," *American Journal of Political Science* 47, no. 4 (2003): 698–713.

24. Neil Malhotra and Alexander G. Kuo, "Attributing Blame: The Public's Response to Hurricane Katrina," *Journal of Politics* 70, no. 1 (2008): 120–35.

25. Saundra Schneider, "Who's to Blame? (Mis)perceptions of the Intergovernmental Response to Disasters," *Publius: Journal of Federalism* 38, no. 4 (2008): 715–38.

26. David Karol and Edward Miguel, "The Electoral Cost of War: Iraq Casualties and the 2004 U.S. Presidential Election," *Journal of Politics* 69, no. 3 (2007): 633–48; Andrew Healy and Neil Malhotra, "Random Events, Economic Losses, and Retrospective Voting: Implications for Democratic Competence," *Quarterly Journal of Political Science* 5, no. 2 (2010): 193–208.

27. Albertson and Gadarian, *Anxious Politics*; Sara Wallace Goodman, *Citizenship in Hard Times: How Ordinary People Respond to Democratic Threat* (New York: Cambridge University Press, 2022).

28. Terry Nguyen, "How the Trump Administration Has Stood in the Way of PPE Distribution," Vox, April 4, 2020.

29. Brian J. Gaines, James H. Kuklinski, Paul J. Quirk, Buddy Peyton, and Jay Verkuilen, "Same Facts, Different Interpretations: Partisan Motivation and Opinion on Iraq," *Journal of Politics* 69, no. 4 (2007): 957–74; Larry Bartels, "Beyond the Running Tally: Partisan Bias in Political Perceptions," *Political Behavior 24*, no. 2 (2002): 117–50.

Chapter 5

1. Ryan Carter, "Long Lines, Big Demand: Still-Limited LA-Area Drive-through Coronavirus Testing Inches Ahead," *Los Angeles Daily News*, March 25, 2020.

2. Melody Petersen and Emily Baumgaertner, "Bottlenecks in Coronavirus Testing Means Excruciating Wait Times for the Sick," *Los Angeles Times*, March 30, 2020.

3. Jack Dolan and Brittny Meija, "LA County Gives Up on Containing Coronavirus, Tells Doctors to Skip Testing of Some Patients," *Los Angeles Times*, March 20, 2020.

4. Lindsey Dawson and Jennifer Kates, "Rapid Home Tests for COVID-19: Issues with Availability and Access in the U.S.," Kaiser Family Foundation, November 4, 2021.

5. Yasmeen Abutaleb, "Biden Administration Looks to Speed Authorization of Rapid Coronavirus Tests," *Washington Post*, October 25, 2021.

6. "What We Know about Delays in Coronavirus Testing," *Washington Post*, March 16, 2020.

7. Ibid.

8. Peter Whoriskey and Neena Satija, "How U.S. Coronavirus Testing Stalled: Flawed Tests, Red Tape and Resistance to Using the Millions of Tests Produced by the WHO," *Washington Post*, March 16, 2020.

9. Farah Stockman, "Sick People across the U.S. Say They Are Being Denied the Coronavirus Test," *New York Times*, March 12, 2020.

10. Alana Wise, "Trump Defends Testing Capacity Despite Experts' Warnings," National Public Radio, April 17, 2020.

11. Data on vaccine allocation are from "Weekly COVID-19 Vaccine Allocations," Kaiser Family Foundation, May 31, 2021, https://www.kff.org/other/state-indicator/weekly-covid-19-vaccine-allocations/?currentTimeframe

=3&selectedRows=%7B%22wrapups%22:%7B%22united-states%22:%7B%7D%7D%7D%7D&sortModel=%7B%22colId%22:%22Location%22,%22sort%22:%22asc%22%7D.

12. David T. Burbach, "Partisan Dimensions of Confidence in the US Military, 1973–2016," *Armed Forces & Society* 45, no. 2 (2019): 211–33.

13. Joseph Turow, Michael Hennessy, Nora Draper, Ope Akanbi, and Diami Virgilio, *Divided We Feel: Partisan Politics Drive Americans' Emotions Regarding Surveillance of Low-Income Populations*. A Report from the Annenberg School for Communication, University of Pennsylvania, 2018.

14. Monica Anderson and Brooke Auxier, "Most Americans Don't Think Cellphone Tracking Will Help Limit COVID-19, Are Divided on Whether It's Acceptable," Pew Research Center, April 16, 2020, https://www.pewresearch.org/fact-tank/2020/04/16/most-americans-dont-think-cellphone-tracking-will-help-limit-covid-19-are-divided-on-whether-its-acceptable/.

15. Samuel Altmann, Luke Milsom, Hannah Zillessen, Raffaele Blasone, Frederic Gerdon, Ruben Bach, Frauke Kreuter, et al., "Acceptability of App-based Contact Tracing for COVID-19: Cross-country Survey Study," *JMIR mHealth and uHealth* 8, no. 8 (2020): e19857; Baobao Zhang, Sarah Kreps, Nina McMurry, and R. Miles McCain, "Americans' Perceptions of Privacy and Surveillance in the COVID-19 Pandemic," *PLOS One* 15, no. 12 (2020): e0242652.

16. M. Guillon and P. Kergall, "Attitudes and Opinions on Quarantine and Support for a Contact-Tracing Application in France during the COVID-19 Outbreak," *Public Health* 188 (2020): 21–31.

17. Craig Timberg and Drew Harwell, "Government Efforts to Track Virus through Phone Location Data Complicated by Privacy Concerns," *Washington Post*, March 19, 2020.

18. E. J. Dionne Jr., *Why Americans Hate Politics* (New York: Simon & Schuster, 1991).

19. Olga Khazan, "The Most American COVID-19 Failure Yet," *The Atlantic*, August 31, 2020.

20. "Top Doctors Give Blistering Assessment of Trump Pandemic Response; Sen. Raphael Warnock (D-GA) Blasts Georgia's Voting Overhaul," CNN, March 29, 2021, http://www.cnn.com/TRANSCRIPTS/2103/29/nday.03.html.

21. Yascha Mounk, "Cancel Everything," *The Atlantic*, March 10, 2020.

22. Ashley Tisdale, one of the stars of Disney's *High School Musical*, even took to TikTok to re-create the choreography from the final song of the movie, "We're all in this together."

23. Kirk Siegler, "Across America, Frustrated Protesters Rally to Reopen the Economy," National Public Radio, April 18, 2020.

24. Economists estimate that these rallies "resulted in more than 30,000 incremental confirmed cases of COVID-19" and "more than 700 deaths (not necessarily among attendees)." Bert Douglas Bernheim, Nina Buchmann, Zach Freitas-Groff, and Sebastián Otero, "The Effects of Large Group Meetings on the Spread of COVID-19: The Case of Trump Rallies," Stanford Institute for Economic Policy Research Working Paper No. 20-043, 2020.

25. Felicia Sonmez, "Texas Lt. Gov. Dan Patrick Comes under Fire for Saying Seniors Should 'Take A Chance' on Their Own Lives for Sake of Grandchildren during Coronavirus Crisis," *Washington Post*, March 24, 2020.

26. "Map: Coronavirus and School Closures in 2019–2020," Education Week, March 6, 2020, https://www.edweek.org/leadership/map-coronavirus-and-school-closures-in-2019-2020/2020/03.

27. Emily Oster, "Parents Can't Wait around Forever," *The Atlantic*, July 2, 2020.

28. Ellen H. Lee, Kelsey L. Kepler, Anita Geevarughese, Rachel Paneth-Pollak, Marie S. Dorsinville, Stephanie Ngai, and Kathleen H. Reilly, "Race/Ethnicity among Children with COVID-19–Associated Multisystem Inflammatory Syndrome," *JAMA Network Open* 3, no. 11 (2020): e2030280.

29. Matt Grossmann, Sarah Reckhow, Katharine O. Strunk, and Meg Turner, "All States Close but Red Districts Reopen: The Politics of In-Person Schooling during the COVID-19 Pandemic," *Educational Researcher* 50, no. 9 (2021): 637–48.

30. Jeremy B. White, "Trump Claims 'Total Authority' over State Decisions," Politico, April 13, 2020.

31. ABC News, "Competition among States, Local Governments Creates Bidding War for Medical Equipment," April 3, 2020.

32. Ella Nilsen, "New York Is in Dire Need of Ventilators. China Just Donated 1,000," Vox, April 4, 2020.

33. Danielle Garrand, "California Received '170 Broken Ventilators' from Federal Government, Governor Says," CBS News, March 29, 2020.

34. Daniel Desrochers, "39 New Kentucky Coronavirus Cases Found. Total is 163. More Businesses Must Close," *Lexington Herald Leader*, March 24, 2020.

35. Mirya R. Holman, Emily M. Farris, and Jane Lawrence Sumner, "Local Political Institutions and First-Mover Policy Responses to COVID-19," *Journal of Political Institutions and Political Economy* 1, no. 4 (2020): 523–41.

36. Guy Grossman, Soojong Kim, Jonah M. Rexer, and Harsha Thirumurthy, "Political Partisanship Influences Behavioral Responses to Governors' Recommendations for COVID-19 Prevention in the United States," *Proceedings of the National Academy of Sciences* 117, no. 39 (2020): 24144–53.

37. Renae Merle, "Trump Says He's 'Stopping Evictions.' Here's Why They're Still Happening," *Washington Post*, August 17, 2020.

38. Gabriel S. Lenz, *Follow the Leader? How Voters Respond to Politicians' Policies and Performance* (Chicago: University of Chicago Press, 2013).

Chapter 6

1. Ruth Simon, "Covid-19's Toll on U.S. Business? 200,000 Extra Closures in Pandemic's First Year," *Wall Street Journal,* April 16, 2021.

2. Yelp, "Local Economic Impact Report," September 2020, https://www.yelpeconomicaverage.com/business-closures-update-sep-2020

3. Nellie Bowles, "Hurt by Lockdowns, California's Small Businesses Push to Recall Governor," *New York Times*, February 19, 2021.

4. "Biden Unveils $1.9 Trillion Economic and Health-Care Relief Package," *Washington Post*, January 14, 2021.

5. "A Torrent of Job Losses Threatens to Overwhelm the U.S. Economy," *New York Times*, March 19, 2020.

6. Unemployment data come from the monthly Current Population Survey and reflect those who are out of work but have been actively looking for work over the past month. It does not include Americans who are not actively looking for work.

7. Thomas B. Pepinsky, "Political Economy and Democratic Capacity to Respond to Pandemics," Social Science Research Council, May 21, 2020, https://items.ssrc.org/covid-19-and-the-social-sciences/democracy-and-pandemics/political-economy-and-democratic-capacity-to-respond-to-pandemics/.

8. "How Germany Saved Its Workforce from Unemployment While Spending Less Per Person Than the U.S," ProPublica, June 3, 2020. https://www.propublica.org/article/how-germany-saved-its-workforce-from-unemployment-while-spending-less-per-person-than-the-u-s; Abi Adams-Prassl, Teodora Boneva, Marta Golin, and Christopher Rauh, "Inequality in the Impact of the Coronavirus Shock: Evidence from Real Time Surveys," *Journal of Public Economics* 189 (2020): 104245.

9. "Bankers Rebuke S.B.A. as Loan System Crashes in Flood of Applications," *New York Times*, April 27, 2020; "Stimulus Cops on Lookout for Fake Employees, Identity Theft," *Wall Street Journal*, May 13, 2020.

10. Randy Albelda, "Gender Impacts of the 'Great Recession' in the United States," in *Women and Austerity*, ed. Maria Karamessini and Jill Rubery, 82–101 (London: Routledge, 2013).

11. "How Millions of Women Became the Most Essential Workers in America," *New York Times*, April 18, 2020.

12. Note that the unemployment rates listed here do not count people who are temporarily providing childcare as unemployed.

13. Titan Alon, Matthias Doepke, Jane Olmstead-Rumsey, and Michèle Tertilt, "This Time It's Different: The Role of Women's Employment in a Pandemic Recession," NBER Working Paper No. 27660, 2020; Stefania Albanesi and Jiyeon Kim, "The Gendered Impact of the COVID-19 Recession on the US Labor Market," NBER Working Paper No. 28505, 2021.

14. Raj Chetty, John Friedman, Nathaniel Hendren, Michael Stepner, and the Opportunity Insights Team, "The Economic Impacts of COVID-19: Evidence from a New Public Database Built Using Private Sector Data," NBER Working Paper No. 26463, 2020; Adams-Prassl et al., "Inequality in the Impact of the Coronavirus Shock."

15. Monica Hake, Adam Dewey, Emily Engelhard, Angela Gallagher, Tom Summerfelt, Corey Malone-Smolla, Tremain Maebry, and Craig Gundersen, "The Impact of the Coronavirus on Local Food Insecurity," Feeding America, March 31, 2021, https://www.feedingamerica.org/research/coronavirus-hunger-research.

16. "As Hunger Swells, Food Stamps Become a Partisan Flash Point," *New York Times*, May 6, 2020.

17. "DeSantis Suspends Work Requirements for Food Stamps until Sept. 1," *Orlando Sentinel*, July 28, 2020.

18. "Federal Judge Strikes Down Trump Plan to Slash Food Stamps for 700,000 Unemployed Americans," *Washington Post*, October 18, 2020.

19. "Trump Floats Economic Stimulus in Response to Coronavirus," *New York Times*, March 9, 2020.

20. "Coronavirus Tests Limits of Central Bank Firepower," *New York Times*, February 29, 2020.

21. João Granja, Christos Makridis, Constantine Yannelis, and Eric Zwick, "Did the Paycheck Protection Program Hit the Target?," NBER Working Paper No. 27095, 2020.

22. "'The Big Guys Get Bailed Out': Restaurants Vie for Relief Funds," *New York Times*, April 20, 2020.

23. Sharon Parrott, Chad Stone, Chye-Ching Huang, Michael Leachman, Peggy Bailey, Aviva Aron-Dine, Stacy Dean, and LaDonna Pavetti, "CARES Act Includes Essential Measures to Respond to Public Health, Economic Crises, but More Will Be Needed," Center on Budget and Policy Priorities, March 27, 2020, https://www.cbpp.org/sites/default/files/atoms/files/3-27-20econ.pdf.

24. "Poultry Worker's Death Highlights Spread of Coronavirus in Meat Plants," *New York Times*, April 19, 2020.

25. Polly Mosendz, Peter Waldman, and Lydia Mulvany, "U.S. Meat Plants Are Deadly as Ever, with No Incentive to Change," Bloomberg, June 18, 2020.

26. "China's Exports Plunge amid Coronavirus Epidemic," *Wall Street Journal*, March 7, 2020.

27. "U.S. Suspends Tariffs for Some Importers Affected by Coronavirus," *Wall Street Journal*, April 19, 2020.

28. Jeffrey A. Frankel, "'No Atheists in Foxholes'? No Libertarians in Financial Crises," Belfer Center, Harvard University, July 17, 2008, https://www.belfercenter.org/publication/no-atheists-foxholes-no-libertarians-financial-crises.

29. Of course, we recognize that these ideological labels are inevitably overly simplistic (and that those particular coalitions can shift by economy policy area, with some libertarians siding with progressives against corporate welfare, for example).

30. Rubrick Biegon, "A Populist Grand Strategy? Trump and the Framing of American Decline," *International Relations* 33, no. 4 (2019): 517–39.

31. Joseph Stiglitz, "Lessons from COVID-19 and Trump for Theory and Policy (Paper)," *Journal of Policy Modeling* 43, no. 4 (2021): 749–60.

32. Jason Kuo and Megumi Naoi, "Individual Attitudes," in *The Oxford Handbook of the Political Economy of International Trade*, ed. Lisa Martin, 99–118 (New York: Oxford University Press, 2015).

33. "Germany Boosts Already Hefty Coronavirus Stimulus," *Wall Street Journal*, August 26, 2020.

Chapter 7

1. "Buy American and Hire American," Executive Order 13788, Federal Register, April 18, 2017, https://www.federalregister.gov/documents/2017/04/21/2017 -08311/buy-american-and-hire-american.

2. Caitlin Dickerson and Michael D. Shear, "Before Covid-19, Trump Aide Sought to Use Disease to Close Borders," *New York Times*, May 3, 2020.

3. Initially, restrictions only applied to the twenty-six countries of the Schengen Area, Europe's free movement zone. It was extended on March 14 to Ireland and the United Kingdom.

4. Hope Yen, "AP FACT CHECK: Trump's Inaccurate Boasts on China Travel Ban," Associated Press, March 26, 2020.

5. Lorenzo Piccoli, Jelena Dzankic, Andreas Perret, Didier Ruedin, and Timothy Craig Jacob-Owens, "International Travel Restrictions in Response to the COVID-19 Outbreak Dataset," EUI Research Data, Robert Schuman Centre for Advanced Studies, 2020, https://hdl.handle.net/1814/68359.

6. Timothy C. Germann, Kai Kadau, Ira M. Longini, and Catherine A. Macken, "Mitigation Strategies for Pandemic Influenza in the United States," *Proceedings of the National Academy of Sciences* 103, no. 15 (2006): 5935–40.

7. Matteo Chinazzi, Jessica T. Davis, Marco Ajelli, Corrado Gioannini, Maria Litvinova, Stefano Merler, Ana Pastore y Piontti, et al., "The Effect of Travel Restrictions on the Spread of the 2019 Novel Coronavirus (COVID-19) Outbreak," *Science* (2020): eaba9757.

8. Reuters, "Germany Treats First Italians as Coronavirus Care Crosses Borders," March 24, 2020.

9. Arne Delfs and Naomi Kresge, "Merkel Says Covid Spike 'Worse Than Anything We've Seen,'" Bloomberg, November 22, 2021.

10. Kim Yi Dionne and Fulya Felicity Turkmen, "The Politics of Pandemic Othering: Putting COVID-19 in Global and Historical Context," *International Organization* 74, no. S1 (2020): E213–E30.

11. Sara Wallace Goodman, "Should U.S. States Be Free to Close Their Borders to Other U.S. Citizens?," *Washington Post*, April 3, 2020.

12. "NSW, Victoria Border Open for Fully Vaccinated at Midnight," *The Age*, November 4, 2021.

13. Andrew Daniller, "Americans' Immigration Policy Priorities: Divisions between—and within—the Two Parties," Pew Research Center, November 11, 2019, https://www.pewresearch.org/fact-tank/2019/11/12/americans-immigration -policy-priorities-divisions-between-and-within-the-two-parties/.

14. Mohamed Younis, "Americans Want More, Not Less, Immigration for First Time," Gallup, July 1, 2020, https://news.gallup.com/poll/313106/americans-not -less-immigration-first-time.aspx.

15. Efrén O. Pérez, "Explicit Evidence on the Import of Implicit Attitudes: The IAT and Immigration Policy Judgments," *Political Behavior* 32, no. 4 (2010): 517–45; Kumar Yogeeswaran and Nilanjana Dasgupta, "Will the 'Real' American

Please Stand Up? The Effect of Implicit National Prototypes on Discriminatory Behavior and Judgments," *Personality and Social Psychology Bulletin* 36, no. 10 (2010): 1332–45.

16. Marisa Abrajano and Zoltan L. Hajnal, *White Backlash: Immigration, Race, and American Politics.* Princeton, NJ: Princeton University Press, 2017.

17. Nicholas A. Valentino, Ted Brader, and Ashley E. Jardina, "Immigration Opposition among US Whites: General Ethnocentrism or Media Priming of Attitudes about Latinos?," *Political Psychology* 34, no. 2 (2013): 149–66.

18. Alexander Kustov, Dillon Laaker, and Cassidy Reller, "The Stability of Immigration Attitudes: Evidence and Implications," *Journal of Politics* 83, no. 4: 1478–94.

19. Mathew J. Creighton, Amaney Jamal, and Natalia C. Malancu, "Has Opposition to Immigration Increased in the United States after the Economic Crisis? An Experimental Approach," *International Migration Review* 49, no. 3 (2015): 727–56.

20. Paul M. Sniderman, Michael Bang Petersen, Rune Slothuus, Rune Stubager, and Philip Petrov, "Reactions to Terror Attacks: A Heuristic Model," *Political Psychology* 40, no. S1 (2019): 245–58; Victoria M. Esses, John F. Dovidio, and Gordon Hodson, "Public Attitudes toward Immigration in the United States and Canada in Response to the September 11, 2001 'Attack on America.'" *Analyses of Social Issues and Public Policy* 2, no. 1 (2002): 69–85.

21. Sara Wallace Goodman, "Immigration Threat, Partisanship, and Democratic Citizenship: Evidence from the US, UK, and Germany," *Comparative Political Studies* (2021): 0010414021997165.

22. Elliot Clissold, Davina Nylander, Cameron Watson, and Antonio Ventriglio, "Pandemics and Prejudice," *International Journal of Social Psychiatry* 66, no. 5 (2020): 421–23. For a general overview, see Dionne and Turkmen, "The Politics of Pandemic Othering."

23. Daniel Straus and Oliver Laughland, "Trump Calls Coronavirus Criticism Democrats' 'New Hoax' and Links It to Immigration," *The Guardian*, February 28, 2020.

24. Thomas J. Bollyky and Jennifer B. Nuzzo, "Trump's 'Early' Travel 'Bans' Weren't Early, Weren't Bans and Didn't Work," *Washington Post*, October 1, 2020.

25. Stephen Braun and Jason Dearen, "Trump's 'Strong Wall' to Block COVID-19 from China Had Holes," Associated Press, July 4, 2020.

26. Steve Eder, Henry Fountain, Michael H. Keller, Muyi Xiao, and Alexandra Stevenson, "430,000 People Have Traveled from China to U.S. since Coronavirus Surfaced," *New York Times*, April 4, 2020.

27. "Cotton, Colleagues Urge Expansion and Extension of Immigration Proclamation," Tom Cotton: Senator for Arkansas, May 7, 2020. https://www.cotton.senate.gov/news/press-releases/cotton-colleagues-urge-expansion-and-extension-of-immigration-proclamation.

28. "Public Health Experts Urge U.S. Officials to Withdraw Order Enabling Mass Expulsion of Asylum Seekers," ReliefWeb, May 19, 2020, https://reliefweb.int/report/united-states-america/public-health-experts-urge-us-officials-withdraw-order-enabling-mass.

29. United States Department of State, "Important Announcement on H2 Visas," March 26, 2020, https://travel.state.gov/content/travel/en/News/visas -news/important-announcement-on-h2-visas.html.

30. Priscilla Alvarez, "Trump Administration Proposes Blocking Asylum Seekers on Public Health Grounds," CNN, July 8, 2020.

31. Candace Norwood, "Trump Restricts Immigration amid the Pandemic. Critics See It as an Excuse to Push His Own Agenda," PBS, July 28, 2020.

32. This search can be repeated at "United States: 1/1/20–4/1/20," Google Trends, https://bit.ly/3q0jUg0.

33. Tali Mendelberg, *The Race Card: Campaign Strategy, Implicit Messages, and the Norm of Equality* (Princeton, NJ: Princeton University Press, 2001).

34. Goodman, "Should U.S. States Be Free to Close Their Borders to Other U.S. Citizens?"

35. Colleen Wilson, "Murphy 'Would Love' to Turn People Away at NJ Borders, but Not Ready to Enforce Quarantine," NorthJersey.com, July 15, 2020.

Chapter 8

1. Ron French and Oralandar Brand-Williams, "Cost of Segregation: Blacks Pay Harsh Price While Whites Suffer Less," *Detroit News*, April 15, 2020; Rashawn Ray, Jane Fran Morgan, Lydia Wildeden, Samantha Elizondo, and Destiny Wiley-Yancy, "Examining and Addressing COVID-19 Racial Disparities in Detroit," Brookings Institution, March 2, 2021, https://www.brookings.edu/research/examining-and -addressing-covid-19-racial-disparities-in-detroit/.

2. Ray et al., "Examining and Addressing COVID-19 Racial Disparities in Detroit."

3. Colin Dwyer, "'Take This Serious': Bus Driver Dies of COVID-19 after Calling Out Coughing Rider," National Public Radio, April 3, 2021.

4. Rashawn Ray, "Why Are Blacks Dying at Higher Rates from COVID-19?," Brookings Institution, March 2, 2020, https://www.brookings.edu/blog/fixgov /2020/04/09/why-are-blacks-dying-at-higher-rates-from-covid-19/.

5. Ruth Igielnik, Scott Keeter, and Hannah Hartig, "Behind Biden's 2020 Victory," Pew Research Center, June 30, 2021, https://www.pewresearch.org/politics /2021/06/30/behind-bidens-2020-victory/.

6. APM Research Lab Staff, "The Color of Coronavirus: COVID-19 Deaths by Race and Ethnicity in the US," March 5, 2021, https://www.apmresearchlab.org /covid/deaths-by-race.

7. The COVID Racial Data Tracker, https://covidtracking.com/race.

8. Sarah Hatcher, Christine Agnew-Brune, Mark Anderson, Laura Zambrando, Charles Rose, Melissa Jim, and Amy Buagher, "COVID-19 among American Indian and Alaska Native Persons—23 States, January 31–July 3, 2020," In *Morbidity and Mortality Weekly Report*, ed. Centers for Disease Control and Prevention, 1166–69 (Washington, DC: U.S. Department of Health and Human Services and Centers for Disease Control and Prevention, 2020).

9. Talha Burki, "COVID-19 among American Indians and Alaska Natives," *Lancet Infectious Diseases* 21, no. 3 (2021): 325–26.

10. Ben Spencer, "'Racist' Oxygen Device May Explain Why Covid Hit Minorities So Hard," *Sunday Times*, November 21, 2021.

11. Yin Paradies, Mandy Truong, and Naomi Priest, "A Systematic Review of the Extent and Measurement of Healthcare Provider Racism," *Journal of General Internal Medicine* 29, no. 2 (2014): 364–87.

12. Merrill Singer, "A Dose of Drugs, a Touch of Violence, a Case of AIDS: Conceptualizing the SAVA Syndemic," *Free Inquiry in Creative Sociology* 28, no. 1 (2000): 13–24.

13. Ruth Petersen, Liping Pan, and Heidi M. Blanck, "Racial and Ethnic Disparities in Adult Obesity in the United States: CDC's Tracking to Inform State and Local Action," *Preventing Chronic Disease* 16 (2019).

14. National Center for Health Statistics, "National Vital Statistics System, Mortality," 2019, https://www.cdc.gov/nchs/nvss/deaths.htm.

15. Christopher W. Tessum, David A. Paolella, Sarah E. Chambliss, Joshua S. Apte, Jason D. Hill, and Julian D. Marshall, "PM2.5 Polluters Disproportionately and Systemically Affect People of Color in the United States," *Science Advances* 7, no. 18 (2021): eabf4491.

16. Raymond Foxworth, Laura E. Evans, Gabriel R. Sanchez, Cheryl Ellenwood, and Carmela M. Roybal, "'I Hope to Hell Nothing Goes Back to the Way It Was Before': COVID-19, Marginalization, and Native Nations," *Perspectives on Politics* (2021): 1–18.

17. Combining racial and ethnic groups together in this last category does mean that we cannot use our data to identify particularities of the Asian American or Native American experience. However, for waves 1–5 of our survey, even with the relatively large sample sizes that we are working with, the number of respondents identifying with one of these groups is simply too small for meaningful statistical comparisons.

18. Using Census Quick Facts to calculate 2019 population, 13.4 percent are Black (one race) out of 328,239,523 Americans, and the population of black Americans is 43,984,096. These data are available at "Population Estimates, July 1 2021, (V2021)," https://www.census.gov/quickfacts/fact/table/US/PST045219. The white-Black gap in good health in our data is 5 percent.

19. Chris Sloan, Robin Duddy-Tenbrunsel, Samantha Ferguson, and Angel Valladares, "COVID-19 Projected to Worsen Racial Disparities in Health Coverage," Avalere, September 16, 2020, https://avalere.com/press-releases/covid-19 -projected-to-worsen-racial-disparities-in-health-coverage.

20. Sabu V. Subramanian and Ichiro Kawachi, "The Association between State Income Inequality and Worse Health Is Not Confounded by Race," *International Journal of Epidemiology* 32, no. 6 (2003): 1022–28.

21. Angus Deaton and Darren Lubotsky, "Mortality, Inequality and Race in American Cities and States," *Social Science & Medicine* 56, no. 6 (2003): 1139–53.

22. Jennifer Valentino-DeVries, Denise Lu, and Gabriel J. X. Dance, "Location Data Says It All: Staying at Home during Coronavirus Is a Luxury," *New York Times*,

April 3, 2020; Annabel X. Tan, Jessica A. Hinman, Hoda S. Abdel Magid, Lorene M. Nelson, and Michelle C. Odden, "Association between Income Inequality and County-Level COVID-19 Cases and Deaths in the US," *JAMA Network Open* 4, no. 5 (2021): e218799; Qinggang Yu, Cristina E. Salvador, Irene Melani, Martha K. Berg, Enrique W. Neblett, and Shinobu Kitayama, "Racial Residential Segregation and Economic Disparity Jointly Exacerbate COVID-19 Fatality in Large American Cities," *Annals of the New York Academy of Sciences* 1494 (2021): 18–34.

23. Elizabeth Barnert, Cyrus Ahalt, and Brie Williams, "Prisons: Amplifiers of the COVID-19 Pandemic Hiding in Plain Sight," *American Journal of Public Health* 110, no. 7 (2020): 964.

24. Ashley Nellis, "The Color of Justice: Racial and Ethnic Disparity in State Prisons," The Sentencing Project, 2016.

25. Elizabeth Barnert, Ada Kwan, and Brie Williams, "Ten Urgent Priorities Based on Lessons Learned from More Than a Half Million Known COVID-19 Cases in US Prisons," *American Journal of Public Health*, 111 no. 6 (2021): 1099–105.

26. Soo Rin Kim, Matthew Vann, Laura Bronner, Grace Manthey, Ryan Best, and Emily Scherer, "Which Cities Have the Biggest Racial Gaps in COVID-19 Testing Access?," FiveThirtyEight, July 22, 2020.

27. Mona N. Fouad, John Ruffin, and Selwyn M. Vickers, "COVID-19 Is Disproportionately High in African Americans. This Will Come as No Surprise . . . ," *American Journal of Medicine* 133, no. 10 (2020): e544–e45.

28. "Risk for COVID-19 Infection, Hospitalization, and Death by Race/Ethnicity," Centers for Disease Control and Prevention, September 9, 2021, https://www.cdc.gov/coronavirus/2019-ncov/covid-data/investigations-discovery/hospitalization-death-by-race-ethnicity.html.

29. Alan M. Kraut, *Silent Travelers: Germs, Genes, and the Immigrant Menace.* Baltimore: Johns Hopkins University Press, 1995.

30. Ben Chapman and Talal Ansari, "Coronavirus Cases Rise as U.S. Marks Holiday Weekend," *Wall Street Journal*, May 23, 2020.

31. "How George Floyd Was Killed in Police Custody," *New York Times*, May 31, 2020.

32. Larry Buchanan, Quoctrung Bui, and Jugal K. Patel, "Black Lives Matter May Be the Largest Movement in U.S. History," *New York Times*, July 3, 2020.

33. Berkeley Lovelace Jr., "CDC Warns George Floyd Protests May Be 'Seeding Event' for More Coronavirus Outbreaks," CNBC, June 4, 2020.

34. Dhaval M. Dave, Andrew I. Friedson, Kyutaro Matsuzawa, Joseph J. Sabia, and Samuel Safford, "Black Lives Matter Protests and Risk Avoidance: The Case of Civil Unrest during a Pandemic," National Bureau of Economic Research, 2020. See also Gregory Neyman and William Dalsey, "Black Lives Matter Protests and COVID-19 Cases: Relationship in Two Databases," *Journal of Public Health* 43, no. 2 (2021): 225–27.

35. "President Trump Calls Coronavirus 'Kung Flu,'" BBC News, June 24, 2020.

36. Katherine J. Roberto, Andrew F. Johnson, and Beth M. Rauhaus, "Stigmatization and Prejudice during the COVID-19 Pandemic," *Administrative Theory & Praxis* 42, no. 3 (2020): 364–78.

37. Peter Romeo, "Half the Nation's Chinese Restaurants Have Closed, Study Finds," Restaurant Business, April 13, 2020.

38. "How the Pandemic and a Rise in Targeted Hate Crimes Has Shifted Spending for Asian Americans," NBC News, June 2, 2021.

39. Yao Li and Harvey L. Nicholson Jr., "When 'Model Minorities' Become 'Yellow Peril'—Othering and the Racialization of Asian Americans in the COVID-19 Pandemic," *Sociology Compass* 15, no. 2 (2021): e12849.

40. Laura Eichelberger, "SARS and New York's Chinatown: The Politics of Risk and Blame during an Epidemic of Fear," *Social Science & Medicine* 65, no. 6 (2007): 1284–95.

41. Tyler T. Reny and Matt A. Barreto, "Xenophobia in the Time of Pandemic: Othering, Anti-Asian Attitudes, and COVID-19," *Politics, Groups, and Identities* (2020): 1–24.

42. Hélène Joffe, *Risk and 'the Other'* (Cambridge: Cambridge University Press, 1999).

43. Pew Research Center, "Many Black and Asian Americans Say They Have Experienced Discrimination amid the COVID-19 Outbreak," June 7, 2020, https://www.pewresearch.org/social-trends/2020/07/01/many-black-and-asian-americans-say-they-have-experienced-discrimination-amid-the-covid-19-outbreak/.

44. Josh Margolin, "FBI Warns of Potential Surge in Hate Crimes against Asian Americans amid Coronavirus," ABC News, March 27, 2020.

45. Katherine Donlevy, "Anti-Asian Hate Crime Jumps 1,900 Percent," Queens Chronicle, 2020.

46. Stop AAPI Hate, "New Data on Anti-Asian Hate Incidents against Elderly and Total National Incidents in 2020," February 9, 2022, https://stopaapihate.org/wp-content/uploads/2021/04/Stop-AAPI-Hate-Press-Statement-Bay-Area-Elderly-Incidents-210209.pdf.

47. Cigdem V. Sirin, Nicholas A. Valentino, and Jose D. Villalobos, *Seeing Us in Them: Social Divisions and the Politics of Group Empathy* (Cambridge: Cambridge University Press, 2021).

48. Neil Ruiz, Khadijah Edwards, and Mark Hugo Lopez, "One-third of Asian Americans Fear Threats, Physical Attacks and Most Say Violence Against Them Is Rising," Pew Research Center, April 21, 2021.

49. The White House, "Executive Order on Advancing Equity, Justice, and Opportunity for Asian Americans, Native Hawaiians, and Pacific Islanders," May 28, 2021, https://www.whitehouse.gov/briefing-room/presidential-actions/2021/05/28/executive-order-on-advancing-equity-justice-and-opportunity-for-asian-americans-native-hawaiians-and-pacific-islanders/.

50. Sean Darling-Hammond, Eli K. Michaels, Amani M. Allen, David H. Chae, Marilyn D. Thomas, Thu T. Nguyen, Mahasin M. Mujahid, and Rucker C. Johnson,

"Covid19? After 'The China Virus' Went Viral: Racially Charged Coronavirus Coverage and Trends in Bias against Asian Americans," *Health Education & Behavior* 47, no. 6 (2020): 870–79.

51. Alexandra Stevenson, "Senator Tom Cotton Repeats Fringe Theory of Coronavirus Origins," *New York Times*, February 17, 2020.

52. Justin Ling, "The Lab Leak Theory Doesn't Hold Up," Foreign Policy, June 15, 2021. To make our position plain, although we remain agnostic about the true origins of the SARS-CoV-2 virus, we are unaware of any affirmative evidence that the virus originated in a lab in China or anywhere else. A zoonotic origin is the most likely scenario.

53. Reny and Barreto, "Xenophobia in the Time of Pandemic."

54. Respondents were given the opportunity in our survey to tell us what their prime sources of news were. We coded answers such as "Fox News," "OAN," "Epoch Times," and "Tucker Carlson" as indicating that the respondent watches right-wing news.

55. Ray et al., "Examining and Addressing COVID-19 Racial Disparities in Detroit"; Fouad, Ruffin, and Vickers, "COVID-19 Is Disproportionately High in African Americans"; Benjamin Seligman, Maddalena Ferranna, and David E. Bloom, "Social Determinants of Mortality from COVID-19: A Simulation Study Using NHANES," *PLOS Medicine* 18, no. 1 (2021): e1003490.

Chapter 9

1. Lazaro Gamio, John Keefe, Denise Lu, and Rich Harris, "Record-Setting Turnout: Tracking Early Voting in the 2020 Election," *New York Times,* November 12, 2020.

2. Tucker Higgins and Nate Rattner, "When Does Vote by Mail and Early Voting Start? A State by State Guide," CNBC, September 4, 2020.

3. "Most Americans Trust Elections Are Fair, but Sharp Divides Exist, a New Poll Finds," National Public Radio, November 1, 2021.

4. "'Pandemic within a Pandemic': Coronavirus and Police Brutality Roil Black Communities," *New York Times*, June 7, 2020.

5. Sara Wallace Goodman, *Citizenship in Hard Times: How Ordinary People Respond to Democratic Threat* (New York: Cambridge University Press, 2022).

6. Nathan P. Kalmoe and Lilliana Mason, "Lethal Mass Partisanship: Prevalence, Correlates, and Electoral Contingencies," Paper presented at the annual meeting of the American Political Science Association Conference, Boston, MA, 2018.

7. Hilde Coffé and Catherine Bolzendahl, "Partisan Cleavages in the Importance of Citizenship Rights and Responsibilities," *Social Science Quarterly* 92, no. 3 (2011): 656–74; Goodman, *Citizenship in Hard Times.*

8. Febriana Firdaus, "How Black Lives Matter Inspired West Papua's Freedom Struggle," Jacobin, July 8, 2020; Guy Sorman, "Black Lives Matter in Paris: An American Movement in France," France-Amerique, September 10, 2020.

9. Ben Zimmer, "Why Trump Is So Obsessed with Antifa," *The Atlantic*, June 4, 2020; "Hard-to-Define 'Antifa' Becomes Election-Year Wedge Issue," *Atlanta Journal-Constitution*, October 9, 2020.

10. Andrew Romano, "Yahoo News/YouGov Coronavirus Poll: Most Americans Reject Anti-Lockdown Protests," Yahoo!News, April 20, 2020.

11. "16 States Have Postponed Primaries during the Pandemic. Here's a List," *New York Times*, August 10, 2020.

12. "Election Highlights: Ohio Judge Rejects Governor's Efforts to Postpone Tuesday's Vote; Biden Wins Washington Primary," *Washington Post*, March 17, 2020.

13. "Trump Attacks an Election He Is at Risk of Losing," *New York Times*, July 30, 2020.

14. For one of many examples, see "Ahead of D.N.C., Trump Digs in on Effort to Undermine Confidence in the Election," *New York Times*, August 17, 2020.

15. It is noteworthy that Trump himself has long voted via absentee ballot.

16. For a review, see Anna Baringer, Michael C. Herron, and Daniel A. Smith, "Voting by Mail and Ballot Rejection: Lessons from Florida for Elections in the Age of the Coronavirus," *Election Law Journal: Rules, Politics, and Policy* 19, no. 3 (2020): 289–320.

17. For a related perspective, see Joshua David Clinton, John S. Lapinski, Sarah Lentz, and Stephen Pettigrew, "Trumped by Trump? Public Support for Vote by Mail Voting in Response to the COVID-19 Pandemic," *SSRN*, June 15, 2020, https://ssrn.com/abstract=3630334.

18. Eric Lutz, "Trump: Mail-in Voting Is 'Horrible' Except When I Do It," *Vanity Fair*, April 8, 2020.

19. Tim Harper, Rachel Orey, and Collier Fernekes, *Counting the Vote during the 2020 Election* (Washington, DC: Bipartisan Policy Center, 2020).

20. Oxford Analytica, "US November Election Could Produce Crisis," September 18, 2020, https://doi.org/10.1108/OXAN-DB256343.

21. Andreas Schedler, "The Menu of Manipulation," *Journal of Democracy* 13, no. 2 (2002): 36–50.

22. Thomas B. Pepinsky, "Why the Impeachment Fight Is Even Scarier Than You Think," Politico, October 31, 2019.

23. "In Torrent of Falsehoods, Trump Claims Election Is Being Stolen," *New York Times*, November 5, 2020.

24. See Tom Pepinsky, "Americans Are Already Set to Conclude That the 2020 Presidential Elections Were Rigged," October 28, 2020, https://tompepinsky.com/2020/10/28/americans-are-already-set-to-conclude-that-the-2020-presidential-elections-were-rigged/.

25. "Trump and His Allies Filed More Than 40 Lawsuits Challenging the 2020 Election Results. All of Them Failed," Business Insider, February 22, 2021.

26. "Rewriting January 6: Republicans and Conservatives Push False and Misleading Accounts of Capitol Riot," *Washington Post*, March 1, 2021.

27. Steven Levitsky and Daniel Ziblatt, *How Democracies Die* (New York: Crown, 2018).

Chapter 10

1. Jonathan Pekar, Michael Worobey, Niema Moshiri, Konrad Scheffler, and Joel O. Wertheim, "Timing the SARS-CoV-2 Index Case in Hubei Province," *Science* 372, no. 6540 (2021): 412–17.

2. Lisa A. Jackson, Evan J. Anderson, Nadine G. Rouphael, Paul C. Roberts, Mamodikoe Makhene, Rhea N. Coler, Michele P. McCullough, et al., "An mRNA Vaccine against SARS-CoV-2—Preliminary Report," *New England Journal of Medicine* 383, no. 20 (2020): 1920–31.

3. Dan Diamond, "The Crash Landing of 'Operation Warp Speed,'" Politico, January 17, 2021.

4. "After Months of Questions, a Key Operation Warp Speed Adviser's Contract Emerges," National Public Radio, October 30, 2020.

5. Jennifer Bleyer, "Divided We Fail," *Scope*, no. 1 (2021), https://www.nyu.edu /about/news-publications/publications/scope-magazine/scope-2021/features /divided-we-fail.html.

6. For a humorous sendup of such claims, see Alexandra Petri, "Opinion: Big Bird is a Communist," *Washington Post*, November 9, 2021.

7. Eliza Relman, "Just 45% of House Republicans Say They've Been Vaccinated While 100% of Congressional Democrats Say They've Gotten the Shot," Business Insider, May 14, 2021.

8. Kayleigh McEnany, *Outnumbered*, Fox News, August 9, 2021.

9. Masha Krupenkin, "Does Partisanship Affect Compliance with Government Recommendations?," *Political Behavior* 43, no. 1 (2021): 451–72.

10. Matthew A. Baum, "Red State, Blue State, Flu State: Media Self-selection and Partisan Gaps in Swine Flu Vaccinations," *Journal of Health Politics, Policy and Law* 36, no. 6 (2011): 1021–59.

11. Samira Sadeque, "Nearly All Fox Staffers Vaccinated for Covid Even as Hosts Cast Doubt on Vaccine," *The Guardian*, September 15, 2021.

12. Ashley Kirzinger, Grace Sparks, and Mollyann Brodie, "KFF Covid-19 Vaccine Monitor: In Their Own Words, Six Months Later," Kaiser Family Foundation, July 13, 2021.

13. Bobby Caina Calvan, "More Governors Publicly Vaccinated, but Florida's Kept Mum," Associated Press, April 7, 2021.

14. Brett Kelman, "Tennessee Abandons Vaccine Outreach to Minors—Not Just for COVID-19," *Tennessean*, July 13, 2021.

15. Tiffany Hsu, "Despite Outbreaks among Unvaccinated, Fox News Hosts Smear Shots," *New York Times,* July 11, 2021.

16. "Biden to Hold July 4 Celebration He Hoped Would Mark 'Independence' from COVID," ABC News, June 15, 2021.

17. The White House, "*National Strategy for the COVID 19 Response and Pandemic Preparedness*," January 2021, https://www.whitehouse.gov/wp-content /uploads/2021/01/National-Strategy-for-the-COVID-19-Response-and-Pandemic -Preparedness.pdf.

18. The same figures made with reference to question about Hispanic and Asian American communities are identical.

19. Centers for Disease Control, "COVID-19 Vaccinations in the United States," 2021, https://www.cdc.gov/coronavirus/2019-ncov/vaccines/reporting-vaccinations.html.

20. Namib Ndugga, Oliva Pham, Latoya Hill, Samantha Artiga, Raisa Alam, and Noah Parker, "Latest Data on COVID-19 Vaccinations Race/Ethnicity," Kaiser Family Foundation, 2021.

21. Latoya Hill and Samantha Artiga, "COVID-19 Vaccination among American Indian and Alaska Native People," Kaiser Family Foundation, April 9, 2021, https://www.kff.org/racial-equity-and-health-policy/issue-brief/covid-19-vaccination-american-indian-alaska-native-people/.

22. @smotus, "Correlation of Biden Vote Share and Adult Covid Vaccination Rate Is Now at .847. (CDC data)," Twitter, June 4, 2021, https://twitter.com/smotus/status/1404483957647831046?s=20.

23. Matthew J. Hornsey, Matthew Finlayson, Gabrielle Chatwood, and Christopher T. Begeny, "Donald Trump and Vaccination: The Effect of Political Identity, Conspiracist Ideation and Presidential Tweets on Vaccine Hesitancy," *Journal of Experimental Social Psychology* 88 (2020): 103947.

24. Carl A. Latkin, Lauren Dayton, Grace Yi, Brian Colon, and Xiangrong Kong, "Mask Usage, Social Distancing, Racial, and Gender Correlates of COVID-19 Vaccine Intentions among Adults in the US," *PLOS One* 16, no. 2 (2021): e0246970; Samantha Artiga, Rachel Garfield, and Kendal Orgera, "Communities of Color at Higher Risk for Health and Economic Challenges due to COVID-19," Kaiser Family Foundation, April 7, 2020, https://www.kff.org/coronavirus-covid-19/issue-brief/communities-of-color-at-higher-risk-for-health-and-economic-challenges-due-to-covid-19/.

25. Rebekah Reuben, Devon Aitken, Jonathan L. Freedman, and Gillian Einstein, "Mistrust of the Medical Profession and Higher Disgust Sensitivity Predict Parental Vaccine Hesitancy," *PLOS One* 15, no. 9 (2020): e0237755.

26. William J. Hall, Mimi V. Chapman, Kent M. Lee, Yesenia M. Merino, Tainayah W. Thomas, B. Keith Payne, Eugenia Eng, Steven H. Day, and Tamera Coyne-Beasley, "Implicit Racial/Ethnic Bias among Health Care Professionals and Its Influence on Health Care Outcomes: A Systematic Review," *American Journal of Public Health* 105, no. 12 (2015): e60–e76; Sandra C. Quinn and Michele P. Andrasik, "Addressing Vaccine Hesitancy in BIPOC Communities—Toward Trustworthiness, Partnership, and Reciprocity," *New England Journal of Medicine* 385 (2021): 97–100.

27. One might ask what explains the reversal in April 2021 of the trend of ever-increasing vaccination rates. We draw particular attention to the April 13, 2021, CDC announcement of adverse side effects from the Johnson & Johnson vaccine, which seems to coincide exactly with the abrupt shift in vaccination trends. See Centers for Disease Control and Prevention, "Joint CDC and FDA Statement on Johnson & Johnson COVID-19 Vaccine," April 13, 2021, https://www.cdc.gov/media/releases/2021/s0413-JJ-vaccine.html.

28. See Centers for Disease Control and Prevention, COVID Data Tracker, https://covid.cdc.gov/covid-data-tracker/#datatracker-home.

29. See U.S. Census Bureau, "County Population by Characteristics: 2010–2019," https://www.census.gov/data/tables/time-series/demo/popest/2010s -counties-detail.html.

30. Rodrigo M. Burgos, Melissa E. Badowski, Emily Drwiega, Samaneh Ghassemi, Nikki Griffith, Fischer Herald, Mikayla Johnson, Renata O. Smith, and Sarah M. Michienzi, "The Race to a COVID-19 Vaccine: Opportunities and Challenges in Development and Distribution," *Drugs in Context* 10 (2021): 2020-12–2.

31. Oxford Analytica, "Vaccine Diplomacy Will Earn China Friends and Money," May 17, 2021, https://doi.org/10.1108/OXAN-DB261517.

32. "Bahrain, Facing a Covid Surge, Starts Giving Pfizer Boosters to Recipients of Chinese Vaccine," *Wall Street Journal*, June 2, 2021; Sui-Wee Lee, "They Relied on Chinese Vaccines. Now They're Battling Outbreaks," *New York Times*, June 22, 2021.

33. Katie Adams, "States Ranked by Percentage of Population Fully Vaccinate: Nov. 22," Becker's Hospital Review, November 22, 2021.

34. NBC 6, "Miami Beach Couple Arrested in Hawaii for Using Fake Vaccination Cards," August 18, 2021, https://www.nbcmiami.com/news/local/miami -beach-couple-arrested-in-hawaii-for-using-fake-vaccination-cards/2531905/.

35. Fox 13, "Seattle Police Says 6 Employees Leaving, 103 Waiting on Exemptions," October 19, 2021, https://www.q13fox.com/news/seattle-police-says-6 -employees-leaving-103-waiting-on-exemptions.

36. Nicole Lyn Pesce, "No, You Can't 'Undo' a COVID Vaccine with a Borax Bath—but You Could Hurt Yourself," MarketWatch, November 12, 2021.

Conclusion

1. Ethan Hauser and Azi Paybarah, "The Governor of Texas Bars Covid Vaccine Mandates," *New York Times*, October 11, 2021.

2. David Kihara, "3rd Conservative Radio Host Who Condemned Vaccines Dies of Covid," Politico, August 29, 2021.

3. Adela Suliman and Paulina Villegas, "Conservative Radio Host and Vaccine Critic Dies of Covid-19 Complications," *Washington Post*, August 12, 2021.

4. Ben Hall, "Outspoken Conservative Radio Host Phil Valentine Dies after Battling COVID-19," NewsChannel 5 Nashville, August 21, 2021.

5. Sharon LaFraniere, "White House Says It Will Narrowly Miss July 4 Vaccination Goal," *New York Times*, June 22, 2021.

6. Berkeley Lovelace, "CDC Reverses Indoor Mask Policy, Saying Fully Vaccinated People and Kids Should Wear Them Indoors," CNBC, July 27, 2021.

7. Benjamin Wallace-Wells, "What Happened to Joe Biden's 'Summer of Freedom' from the Pandemic?," *New Yorker*, August 12, 2021.

8. Centers for Disease Control and Prevention, "Rates of COVID-19 Cases and Deaths by Vaccination Status," https://covid.cdc.gov/covid-data-tracker/#rates -by-vaccine-status.

9. Rachel Treisman, "Fox Anchor Neil Cavuto Urged Viewers to Get Vaccinated. Then Came the Death Threats," National Public Radio, October 27, 2021.

10. Allan Smith, "Trump Booed at Alabama Rally after Telling Supporters to Get Vaccinated," NBC News, August 22, 2021.

11. Cary Funk and John Gramlich, "10 Facts about Americans and Coronavirus Vaccines," Pew Research Center, September 20, 2021, https://www.pewresearch.org/fact-tank/2021/09/20/10-facts-about-americans-and-coronavirus-vaccines/.

12. Ashley Kirzinger, Audrey Kearney, Liz Hamel, and Mollyann Brodie, "KFF COVID-19 Vaccine Monitor: The Increasing Importance of Partisanship in Predicting COVID-19 Vaccination Status," Kaiser Family Foundation, November 16, 2021.

13. David Leonhardt, "U.S. Covid Deaths Get Even Redder," *New York Times*, November 8, 2021.

14. Chico Harlan, Stefano Pitrelli, and Rick Noack, "Vaccine Mandates Are Spreading. Italy Shows What to Expect," *Washington Post*, November 12, 2021; Manuela Andreoni, "Brazil Surpasses the U.S. in Getting People Fully Vaccinated," *New York Times*, November 14, 2021.

15. Andrea Schneiker, "Populist Leadership: The Superhero Donald Trump as Savior in Times of Crisis," *Political Studies* 68, no. 4 (2020): 857–74.

16. Ibid.

17. Paulina Villegas, "Birx Says Trump's Idea to Inject Disinfectant Haunts Her: 'I Still Think about It Every Day,'" *Washington Post,* March 16, 2021, https://www.washingtonpost.com/health/2021/03/16/deborah-birx-disinfectant-injection-moment-interview/.

18. Paul Goren, "Party Identification and Core Political Values," *American Journal of Political Science* 49, no. 4 (2005): 881–96.

19. John A. Terrizzi, Natalie J. Shook, and Michael A. McDaniel, "The Behavioral Immune System and Social Conservatism: A Meta-analysis," *Evolution and Human Behavior* 34, no. 2 (2013): 99–108.

20. Jay J. Van Bavel, Katherine Baicker, Paulo S. Boggio, Valerio Capraro, Aleksandra Cichocka, Mina Cikara, Molly J. Crockett, et al., "Using Social and Behavioural Science to Support COVID-19 Pandemic Response," *Nature Human Behaviour* 4, no. 5 (2020): 460–71.

21. Grace Dean and Andrew Dunn, "Donald Trump and His Son Donald Trump Jr., without Evidence, Accuse Pfizer of Deliberately Waiting until after Election Day to Release Its COVID-19 Vaccine Trial Results," Business Insider, November 10, 2020.

22. Elaine Kamarck, "Pandemic Politics: Red State Governors Are in Trouble for Their Covid Leadership," Brookings Institution, October 19, 2021.

23. Jowei Chen, "Voter Partisanship and the Effect of Distributive Spending on Political Participation," *American Journal of Political Science* 57, no. 1 (2013): 200–17.

24. Andrew Soergel, "States Competing in 'Global Jungle' for PPE," *US News and World Report*, April 7, 2020.

25. Katherine Eban, "How Jared Kushner's Secret Testing Plan 'Went Poof into Thin Air'," *Vanity Fair*, July 30, 2020.

26. David E. Lewis, "Is the Failed Pandemic Response a Symptom of a Diseased Administrative State?," *Daedalus* 150, no. 3 (2021): 68–88.

27. Jamie Gumbrecht and Jessica Small, "House Committee Releases New Evidence from Investigation into Trump Administration Interference with CDC during Covid-19 Pandemic," CNN, November 12, 2021.

28. Larry Buchanan, Quoctrung Bui, and Jugal K. Patel, "Black Lives Matter May Be the Largest Movement in U.S. History," *New York Times*, July 3, 2020.

29. United States Elections Project, "National General Election VEP Turnout Rates, 1789–Present," http://www.electproject.org/national-1789-present.

30. Amy E. Lerman and Katherine T. McCabe, "Personal Experience and Public Opinion: A Theory and Test of Conditional Policy Feedback," *Journal of Politics* 79, no. 2 (2017): 624–41.

31. For a related argument about how successful policies become self-undermining because they are so effective and invisible, see Suzanne Mettler, *The Submerged State: How Invisible Government Policies Undermine American Democracy* (Chicago: University of Chicago Press, 2011).

32. Michael Bang Petersen, "COVID Lesson: Trust the Public with Hard Truths," *Nature* 598, no. 7880 (2021): 237–37; Julie Hassing Nielsen and Johannes Lindvall, "Trust in Government in Sweden and Denmark during the COVID-19 Epidemic," *West European Politics* 44, no. 5–6 (2021): 1180–204.

33. This is also a theme in Steven Levitsky and Daniel Ziblatt, *How Democracies Die* (New York: Crown, 2018).

34. See Bo Rothstein and Jan Teorell, "What Is Quality of Government? A Theory of Impartial Government Institutions," *Governance* 21, no. 2 (2008): 165–90.

Epilogue

1. Alison Tyson and Cary Funk, "Increasing Public Criticism, Confusion over COVID-19 Response in U.S.," Pew Research Center, February 9, 2022, https://www.pewresearch.org/science/2022/02/09/increasing-public-criticism-confusion-over-covid-19-response-in-us/?utm_content=buffer8b954&utm_medium=social&utm_source=twitter.com&utm_campaign=buffer.

2. Ashley Kirzinger, Audrey Kearney, Liz Hamel, and Mollyann Brodie, "KFF COVID-19 Vaccine Monitor: The Increasing Importance of Partisanship in Predicting COVID-19 Vaccination Status," Kaiser Family Foundation, November 16, 2021, https://www.kff.org/coronavirus-covid-19/poll-finding/importance-of-partisanship-predicting-vaccination-status/.

Appendix

1. Andrew Gelman and Jennifer Hill, *Data Analysis Using Regression and Multilevel/Hierarchical Models* (New York: Cambridge University Press, 2006).

BIBLIOGRAPHY

Aarøe, Lene, Michael Bang Petersen, and Kevin Arceneaux. "The Behavioral Immune System Shapes Political Intuitions: Why and How Individual Differences in Disgust Sensitivity Underlie Opposition to Immigration." *American Political Science Review* 111, no. 2 (2017): 277–94.

Abrajano, Marisa, and Zoltan L. Hajnal. *White Backlash: Immigration, Race, and American Politics.* Princeton, NJ: Princeton University Press, 2017.

Abramowitz, Alan I. "Peak Polarization? The Rise of Partisan-Ideological Consistency and Its Consequences." Prepared for delivery at the State of the Parties Conference, Ray Bliss Institute, University of Akron, November 4–5, 2021. https://uakron.edu/bliss/docs/State-of-the-Parties-2021/abramowitz-sop21 .pdf.

Abramowitz, Alan I., and Steven Webster. "The Rise of Negative Partisanship and the Nationalization of US Elections in the 21st Century." *Electoral Studies* 41 (2016): 12–22.

Abutaleb, Yasmeen. "Biden Administration Looks to Speed Authorization of Rapid Coronavirus Tests." *Washington Post*, October 25, 2021.

Abutaleb, Yasmeen, Ashley Parker, Josh Dawsey, and Philip Rucker. "The Inside Story of How Trump's Denial, Mismanagement and Magical Thinking Led to the Pandemic's Dark Winter." *Washington Post*, December 19, 2020.

Acharya, Avidit, Matthew Blackwell, and Maya Sen. *Deep Roots: How Slavery Still Shapes Southern Politics.* Princeton, NJ: Princeton University Press, 2018.

Achen, Christopher H., and Larry M. Bartels. *Democracy for Realists: Why Elections Do Not Produce Responsive Government.* Princeton, NJ: Princeton University Press, 2017.

Adams, Katie. "States Ranked by Percentage of Population Fully Vaccinate: Nov. 22." *Becker's Hospital Review*, November 22, 2021.

Adams-Prassl, Abi, Teodora Boneva, Marta Golin, and Christopher Rauh. "Inequality in the Impact of the Coronavirus Shock: Evidence from Real Time Surveys." *Journal of Public Economics* 189 (2020): 104245.

Adolph, Christopher, Kenya Amano, Bree Bang-Jensen, Nancy Fullman, and John Wilkerson. "Pandemic Politics: Timing State-Level Social Distancing Responses to COVID-19." *Journal of Health Politics, Policy and Law* 46, no. 2 (2021): 211–33.

Albanesi, Stefania, and Jiyeon Kim. "The Gendered Impact of the COVID-19 Recession on the US Labor Market." NBER Working Paper No. 28505, 2021.

Albelda, Randy. "Gender Impacts of the 'Great Recession' in the United States." In *Women and Austerity: The Economic Crisis and the Future for Gender Equality*, ed. Maria Karamessini and Jill Rubery, 82–101. London: Routledge, 2013.

Albertson, Bethany, and Shana Kushner Gadarian. *Anxious Politics: Democratic Citizenship in a Threatening World*. New York: Cambridge University Press, 2015.

Adlerman, Liz. "As Coronavirus Spreads, Face Mask Makers Go into Overdrive." *New York Times*, February 6, 2020.

"Ahead of D.N.C., Trump Digs in on Effort to Undermine Confidence in the Election." *New York Times*, August 17, 2020.

Alltucker, Ken, and Grace Hauck. "Trump Addressed the Nation on Coronavirus. We Checked the Facts." *USA Today*, February 26, 2020.

Alon, Titan, Matthias Doepke, Jane Olmstead-Rumsey, and Michèle Tertilt. "This Time It's Different: The Role of Women's Employment in a Pandemic Recession." NBER Working Paper No. 27660, 2020.

Alsan, Marcella, Stefanie Stantcheva, David Yang, and David Cutler. "Disparities in Coronavirus 2019 Reported Incidence, Knowledge, and Behavior among US Adults." *JAMA Network Open* 3, no. 6 (2020): e2012403–e03.

Alter, Charlotte. "How the Anti-Trump Resistance Is Organizing Its Outrage." *Time*, October 18, 2018.

Altmann, Samuel, Luke Milsom, Hannah Zillessen, Raffaele Blasone, Frederic Gerdon, Ruben Bach, Frauke Kreuter, et al. "Acceptability of App-Based Contact Tracing for COVID-19: Cross-country Survey Study." *JMIR mHealth and uHealth* 8, no. 8 (2020): e19857.

Alvarez, Priscilla. "Trump Administration Proposes Blocking Asylum Seekers on Public Health Grounds." CNN, July 8, 2020.

Amato, Fábio. "Coronavírus: MP concentra no governo federal poder para restringir circulação de pessoas." *G1*, March 21, 2020.

Ananyev, Maxim, Michael Poyker, and Yuan Tian. "The Safest Time to Fly: Pandemic Response in the Era of Fox News." *Journal of Population Economics* 34, no. 3 (2021): 775–802.

Anderson, Bryan, Gary D. Robertson, and Jill Colvin. "Trump Says GOP Is Pulling Convention from North Carolina." Associated Press, June 2, 2020.

Anderson, Monica, and Brooke Auxier. "Most Americans Don't Think Cellphone Tracking Will Help Limit COVID-19, Are Divided on Whether It's Acceptable." Pew Research Center, April 16, 2020. https://www.pewresearch.org/fact-tank /2020/04/16/most-americans-dont-think-cellphone-tracking-will-help-limit -covid-19-are-divided-on-whether-its-acceptable/.

Anderton, Robert, Vasco Botelho, Agostino Consolo, António Dias da Silva, Claudia Foroni, Matthias Mohr, and Lara Vivian. "The Impact of the COVID-19 Pandemic on the Euro Area Labour Market." *ECB Economic Bulletin* 8 (2020).

Andreoni, Manuela. "Brazil Surpasses the U.S. in Getting People Fully Vaccinated." *New York Times*, November 14, 2021.

APM Research Lab Staff. "The Color of Coronavirus: COVID-19 Deaths by Race and Ethnicity in the US." APM Research Lab, March 5, 2021. https://www.apmresearchlab.org/covid/deaths-by-race.

Ariadne Labs. "Global Learnings from South Korea: Protecting Health Care Workers from COVID-19." March 12, 2020. https://covid19.ariadnelabs.org/global-learnings-south-korea/.

Arrow, Kenneth J. "Uncertainty and the Welfare Economics of Medical Care." *American Economic Review* 53, no. 5 (1963): 941–73.

Artiga, Samantha, Rachel Garfield, and Kendal Orgera. "Communities of Color at Higher Risk for Health and Economic Challenges Due to COVID-19." Kaiser Family Foundation, April 7, 2020. https://www.kff.org/coronavirus-covid-19/issue-brief/communities-of-color-at-higher-risk-for-health-and-economic-challenges-due-to-covid-19/.

Ash, Elliott, Sergio Galletta, Dominik Hangartner, Yotam Margalit, and Matteo Pinna. "The Effect of Fox News on Health Behavior during COVID-19." *SSRN* 3636762, June 28, 2020.

Azari, Julia. "Weak Parties and Strong Partisanship Are a Bad Combination." Vox, November 3, 2016.

Baker, Peter, and Maggie Haberman. "In Torrent of Falsehoods, Trump Claims Election Is Being Stolen." *New York Times*, November 5, 2020.

Baker, Peter, Maggie Haberman, and Annie Karni. "Trump Floats Economic Stimulus in Response to Coronavirus." *New York Times*, March 9, 2020.

Baker, William D., and John R. Oneal. "Patriotism or Opinion Leadership? The Nature and Origins of the "Rally 'Round the Flag" Effect." *Journal of Conflict Resolution* 45, no. 5 (2001): 661–87.

Baringer, Anna, Michael C. Herron, and Daniel A. Smith. "Voting by Mail and Ballot Rejection: Lessons from Florida for Elections in the Age of the Coronavirus." *Election Law Journal: Rules, Politics, and Policy* 19, no. 3 (2020): 289–320.

Barnert, Elizabeth, Cyrus Ahalt, and Brie Williams. "Prisons: Amplifiers of the COVID-19 Pandemic Hiding in Plain Sight." *American Journal of Public Health* 110, no. 7 (2020): 964–66.

Barnert, Elizabeth, Ada Kwan, and Brie Williams. "Ten Urgent Priorities Based on Lessons Learned from More Than a Half Million Known COVID-19 Cases in US Prisons." *American Journal of Public Health* 111, no. 6 (2021): 1099–105.

Bartels, Larry. "Beyond the Running Tally: Partisan Bias in Political Perceptions." *Political Behavior* 24, no. 2 (2002): 117–50.

Baum, Matthew A. "Red State, Blue State, Flu State: Media Self-selection and Partisan Gaps in Swine Flu Vaccinations." *Journal of Health Politics, Policy and Law* 36, no. 6 (2011): 1021–59.

Bavel, Jay J. Van, Katherine Baicker, Paulo S. Boggio, Valerio Capraro, Aleksandra Cichocka, Mina Cikara, Molly J. Crockett, et al. "Using Social and Behavioural Science to Support COVID-19 Pandemic Response." *Nature Human Behaviour* 4, no. 5 (2020): 460–71.

Bazzi, Samuel, Martin Fiszbein, and Mesay Gebresilasse. "'Rugged Individualism' and Collective (in)Action during the COVID-19 Pandemic." *Journal of Public Economics* 195 (2021): 104357.

Benoit, Bertrand, and Tom Fairless. "Germany Boosts Already Hefty Coronavirus Stimulus." *Wall Street Journal*, August 26, 2020.

Berelson, Bernard, Paul Lazarsfeld, and William McPhee. *Voting: A Study of Opinion Formation in a Presidential Campaign.* Chicago: University of Chicago Press, 1954.

Berinsky, Adam "Assuming the Costs of War: Events, Elites, and American Public Support for Military Conflict." *Journal of Politics* 69, no. 4 (2007): 975–97.

Bernheim, Bert Douglas, Nina Buchmann, Zach Freitas-Groff, and Sebastián Otero. "The Effects of Large Group Meetings on the Spread of COVID-19: The Case of Trump Rallies." Stanford Institute for Economic Policy Research Working Paper No. 20-043, 2020.

Biden, Joe. "FLASHBACK by Joe Biden: Trump Is Worst Possible Leader to Deal with Coronavirus Outbreak." *USA Today*, January 27, 2020.

"Biden to Hold July 4 Celebration He Hoped Would Mark 'Independence' from COVID." ABC News, June 15, 2021.

Biegon, Rubrick. "A Populist Grand Strategy? Trump and the Framing of American Decline." *International Relations* 33, no. 4 (2019): 517–39.

Bishop, Bill. *The Big Sort: Why the Clustering of Like-Minded America Is Tearing Us Apart.* Boston: Houghton Mifflin Harcourt, 2009.

Blake, Aaron. "The Trump Administration Just Changed Its Description of the National Stockpile to Jibe with Jared Kushner's Controversial Claim." *Washington Post*, April 3, 2020.

Bleyer, Jennifer. "Divided We Fail." *Scope*, no. 1 (2021). https://www.nyu.edu /about/news-publications/publications/scope-magazine/scope-2021/features /divided-we-fail.html.

Blinder, Alan. "In Rural Alabama, a Longtime Mistrust of Medicine Fuels a Tuberculosis Outbreak." *New York Times*, January 17, 2016.

Boburg, Shawn, Robert O'Harrow Jr., Neena Satija, and Amy Goldstein. "Inside the Coronavirus Testing Failure: Alarm and Dismay among the Scientists Who Sought to Help." *Washington Post*, April 3, 2020.

Bohn, Kevin. "US Surgeon General Says He Thinks Coronavirus Is Contained in Certain Areas of the Country." CNN, March 8, 2020.

Bollyky, Thomas J., and Jennifer B. Nuzzo. "Trump's 'Early' Travel 'Bans' Weren't Early, Weren't Bans and Didn't Work." *Washington Post*, October 1, 2020.

Bolton, Alexander. "GOP Senators Tell Trump to Make Fauci Face of Government's Coronavirus Response." The Hill, March 10, 2020.

Bowles, Nellie. "Hurt by Lockdowns, California's Small Businesses Push to Recall Governor." *New York Times*, February 19, 2021.

Brader, Ted. *Campaigning for Hearts and Minds: How Emotional Appeals in Political Ads Work.* Chicago: University of Chicago Press, 2006.

Brader, Ted, and Nicholas A. Valentino. "Identities, Interests, and Emotions: Symbolic versus Material Wellsprings of Fear, Anger, and Enthusiasm." In *The Affect*

Effect: Dynamics of Emotion in Political Thinking and Behavior, ed. W. Russell Neuman, George E. Marcus, Ann N. Crigler and Michael MacKuen, 180–201. Chicago: University of Chicago Press, 2007.

Bradner, Eric, and Phil Mattingly. "McCain, Graham Lead in GOP Criticism of Trump Ban, Many Others Stay Mum." CNN, January 29, 2017.

Branswell, Helen. "Coronavirus Concerns Trigger Global Run on Supplies for Health Workers, Causing Shortages." Statnews, February 7, 2020.

Braun, Stephen, and Jason Dearen. "Trump's 'Strong Wall' to Block COVID-19 from China Had Holes." Associated Press, July 4, 2020.

Brookings Institution. "The Replacements: Why and How 'Acting' Officials Are Making Senate Confirmation Obsolete." September 23, 2020. https://ourpublicservice.org/publications/the-replacements/.

Brown, Nadia E., Ray Block, and Christopher T. Stout, eds. *The Politics of Protest: Readings on the Black Lives Matter Movement*. New York: Routledge, 2021.

Buchanan, Larry, Quoctrung Bui, and Jugal K. Patel. "Black Lives Matter May Be the Largest Movement in U.S. History." *New York Times*, July 3, 2020.

Burbach, David T. "Partisan Dimensions of Confidence in the US Military, 1973–2016." *Armed Forces & Society* 45, no. 2 (2019): 211–33.

Bureau of Labor Statistics. "Labor Force Statistics from the Current Population Survey." https://www.bls.gov/web/empsit/cpsee_e16.htm.

Burgos, Rodrigo M., Melissa E. Badowski, Emily Drwiega, Samaneh Ghassemi, Nikki Griffith, Fischer Herald, Mikayla Johnson, Renata O. Smith, and Sarah M. Michienzi. "The Race to a COVID-19 Vaccine: Opportunities and Challenges in Development and Distribution." *Drugs in Context* 10 (2021): 2020-12-2.

Burki, Talha. "COVID-19 among American Indians and Alaska Natives." *Lancet Infectious Diseases* 21, no. 3 (2021): 325–26.

Burns, Alexander. "Trump Attacks an Election He Is at Risk of Losing." *New York Times*, July 30, 2020.

Bursztyn, Leonardo, Aakaash Rao, Christopher Roth, and David Yanagizawa-Drott. "Misinformation during a Pandemic." NBER Working Paper No. 27417, 2020.

Calvan, Bobby Caina. "More Governors Publicly Vaccinated, but Florida's Kept Mum." Associated Press, April 7, 2021.

Campbell, Angus, Philip Converse, Warren E. Miller, and Donald Stokes. *The American Voter*. Chicago: University of Chicago Press, 1960.

Carpenter, Daniel. "Is Health Politics Different?" *Annual Review of Political Science* 15, no. 2012 (2012): 287–311.

Carter, Ryan. "Long Lines, Big Demand: Still-Limited LA-Area Drive-through Coronavirus Testing Inches Ahead." *Los Angeles Daily News*, March 25, 2020.

Cassese, Erin C. "Straying from the Flock? A Look at How Americans' Gender and Religious Identities Cross-Pressure Partisanship." *Political Research Quarterly* 73, no. 1 (2019): 169–83.

Cassino, Dan, and Yasemin Besen-Cassino. "Of Masks and Men? Gender, Sex, and Protective Measures during COVID-19." *Politics & Gender* 16, no. 4 (2020): 1052–62.

Centers for Disease Control and Prevention. "CDC Confirms Possible Instance of Community Spread of COVID-19 in U.S." February 26, 2020. https://www.cdc.gov/media/releases/2020/s0226-Covid-19-spread.html.

———. COVID Data Tracker. https://covid.cdc.gov/covid-data-tracker/#datatracker-home.

———. "COVID-19 Vaccinations in the United States." 2021, https://www.cdc.gov/coronavirus/2019-ncov/vaccines/reporting-vaccinations.html.

———. "Disease Burden of Flu." 2022. https://www.cdc.gov/flu/about/burden/index.html.

———. "Joint CDC and FDA Statement on Johnson & Johnson COVID-19 Vaccine." April 13, 2021. https://www.cdc.gov/media/releases/2021/s0413-JJ-vaccine.html.

———. "Public Health Screening to Begin at 3 U.S. Airports for 2019 Novel Coronavirus ('2019-nCoV')." January 17, 2020. https://www.cdc.gov/media/releases/2020/p0117-coronavirus-screening.html.

———. "Rates of COVID-19 Cases and Deaths by Vaccination Status." https://covid.cdc.gov/covid-data-tracker/#rates-by-vaccine-status.

———. "Risk for COVID-19 Infection, Hospitalization, and Death by Race/Ethnicity." September 9, 2021. https://www.cdc.gov/coronavirus/2019-ncov/covid-data/investigations-discovery/hospitalization-death-by-race-ethnicity.html.

———. "Transcript for the CDC Telebriefing Update on COVID-19." February 26, 2020. https://www.cdc.gov/media/releases/2020/t0225-cdc-telebriefing-covid-19.html.

Chait, Jonathan. "Trump: I Was Right, Coronavirus Cases 'Will Go Down to Zero, Ultimately.'" *New York Magazine*, April 28, 2020.

Chapman, Ben, and Talal Ansari. "Coronavirus Cases Rise as U.S. Marks Holiday Weekend." *Wall Street Journal*, May 23, 2020.

Chen, Jowei. "Voter Partisanship and the Effect of Distributive Spending on Political Participation." *American Journal of Political Science* 57, no. 1 (2013): 200–17.

Cheng, Vincent Chi-Chung, Shuk-Ching Wong, Vivien Wai-Man Chuang, Simon Yung-Chun So, Jonathan Hon-Kwan Chen, Siddharth Sridhar, Kelvin Kai-Wang To, et al. "The Role of Community-wide Wearing of Face Mask for Control of Coronavirus Disease 2019 (COVID-19) Epidemic Due to SARS-CoV-2." *Journal of Infection* 81, no. 1 (2020): 107–14.

Chetty, Raj, John Friedman, Nathaniel Hendren, Michael Stepner, and the Opportunity Insights Team. "The Economic Impacts of COVID-19: Evidence from a New Public Database Built Using Private Sector Data." NBER Working Paper No. 26463, 2020.

"China's Exports Plunge amid Coronavirus Epidemic." *Wall Street Journal*, March 7, 2020.

Chinazzi, Matteo, Jessica T. Davis, Marco Ajelli, Corrado Gioannini, Maria Litvinova, Stefano Merler, Ana Pastore y Piontti, et al. "The Effect of Travel Restrictions on the Spread of the 2019 Novel Coronavirus (COVID-19) Outbreak." *Science* (2020): eaba9757.

Chitale, Radha. "The Best and Worst States for Heart Attack." ABC News, July 9, 2009.

Chong, Dennis, Jack Citrin, and Patricia Conley. "When Self-Interest Matters." *Political Psychology* 22, no. 3 (2001): 541–70.

Chu, Derek K., Elie A. Akl, Stephanie Duda, Karla Solo, Sally Yaacoub, Holger J. Schünemann, Amena El-harakeh, et al. "Physical Distancing, Face Masks, and Eye Protection to Prevent Person-to-Person Transmission of SARS-CoV-2 and COVID-19: A Systematic Review and Meta-analysis." *The Lancet* 395, no. 10242 (2020): 1973–87.

Clinton, Joshua David, John S. Lapinski, Sarah Lentz, and Stephen Pettigrew. "Trumped by Trump? Public Support for Vote by Mail Voting in Response to the COVID-19 Pandemic." *SSRN*, June 15, 2020. https://ssrn.com/abstract=3630334.

Clissold, Elliot, Davina Nylander, Cameron Watson, and Antonio Ventriglio. "Pandemics and Prejudice." *International Journal of Social Psychiatry* 66, no. 5 (2020): 421–23.

CNBC. "First on CNBC: CNBC Transcript; National Economic Council Director Larry Kudlow Speaks with CNBC's Kelly Evans on CNBC's 'The Exchange' Today." September 22, 2020.

CNN. "Top Doctors Give Blistering Assessment of Trump Pandemic Response; Sen. Raphael Warnock (D-GA) Blasts Georgia's Voting Overhaul." March 29, 2021. http://www.cnn.com/TRANSCRIPTS/2103/29/nday.03.html.

Coffé, Hilde, and Catherine Bolzendahl. "Partisan Cleavages in the Importance of Citizenship Rights and Responsibilities." *Social Science Quarterly* 92, no. 3 (2011): 656–74.

Cohen, Patricia. "'Still Catching Up': Jobless Numbers May Not Tell Full Story." *New York Times*, May 28, 2020.

———. "A Torrent of Job Losses Threatens to Overwhelm the U.S. Economy." *New York Times*, March 19, 2020.

"Competition among States, Local Governments Creates Bidding War for Medical Equipment," ABC News, April 3, 2020.

Connaughton, Aidan. "Those on Ideological Right Favor Fewer COVID-19 Restrictions in Most Advanced Economies." Pew Research Center, July 30, 2021. https://www.pewresearch.org/fact-tank/2021/07/30/those-on-ideological-right-favor-fewer-covid-19-restrictions-in-most-advanced-economies/.

Cook, Nancy, and Matthew Choi. "Trump Rallies His Base to Treat Coronavirus as a 'Hoax.'" Politico, February 28, 2020.

Corasaniti, Nick, and Stephanie Saul. "16 States Have Postponed Primaries during the Pandemic. Here's a List." *New York Times*, August 10, 2020.

Corman, Juliane, and David Levin. "Support for Government Provision of Health Care and the Patient Protection and Affordable Care Act." *Public Opinion Quarterly* 80, no. 1 (2016): 114–79.

"Coronavirus: Bolsonaro Downplays Threat of Pandemic to Brazil." BBC, March 25, 2020.

"Coronavirus: Northern Italy Quarantines 16 Million People." BBC, March 8, 2020.

"Cost to Treat Ebola: $1 Million For Two Patients." NBC News, November 18, 2014. https://www.nbcnews.com/storyline/ebola-virus-outbreak/cost-treat-ebola-1-million-two-patients-n250986.

Cotton, Tom. "Cotton, Colleagues Urge Expansion and Extension of Immigration Proclamation." Tom Cotton: Senator for Arkansas, May 7, 2020. https://www.cotton.senate.gov/news/press-releases/cotton-colleagues-urge-expansion-and-extension-of-immigration-proclamation.

COVID Tracking Project. "US Daily Reported Tests, Mar 1–Mar 7." covidtracking.com.

Cowley, Stacy. "Bankers Rebuke S.B.A. as Loan System Crashes in Flood of Applications." *New York Times*, April 27, 2020.

Cramer, Kathy J. *The Politics of Resentment: Rural Consciousness in Wisconsin and the Rise of Scott Walker.* Chicago: University of Chicago Press, 2016.

Creighton, Mathew J., Amaney Jamal, and Natalia C. Malancu. "Has Opposition to Immigration Increased in the United States after the Economic Crisis? An Experimental Approach." *International Migration Review* 49, no. 3 (2015): 727–56.

Crump, James. "'It Was a Government of Chaos': Kushner's Coronavirus Task Force Whistleblower Says He Was Pressured to 'Fudge' Death Data Model." *The Independent*, September 23, 2020.

Daniller, Andrew. "Americans' Immigration Policy Priorities: Divisions between—and within—the Two Parties." Pew Research Center, November 11, 2019. https://www.pewresearch.org/fact-tank/2019/11/12/americans-immigration-policy-priorities-divisions-between-and-within-the-two-parties/.

Darling-Hammond, Sean, Eli K. Michaels, Amani M. Allen, David H. Chae, Marilyn D. Thomas, Thu T. Nguyen, Mahasin M. Mujahid, and Rucker C. Johnson. "Covid19? After 'The China Virus' Went Viral: Racially Charged Coronavirus Coverage and Trends in Bias against Asian Americans." *Health Education & Behavior* 47, no. 6 (2020): 870–79.

Dave, Dhaval M., Andrew I. Friedson, Kyutaro Matsuzawa, Joseph J. Sabia, and Samuel Safford. "Black Lives Matter Protests and Risk Avoidance: The Case of Civil Unrest during a Pandemic." National Bureau of Economic Research, 2020.

Dawson, Lindsey, and Jennifer Kates. "Rapid Home Tests for COVID-19: Issues with Availability and Access in the U.S." Kaiser Family Foundation, November 4, 2021.

Dean, Grace and Andrew Dunn. "Donald Trump and His Son Donald Trump Jr., without Evidence, Accuse Pfizer of Deliberately Waiting until after Election Day to Release Its COVID-19 Vaccine Trial Results." Business Insider, November 10, 2020.

Deaton, Angus, and Darren Lubotsky. "Mortality, Inequality and Race in American Cities and States." *Social Science & Medicine* 56, no. 6 (2003): 1139–53.

DeBonis, Mike, and Jeremy Barr. "Rewriting January 6: Republicans and Conservatives Push False and Misleading Accounts of Capitol Riot." *Washington Post*, March 1, 2021.

Delfs, Arne, and Naomi Kresge. "Merkel Says Covid Spike 'Worse Than Anything We've Seen.'" Bloomberg, November 22, 2021.

Delli Carpini, Michael X., and Scott Keeter. *What Americans Know about Politics and Why It Matters*. New Haven, CT: Yale University Press, 1996.

DeParle, Jason. "As Hunger Swells, Food Stamps Become a Partisan Flash Point." *New York Times*, May 6, 2020.

Desrochers, Daniel. "39 New Kentucky Coronavirus Cases Found. Total Is 163. More Businesses Must Close." *Lexington Herald Leader*, March 24, 2020.

Diamond, Dan. "The Crash Landing of 'Operation Warp Speed.'" Politico, January 17, 2021.

———. "Trump Advisers Privately Warned of 'Critical Mistakes' as Pandemic Loomed." *Washington Post*, September 14, 2021.

Dickerson, Caitlin, and Michael D. Shear. "Before Covid-19, Trump Aide Sought to Use Disease to Close Borders." *New York Times*, May 3, 2020.

Dimock, Michael, and Richard Wike. "America Is Exceptional in the Nature of Its Political Divide." Pew Research Center, November 13, 2020. https://www .pewresearch.org/fact-tank/2020/11/13/america-is-exceptional-in-the-nature -of-its-political-divide/.

Dionne, E. J., Jr. *Why Americans Hate Politics*. New York: Simon & Schuster, 1991.

Dionne, Kim Yi, and Fulya Felicity Turkmen. "The Politics of Pandemic Othering: Putting COVID-19 in Global and Historical Context." *International Organization* 74, no. S1 (2020): E213–E30.

Dolan, Jack, and Brittny Meija. "LA County Gives Up on Containing Coronavirus, Tells Doctors to Skip Testing of Some Patients." *Los Angeles Times*, March 20, 2020.

Donlevy, Katherine. "Anti-Asian Hate Crime Jumps 1,900 Percent." *Queens Chronicle*, 2020.

Druckman, James N., Jordan Fein, and Thomas J. Leeper. "A Source of Bias in Public Opinion Stability." *American Political Science Review* (2012): 430–54.

Duehren, Andrew. "Stimulus Cops on Lookout for Fake Employees, Identity Theft." *Wall Street Journal*, May 13, 2020.

Dwyer, Colin. "'Take This Serious': Bus Driver Dies of COVID-19 after Calling Out Coughing Rider." National Public Radio, April 3, 2021.

Eban, Katherine. "How Jared Kushner's Secret Testing Plan 'Went Poof into Thin Air'." *Vanity Fair*, July 30, 2020.

———. "'That's Their Problem': How Jared Kushner Let the Markets Decide America's COVID-19 Fate." *Vanity Fair*, September 17, 2020.

EdBuild. "Nonwhite School Districts Get $23 Billion Less Than White Districts Despite Serving the Same Number of Students." https://edbuild.org/content /23-billion.

Eder, Steve, Henry Fountain, Michael H. Keller, Muyi Xiao, and Alexandra Stevenson. "430,000 People Have Traveled from China to U.S. since Coronavirus Surfaced." *New York Times*, April 4, 2020.

EducationWeek. "Map: Coronavirus and School Closures in 2019–2020." Education Week, March 6, 2020. https://www.edweek.org/leadership/map -coronavirus-and-school-closures-in-2019-2020/2020/03.

Edwards, Frank, Hedwig Lee, and Michael Esposito. "Risk of Being Killed by Police Use of Force in the United States by Age, Race-Ethnicity, and Sex." *Proceedings of the National Academy of Sciences* 116, no. 34 (2019): 16793–98.

Edwards, George C., and B. Dan Wood. "Who Influences Whom? The President, Congress, and the Media." *American Political Science Review* 93, no. 2 (1999): 327–44.

Eichelberger, Laura. "SARS and New York's Chinatown: The Politics of Risk and Blame during an Epidemic of Fear." *Social Science & Medicine* 65, no. 6 (2007): 1284–95.

Eichenberg, Richard C., Richard J. Stoll, and Matthew Lebo. "War President: The Approval Ratings of George W. Bush." *Journal of Conflict Resolution* 50, no. 6 (2006): 783–808.

Enten, Harry. "Flu Shots Uptake Is Now Partisan. It Didn't Use to Be." CNN, November 14, 2021.

Erikson, Robert S., and Laura Stoker. "Caught in the Draft: The Effects of Vietnam Draft Lottery Status on Political Attitudes." *American Political Science Review* (2011): 221–37.

Esses, Victoria M., John F. Dovidio, and Gordon Hodson. "Public Attitudes toward Immigration in the United States and Canada in Response to the September 11, 2001 'Attack on America.'" *Analyses of Social Issues and Public Policy* 2, no. 1 (2002): 69–85.

Falconbridge, Guy, and Kate Holton. "Healthy Again, British PM Says Too Risky to Relax Lockdown Yet." Reuters, April 26, 2020.

Farr, Christina. "Germany's Coronavirus Response Is a Master Class in Science Communication." CNBC, July 21, 2020.

Finkel, Eli J., Christopher A. Bail, Mina Cikara, Peter H. Ditto, Shanto Iyengar, Samara Klar, Lilliana Mason, et al. "Political Sectarianism in America." *Science* 370, no. 6516 (2020): 533–36.

Fiorina, Morris. *Retrospective Voting in American National Elections.* New Haven, CT: Yale University Press, 1981.

Fiorina, Morris P., and Samuel J. Abrams. "Political Polarization in the American Public." *Annual Review of Political Science* 11 (2008): 563–88.

Firdaus, Febriana. "How Black Lives Matter Inspired West Papua's Freedom Struggle." *Jacobin*, July 8, 2020.

Fisher, Max, and Choe Sang-Hun. "How South Korea Flattened the Curve." *New York Times*, April 10, 2020.

Folha de S.Paulo. "Ministério da Saúde pressiona Manaus e diz ser 'inadmissível' não usar cloroquina contra Covid-19." January 1, 2021.

Folkman, Susan, and Richard S. Lazarus. "Coping as a Mediator of Emotion." *Journal of Personality and Social Psychology* 54, no. 3 (1988): 466–75.

Forde, Allana T., Danielle M. Crookes, Shakira F. Suglia, and Ryan T. Demmer. "The Weathering Hypothesis as an Explanation for Racial Disparities in Health: A Systematic Review." *Annals of Epidemiology* 33 (2019): 66–75.

Forgey, Quint. "Trump Floats His Own Coronavirus Hunches on 'Hannity.'" March 5, 2020.

Fouad, Mona N., John Ruffin, and Selwyn M. Vickers. "COVID-19 Is Disproportionately High in African Americans. This Will Come as No Surprise." *American Journal of Medicine* 133, no. 10 (2020): e544–e45.

Fox News. *Hannity*. April 7, 2020.

Fox 13. "Seattle Police Says 6 Employees Leaving, 103 Waiting on Exemptions." October 19, 2021. https://www.q13fox.com/news/seattle-police-says-6-employees -leaving-103-waiting-on-exemptions.

Foxworth, Raymond, Laura E. Evans, Gabriel R. Sanchez, Cheryl Ellenwood, and Carmela M. Roybal. "'I Hope to Hell Nothing Goes Back to the Way It Was Before': COVID-19, Marginalization, and Native Nations." *Perspectives on Politics* (2021): 1–18.

Frankel, Jeffrey A. "'No Atheists in Foxholes'? No Libertarians in Financial Crises." Belfer Center, Harvard University, July 17, 2008. https://www.belfercenter.org /publication/no-atheists-foxholes-no-libertarians-financial-crises.

French, Ron, and Oralandar Brand-Williams. "Cost of Segregation: Blacks Pay Harsh Price While Whites Suffer Less." *Detroit News*, April 15, 2020.

Frum, David. "This Is Trump's Fault." *The Atlantic*, April 7, 2020.

Funk, Cary, and John Gramlich. "10 Facts about Americans and Coronavirus Vaccines." Pew Research Center, September 20, 2021. https://www.pewresearch.org /fact-tank/2021/09/20/10-facts-about-americans-and-coronavirus-vaccines/.

Gabriel, Trip. "Ohio's G.O.P. Governor Splits from Trump, and Rises in Popularity." *New York Times*, April 28, 2020.

Gadarian, Shana Kushner. "Scary Pictures: How Terrorism Imagery Affects Voter Evaluations." *Political Communication* 31, no. 2 (2014): 282–302.

Gaines, Brian J., James H. Kuklinski, Paul J. Quirk, Buddy Peyton, and Jay Verkuilen. "Same Facts, Different Interpretations: Partisan Motivation and Opinion on Iraq." *Journal of Politics* 69, no. 4 (2007): 957–74.

Galasso, Vincenzo, Vincent Pons, Paola Profeta, Michael Becher, Sylvain Brouard, and Martial Foucault. "Gender Differences in COVID-19 Attitudes and Behavior: Panel Evidence from Eight Countries." *Proceedings of the National Academy of Sciences* 117, no. 44 (2020): 27285–91.

Gamio, Lazaro, John Keefe, Denise Lu, and Rich Harris. "Record-Setting Turnout: Tracking Early Voting in the 2020 Election." *New York Times*, November 12, 2020.

Garrand, Danielle. "California Received '170 Broken Ventilators' from Federal Government, Governor Says." CBS News, March 29, 2020.

Gelman, Andrew, and Jennifer Hill. *Data Analysis Using Regression and Multilevel/ Hierarchical Models*. New York: Cambridge University Press, 2006.

Germann, Timothy C., Kai Kadau, Ira M. Longini, and Catherine A. Macken. "Mitigation Strategies for Pandemic Influenza in the United States." *Proceedings of the National Academy of Sciences* 103, no. 15 (2006): 5935–40.

Gidron, Noam, James Adams, and Will Horne. *American Affective Polarization in Comparative Perspective*. Cambridge: Cambridge University Press, 2020.

Goldberg, Carey. "Got Extra Masks or Goggles? Mass. Hospitals Already Running Short, Ask for Donations." *WBUR News*, March 17, 2020.

Gollust, Sarah E., Rebekah H. Nagler, and Erika Franklin Fowler. "The Emergence of COVID-19 in the US: A Public Health and Political Communication Crisis." *Journal of Health Politics, Policy and Law* 45, no. 6 (2020): 967–81.

Goodman, Sara Wallace. *Citizenship in Hard Times: How Ordinary People Respond to Democratic Threat.* New York: Cambridge University Press, 2022.

———. "Immigration Threat, Partisanship, and Democratic Citizenship: Evidence from the US, UK, and Germany." *Comparative Political Studies* 54, no. 11 (2021): 2052–83.

———. "Should U.S. States Be Free to Close Their Borders to Other U.S. Citizens?" *Washington Post,* April 3, 2020.

Goolsbee, Austan, and Chad Syverson. "Fear, Lockdown, and Diversion: Comparing Drivers of Pandemic Economic Decline 2020." *Journal of Public Economics* 193 (2021): 104311.

Goren, Paul. "Party Identification and Core Political Values." *American Journal of Political Science* 49, no. 4 (2005): 881–96.

Granja, João, Christos Makridis, Constantine Yannelis, and Eric Zwick. "Did the Paycheck Protection Program Hit the Target?" NBER Working Paper No. 27095, 2020.

Green, Donald P., Bradley Palmquist, and Eric Schickler. *Partisan Hearts and Minds: Political Parties and the Social Identities of Voters.* New Haven, CT: Yale University Press, 2004.

Green, Jon, Jared Edgerton, Daniel Naftel, Kelsey Shoub, and Skyler J. Cranmer. "Elusive Consensus: Polarization in Elite Communication on the COVID-19 Pandemic." *Science Advances* 6, no. 28 (2020): eabc2717.

Greer, Scott L., and Peter D. Jacobson. "Health Care Reform and Federalism." *Journal of Health Politics, Policy and Law* 35, no. 2 (2010): 203–26.

Greer, Scott L., and Phillip M. Singer. "The United States Confronts Ebola: Suasion, Executive Action and Fragmentation." *Health Economics Policy and Law* 12, no. 1 (2017): 81–104.

Groenendyk, Eric. "Current Emotion Research in Political Science: How Emotions Help Democracy Overcome Its Collective Action Problem." *Emotion Review* 3, no. 4 (2011): 455–63.

Groenendyk, Eric, Ted Brader, and Nicholas Valentino. "Appraising Political Emotions: Appraisals, Emotions, and Behavior in Response to Threatening News." ResearchGate, January 2011.

Gross, James, and Ross Thompson. "Emotion Regulation: Conceptual Foundations." In *Handbook of Emotion Regulation,* ed. James Gross, 3–26. New York: Guilford, 2009.

Grossman, Guy, Soojong Kim, Jonah M. Rexer, and Harsha Thirumurthy. "Political Partisanship Influences Behavioral Responses to Governors' Recommendations for COVID-19 Prevention in the United States." *Proceedings of the National Academy of Sciences* 117, no. 39 (2020): 24144–53.

Grossmann, Matt, Sarah Reckhow, Katharine O. Strunk, and Meg Turner. "All States Close but Red Districts Reopen: The Politics of In-Person Schooling during the COVID-19 Pandemic." *Educational Researcher* 50, no. 9 (2021): 637–48.

Guillon, M., and P. Kergall. "Attitudes and Opinions on Quarantine and Support for a Contact-Tracing Application in France during the COVID-19 Outbreak." *Public Health* 188 (2020): 21–31.

Gumbrecht, Jamie, and Jessica Small. "House Committee Releases New Evidence from Investigation into Trump Administration Interference with CDC during Covid-19 Pandemic." CNN, November 12, 2021.

Haberman, Maggie. "Trade Adviser Warned White House in January of Risks of a Pandemic." *New York Times*, April 6, 2020.

Hake, Monica, Adam Dewey, Emily Engelhard, Angela Gallagher, Tom Summerfelt, Corey Malone-Smolla, Tremain Maebry, and Craig Gundersen. "The Impact of the Coronavirus on Local Food Insecurity." Feeding America, March 31, 2021. https://www.feedingamerica.org/research/coronavirus-hunger-research.

Hall, Ben. "Outspoken Conservative Radio Host Phil Valentine Dies after Battling COVID-19." NewsChannel 5 Nashville, August 21, 2021.

Hall, William J., Mimi V. Chapman, Kent M. Lee, Yesenia M. Merino, Tainayah W. Thomas, B. Keith Payne, Eugenia Eng, Steven H. Day, and Tamera Coyne-Beasley. "Implicit Racial/Ethnic Bias among Health Care Professionals and Its Influence on Health Care Outcomes: A Systematic Review." *American Journal of Public Health* 105, no. 12 (2015): e60–e76.

Hallal, Pedro C. "SOS Brazil: Science under Attack." *The Lancet* 397, no. 10272 (2021): 373–74.

Harlan, Chico, Stefano Pitrelli, and Rick Noack. "Vaccine Mandates Are Spreading. Italy Shows What to Expect." *Washington Post*, November 12, 2021.

Harper, Tim, Rachel Orey, and Collier Fernekes. *Counting the Vote during the 2020 Election.* Washington, DC: Bipartisan Policy Center, 2020.

Hartfield, Matthew, and Samuel Alizon. "Introducing the Outbreak Threshold in Epidemiology." *PLOS Pathogens* 9, no. 6 (2013): e1003277–e77.

Hatcher, Sarah, Christine Agnew-Brune, Mark Anderson, Laura Zambrando, Charles Rose, Melissa Jim, and Amy Buagher. "COVID-19 among American Indian and Alaska Native Persons—23 States, January 31–July 3, 2020." In *Morbidity and Mortality Weekly Report*, ed. Centers for Disease Control and Prevention, 1166–69. Washington, DC: U.S. Department of Health and Human Services and Centers for Disease Control and Prevention, 2020.

Hauser, Ethan, and Azi Paybarah. "The Governor of Texas Bars Covid Vaccine Mandates." *New York Times*, October 11, 2021.

Healy, Andrew, and Neil Malhotra. "Random Events, Economic Losses, and Retrospective Voting: Implications for Democratic Competence." *Quarterly Journal of Political Science* 5, no. 2 (2010): 193–208.

Healy, Beth. "Miscommunication, Missing Supplies Strain COVID-19 Coordination between Mass. And FEMA." *WBUR News*, April 12, 2020.

Heath, Brad. "Americans Divided on Party Lines over Risk from Coronavirus: Reuters/Ipsos Poll." Reuters, March 6.

Hernandez, Joe. "The FAA Has Seen A 'Significantly Higher' Number of Unruly Passenger Reports in 2021." National Public Radio, May 28, 2021.

Hetherington, Marc J. "Resurgent Mass Partisanship: The Role of Elite Polarization." *American Political Science Review* 95, no. 3 (2001): 619–31.

Higgins, Tucker, and Nate Rattner. "When Does Vote by Mail and Early Voting Start? A State by State Guide." CNBC, September 4, 2020.

Hill, Evan, Ainara Tiefenthäler, Christiaan Triebert, Drew Jordan, Haley Willis, and Robin Stein. "How George Floyd Was Killed in Police Custody." *New York Times*, May 31, 2020.

Hill, Latoya, and Samantha Artiga. "COVID-19 Vaccination among American Indian and Alaska Native People." Kaiser Family Foundation, April 9, 2021. https://www.kff.org/racial-equity-and-health-policy/issue-brief/covid-19-vaccination-american-indian-alaska-native-people/.

Holman, Mirya R., Emily M. Farris, and Jane Lawrence Sumner. "Local Political Institutions and First-Mover Policy Responses to COVID-19." *Journal of Political Institutions and Political Economy* 1, no. 4 (2020): 523–41.

Holmes, Kristen, Carma Hassan, and David Williams. "New England Patriots Team Plane with 1.2 Million N95 Masks Arrives from China to Help Ease Shortages." CNN, April 3, 2020.

Hornsey, Matthew J., Matthew Finlayson, Gabrielle Chatwood, and Christopher T. Begeny. "Donald Trump and Vaccination: The Effect of Political Identity, Conspiracist Ideation and Presidential Tweets on Vaccine Hesitancy." *Journal of Experimental Social Psychology* 88 (2020): 103947.

Howard, Marc Morjé. *Unusually Cruel: Prisons, Punishment, and the Real American Exceptionalism.* Oxford: Oxford University Press, 2017.

Hsu, Spencer S. "Federal Judge Strikes Down Trump Plan to Slash Food Stamps for 700,000 Unemployed Americans." *Washington Post*, October 18, 2020.

Hsu, Tiffany. "Despite Outbreaks among Unvaccinated, Fox News Hosts Smear Shots." *New York Times*, July 11, 2021.

Huberfeld, Nicole, Sarah H. Gordon, and David K. Jones. "Federalism Complicates the Response to the COVID-19 Health and Economic Crisis: What Can Be Done?" *Journal of Health Politics, Policy and Law* 45 (6) (2020): 951–65.

Hutchinson, Bill. "'Incomprehensible': Confrontations over Masks Erupt amid COVID-19 Crisis." ABC News, May 7, 2020.

Igielnik, Ruth, Scott Keeter, and Hannah Hartig. "Behind Biden's 2020 Victory." Pew Research Center, June 30, 2021. https://www.pewresearch.org/politics/2021/06/30/behind-bidens-2020-victory/.

"Interview: Bret Baier and Martha MacCallum Host a Town Hall with Donald Trump." YouTube, March 5, 2020. https://www.youtube.com/watch?v=cukyV5UGuEE.

Iyengar, Shanto, and Masha Krupenkin. "Partisanship as Social Identity: Implications for the Study of Party Polarization." Paper presented at The Forum, 2018.

Iyengar, Shanto, Yphtach Lelkes, Matthew Levendusky, Neil Malhotra, and Sean J. Westwood. "The Origins and Consequences of Affective Polarization in the United States." *Annual Review of Political Science* 22 (2019): 129–46.

Iyengar, Shanto, Gaurav Sood, and Yphtach Lelkes. "Affect, Not Ideology: A Social Identity Perspective on Polarization." *Public Opinion Quarterly* 76, no. 3 (2012): 405–31.

Jackson, Lisa A., Evan J. Anderson, Nadine G. Rouphael, Paul C. Roberts, Mamo-dikoe Makhene, Rhea N. Coler, Michele P. McCullough, et al. "An mRNA Vaccine against SARS-CoV-2—Preliminary Report." *New England Journal of Medicine* 383, no. 20 (2020): 1920–31.

Joffe, Hélène. *Risk and "The Other."* Cambridge: Cambridge University Press, 1999.

Jones, Christina L., Jakob D. Jensen, Courtney L. Scherr, Natasha R. Brown, Kath-eryn Christy, and Jeremy Weaver. "The Health Belief Model as an Explanatory Framework in Communication Research: Exploring Parallel, Serial, and Mod-erated Mediation." *Health Communication* 30, no. 6 (2015): 566–76.

Jones, Jeffrey M. "Trump Job Approval at Personal Best 49%." Gallup, February 4, 2020.

Jordan, Miriam, and Caitlin Dickerson. "Poultry Worker's Death Highlights Spread of Coronavirus in Meat Plants." *New York Times*, April 19, 2020.

Jurkowitz, Mark, and Amy Mitchell. "Cable TV and COVID-19: How Americans Perceive the Outbreak and View Media Coverage Differ by Main News Source." Pew Research Center for Journalism and Media, April 1, 2020. https://www .journalism.org/2020/04/01/cable-tv-and-covid-19-how-americans-perceive -the-outbreak-and-view-media-coverage-differ-by-main-news-source/.

Kaiser Family Foundation. "Weekly COVID-19 Vaccine Allocations." May 31, 2021. https://www.kff.org/other/state-indicator/weekly-covid-19-vaccine-allocations /?currentTimeframe=3&selectedRows=%7B%22wrapups%22:%7B%22united -states%22:%7B%7D%7D%7D&sortModel=%7B%22colId%22:%22Location %22,%22sort%22:%22asc%22%7D.

Kalmoe, Nathan P., and Lilliana Mason. "Lethal Mass Partisanship: Prevalence, Correlates, and Electoral Contingencies." Presented at the annual meeting of the American Political Science Association Conference, Boston, MA, 2018.

Kam, Cindy D. "'And Why Is That a Partisan Issue?' Source Cues, Persuasion, and School Lunches." *Journal of Politics* 82, no. 1 (2020): 361–66.

Kamarck, Elaine. "Pandemic Politics: Red State Governors Are in Trouble for Their Covid Leadership." Brookings Institution, October 19, 2021.

Karol, David, and Edward Miguel. "The Electoral Cost of War: Iraq Casualties and the 2004 U.S. Presidential Election." *Journal of Politics* 69, no. 3 (2007): 633–48.

Kelman, Brett. "Tennessee Abandons Vaccine Outreach to Minors—Not Just for COVID-19." *Tennessean*, July 13, 2021.

Kenen, Joanne. "How Testing Failures Allowed Coronavirus to Sweep the U.S." Politico, March 8, 2020.

Khazan, Olga. "The Most American COVID-19 Failure Yet." *The Atlantic*, August 31, 2020.

Kihara, David. "3rd Conservative Radio Host Who Condemned Vaccines Dies of Covid." Politico, August 29, 2021.

Kim, June-Ho, Julia Ah-Reum An, SeungJu Jackie Oh, Juhwan Oh, and Jong-Koo Lee. "Emerging COVID-19 Success Story: South Korea Learned the Lessons of MERS." Our World in Data, March 5, 2021. https://ourworldindata.org/covid -exemplar-south-korea.

Kim, Naeun Lauren, and Hyunjoo Im. "Do Liberals Want Curbside Pickup More Than Conservatives? Contactless Shopping as Protectionary Action against the COVID-19 Pandemic." *International Journal of Consumer Studies*, May 7, 2021.

Kim, Soo Rin, Matthew Vann, Laura Bronner, Grace Manthey, Ryan Best, and Emily Scherer. "Which Cities Have the Biggest Racial Gaps in COVID-19 Testing Access?" FiveThirtyEight, July 22, 2020.

King, Jamilah. "Eight Trump Campaign Staffers Test Positive for Coronavirus after Tulsa Rally." *Mother Jones*, June 27, 2020.

Kirzinger, Ashley, Audrey Kearney, Liz Hamel, and Mollyann Brodie. "KFF COVID-19 Vaccine Monitor: The Increasing Importance of Partisanship in Predicting COVID-19 Vaccination Status." Kaiser Family Foundation, November 16, 2021.

Kirzinger, Ashley, Grace Sparks, and Mollyann Brodie. "KFF Covid-19 Vaccine Monitor: In Their Own Words, Six Months Later." Kaiser Family Foundation, July 13, 2021.

Kitschelt, Herbert. "Formation of Party Cleavages in Post-Communist Democracies: Theoretical Propositions." *Party Politics* 1, no. 4 (1995): 447–72.

———. "Linkages between Citizens and Politicians in Democratic Polities." *Comparative Political Studies* 33, no. 6–7 (2000): 845–79.

Klar, Samara, and Yanna Krupnikov. *Independent Politics: How American Disdain for Parties Leads to Political Inaction.* New York: Cambridge University Press, 2016.

Klein, Ezra. *Why We're Polarized.* New York: Simon & Schuster, 2020.

Kraut, Alan M. *Silent Travelers: Germs, Genes, and the Immigrant Menace.* Baltimore: Johns Hopkins' University Press, 1995.

Krupenkin, Masha. "Does Partisanship Affect Compliance with Government Recommendations?" *Political Behavior* 43, no. 1 (2021): 451–72.

Kumar, Anita. "Trump Fears Emergency Declaration Would Contradict Coronavirus Message." Politico, March 11, 2020.

Kuo, Jason, and Megumi Naoi. "Individual Attitudes." In *The Oxford Handbook of the Political Economy of International Trade*, ed. Lisa Martin, 99–118. New York: Oxford University Press, 2015.

Kustov, Alexander, Dillon Laaker, and Cassidy Reller. "The Stability of Immigration Attitudes: Evidence and Implications." *Journal of Politics* 83, no. 4: 1478–94.

LaFraniere, Sharon. "White House Says It Will Narrowly Miss July 4 Vaccination Goal." *New York Times*, June 22, 2021.

Latkin, Carl A., Lauren Dayton, Grace Yi, Brian Colon, and Xiangrong Kong. "Mask Usage, Social Distancing, Racial, and Gender Correlates of COVID-19 Vaccine Intentions among Adults in the US." *PLOS One* 16, no. 2 (2021): e0246970.

Lau, Richard R., and David P. Redlawsk. *How Voters Decide: Information Processing in Election Campaigns.* New York: Cambridge University Press, 2006.

Lazarus, Richard S. "Cognition and Motivation in Emotion." *American Psychologist* 46, no. 4 (1991): 352–67.

Lee, Ellen H., Kelsey L. Kepler, Anita Geevarughese, Rachel Paneth-Pollak, Marie S. Dorsinville, Stephanie Ngai, and Kathleen H. Reilly. "Race/Ethnicity among Children with COVID-19–Associated Multisystem Inflammatory Syndrome." *JAMA Network Open* 3, no. 11 (2020): e2030280.

Lee, Sui-Wee. "They Relied on Chinese Vaccines. Now They're Battling Outbreaks." *New York Times*, June 22, 2021.

Lenz, Gabriel S. *Follow the Leader? How Voters Respond to Politicians' Policies and Performance.* Chicago: University of Chicago Press, 2013.

Leonhardt, David. "A Complete List of Trump's Attempts to Play Down Coronavirus." *New York Times*, March 15, 2020.

———. "U.S. Covid Deaths Get Even Redder." *New York Times*, November 8, 2021.

Lerman, Amy E., and Katherine T. McCabe. "Personal Experience and Public Opinion: A Theory and Test of Conditional Policy Feedback." *Journal of Politics* 79, no. 2 (2017): 624–41.

Levendusky, Matthew. *The Partisan Sort: How Liberals Became Democrats and Conservatives Became Republicans.* Chicago: University of Chicago Press, 2009.

Levitsky, Steven, and Daniel Ziblatt. *How Democracies Die.* New York: Crown, 2018.

Levey, Noam M. "Hospitals Say Feds Are Seizing Masks and Other Coronavirus Supplies without a Word." *Los Angeles Times*, April 7, 2020.

Lewis, David E. "Is the Failed Pandemic Response a Symptom of a Diseased Administrative State?" *Daedalus* 150, no. 3 (2021): 68–88.

Li, Yao, and Harvey L. Nicholson Jr. "When 'Model Minorities' become 'Yellow Peril'—Othering and the Racialization of Asian Americans in the COVID-19 Pandemic." *Sociology Compass* 15, no. 2 (2021): e12849.

Lipton, Eric. "The 'Red Dawn' Emails: 8 Key Exchanges on the Faltering Response to the Coronavirus." *New York Times*, April 11, 2020.

Lipton, Eric, David E. Sanger, Maggie Haberman, Michael D. Shear, Mark Mazzetti, and Julian E. Barnes. "He Could Have Seen What Was Coming: Behind Trump's Failure on the Virus." *New York Times*, April 11, 2020.

Lodge, Milton, and Charles S. Taber. *The Rationalizing Voter.* New York: Cambridge University Press, 2013.

Lorenz, Taylor, Kellen Browning, and Sheera Frenkel. "TikTok Teens and K-Pop Stans Say They Sank Trump Rally." *New York Times*, June 21, 2020.

Lovelace, Berkeley, Jr. "CDC Reverses Indoor Mask Policy, Saying Fully Vaccinated People and Kids Should Wear Them Indoors." CNBC, July 27, 2021.

———. "CDC Warns George Floyd Protests May Be 'Seeding Event' for More Coronavirus Outbreaks." CNBC, June 4, 2020.

Lozano, Alicia Victoria. "Southwest Airlines Employee Hospitalized after Passenger Punched Her, Police Say." NBC News, November 13, 2021.

Lupia, Arthur. *Uninformed: Why People Know So Little about Politics and What We Can Do about It.* New York: Oxford University Press, 2016.

Lupia, Arthur, and Jesse Menning. "Politics and the Equilibrium of Fear: Can Strategies and Emotions Interact?" In *The Affect Effect: Dynamics of Emotion in*

Political Thinking and Behavior, ed. George E. Marcus, W. Russell Neuman, and Michael MacKuen, 337–56. Chicago: University of Chicago Press, 2008.

Lutz, Eric. "Trump: Mail-in Voting Is 'Horrible' Except When I Do It." *Vanity Fair*, April 8, 2020.

MacGillis, Alec. "How Germany Saved Its Workforce from Unemployment While Spending Less Per Person Than the U.S." ProPublica, June 3, 2020. https://www.propublica.org/article/how-germany-saved-its-workforce-from-unemployment-while-spending-less-per-person-than-the-u-s.

Malhotra, Neil, and Alexander G. Kuo. "Attributing Blame: The Public's Response to Hurricane Katrina." *Journal of Politics* 70, no. 1 (2008): 120–35.

Marcus, George, W. Russell Neuman, and Michael MacKuen. *Affective Intelligence and Political Judgment.* Chicago: University of Chicago Press, 2000.

Margolin, Josh. "FBI Warns of Potential Surge in Hate Crimes against Asian Americans amid Coronavirus." ABC News, March 27, 2020.

Mason, Lilliana. "A Cross-cutting Calm: How Social Sorting Drives Affective Polarization." *Public Opinion Quarterly* 80, no. S1 (2016): 351–77.

———. *Uncivil Agreement: How Politics Became Our Identity.* Chicago: University of Chicago Press, 2018.

Matoso, Filipe, and Mateus Rodrigues. "Coronavírus: Bolsonaro diz na TV que não há razão para pânico ainda que problema se agrave." G1, June 3, 2020.

Mauldin, William. "U.S. Suspends Tariffs for Some Importers Affected by Coronavirus." *Wall Street Journal*, April 19, 2020.

McCarty, Nolan, Keith T. Poole, and Howard Rosenthal. *Polarized America: The Dance of Ideology and Unequal Riches.* Cambridge, MA: MIT Press, 2016.

McCoy, Jennifer, and Murat Somer. "Toward a Theory of Pernicious Polarization and How It Harms Democracies: Comparative Evidence and Possible Remedies." *ANNALS of the American Academy of Political and Social Science* 681, no. 1 (2019): 234–71.

McEnany, Kayleigh. "Outnumbered." *Fox News*, August 9, 2021.

Mehta, Dhrumil. "The Media Really Has Neglected Puerto Rico." FiveThirtyEight, September 28, 2017.

Melton, Marissa. "Is 'Make America Great Again' Racist?." VOA, August 31, 2017.

Mendelberg, Tali. *The Race Card: Campaign Strategy, Implicit Messages, and the Norm of Equality.* Princeton, NJ: Princeton University Press, 2001.

Merle, Renae. "Trump Says He's 'Stopping Evictions.' Here's Why They're Still Happening." *Washington Post*, August 17, 2020.

Merolla, Jennifer L., and Elizabeth J. Zechmeister. *Democracy at Risk: How Terrorist Threats affect the Public.* Chicago: University of Chicago Press, 2009.

Mettler, Suzanne. *The Submerged State: How Invisible Government Policies Undermine American Democracy.* Chicago: University of Chicago Press, 2011.

Meyersohn, Nathaniel. "CVS and Walgreens Warn There Could Be a Shortage of Hand Sanitizer." CNN, February 28, 2020.

Miao, Hannah. "White House Abandoned Plan to Send 650 Million Face Masks across the U.S. in April, Report Says." CNBC, September 17, 2020.

Michener, Jamila. *Fragmented Democracy: Medicaid, Federalism, and Unequal Politics.* New York: Cambridge University Press, 2018.

———. "Race, Politics, and the Affordable Care Act." *Journal of Health Politics, Policy and Law* 45, no. 4 (2020): 547–66.

Miller, Greg, and Ellen Nakashima. "President's Intelligence Briefing Book Repeatedly Cited Virus Threat." *Washington Post*, April 27, 2020.

Mishra, Swapnil, James A. Scott, Daniel J. Laydon, Seth Flaxman, Axel Gandy, Thomas A. Mellan, H. Juliette T. Unwin, et al. "Comparing the Responses of the UK, Sweden and Denmark to COVID-19 Using Counterfactual Modelling." *Scientific Reports* 11, no. 1 (2021): 1–9.

Mohammed, Anwar, Regan M. Johnston, and Clifton van der Linden. "Public Responses to Policy Reversals: The Case of Mask Usage in Canada during COVID-19." *Canadian Public Policy* 46, no. S2 (2020): S119–26.

Monmouth University Polling Institute. "Majority Support Trump Impeachment." January 25, 2021. https://www.monmouth.edu/polling-institute/reports /monmouthpoll_US_012521/.

Montez, Jennifer Karas, Jason Beckfield, Julene Kemp Cooney, Jacob M. Grumbach, Mark D. Hayward, Huseyin Zeyd Koytak, Steven H. Woolf, and Anna Zajacova. "US State Policies, Politics, and Life Expectancy." *Milbank Quarterly* 98, no. 3 (2020): 668–99.

Moreland, Amanda, Christine Herlihy, Michael A. Tynan, Gregory Sunshine, Russell F. McCord, Charity Hilton, Jason Poovey, et al. "Timing of State and Territorial COVID-19 Stay-at-Home Orders and Changes in Population Movement—United States, March 1–May 31, 2020." *Morbidity and Mortality Weekly Report* 69, no. 35 (2020): 1198.

Mosendz, Polly, Peter Waldman, and Lydia Mulvany. "U.S. Meat Plants Are Deadly as Ever, with No Incentive to Change." Bloomberg, June 18, 2020.

Mounk, Yascha. "Cancel Everything." *The Atlantic*, March 10, 2020.

Moussaoui, Lisa S., Nana D. Ofosu, and Olivier Desrichard. "Social Psychological Correlates of Protective Behaviours in the COVID-19 Outbreak: Evidence and Recommendations from a Nationally Representative Sample." *Applied Psychology: Health and Well-Being* 12, no. 4 (2020): 1183–204.

Moyer, Melinda Wenner. "Pods, Microschools and Tutors: Can Parents Solve the Education Crisis on Their Own?" *New York Times*, July 22, 2020.

Mueller, John E. "Presidential Popularity from Truman to Johnson." *American Political Science Review* 64, no. 1 (1970): 18–34.

Murphy, Sean. "Health Official: Trump Rally 'Likely' Source of Virus Surge." Associated Press, July 8, 2020.

Mutz, Diana. "Effects of 'In-Your-Face' Television Discourse on Perceptions of a Legitimate Opposition." *American Political Science Review* 101, no. 4 (2007): 621–35.

Narlikar, Amrita. "In Brief: The Coronavirus and Germany." German Institute for Global and Area Studies, March 12, 2020.

National Alliance to End Homelessness. "Racial Inequalities in Homelessness, by the Numbers." June 1, 2020. https://endhomelessness.org/resource/racial -inequalities-homelessness-numbers/.

National Center for Health Statistics. "National Vital Statistics System, Mortality." 2019. https://www.cdc.gov/nchs/nvss/deaths.htm.

National Public Radio. "After Months of Questions, a Key Operation Warp Speed Adviser's Contract Emerges." October 30, 2020.

———. "Trump Tells Woodward He Deliberately Downplayed Coronavirus Threat." September 10, 2020.

———. "A 'War' for Medical Supplies: States Say FEMA Wins by Poaching Orders." April 15, 2020.

———. "Writer Michael Anton Makes the Case for Why Trump Should Be Reelected." National Public Radio, October 20, 2020.

NBC 6. "Miami Beach Couple Arrested in Hawaii for Using Fake Vaccination Cards." August 18, 2021. https://www.nbcmiami.com/news/local/miami -beach-couple-arrested-in-hawaii-for-using-fake-vaccination-cards/2531905/.

Ndugga, Namib, Oliva Pham, Latoya Hill, Samantha Artiga, Raisa Alam, Noah Parker. "Latest Data on COVID-19 Vaccinations Race/Ethnicity." Kaiser Family Foundation, January 12, 2021.

Neelon, Brian, Fedelis Mutiso, Noel T. Mueller, John L. Pearce, and Sara E. Benjamin-Neelon. "Associations between Governor Political Affiliation and COVID-19 Cases, Deaths, and Testing in the US." *American Journal of Preventive Medicine*, March 9, 2021.

Nellis, Ashley. "The Color of Justice: Racial and Ethnic Disparity in State Prisons." The Sentencing Project, 2016.

Nelson, Thomas E., and Donald R. Kinder. "Issue Frames and Group-Centrism in American Public Opinion." *Journal of Politics* 58, no. 4 (1996): 1055–78.

Neuman, W. Russell, George Marcus, Ann N. Crigler, and Michael MacKuen, eds. *The Affect Effect: Dynamics of Emotion in Political Thinking and Behavior*. Chicago: University of Chicago Press, 2007.

Neyman, Gregory, and William Dalsey. "Black Lives Matter Protests and COVID-19 Cases: Relationship in Two Databases." *Journal of Public Health* 43, no. 2 (2021): 225–27.

Nguyen, Terry. "How the Trump Administration Has Stood in the Way of PPE Distribution." Vox, April 4, 2020.

Nielsen, Julie Hassing, and Johannes Lindvall. "Trust in Government in Sweden and Denmark during the COVID-19 Epidemic." *West European Politics* 44, no. 5–6 (2021): 1180–204.

Nilsen, Ella. "New York Is in Dire Need of Ventilators. China Just Donated 1,000." Vox, April 4, 2020.

Norwood, Candace. "Trump Restricts Immigration amid the Pandemic. Critics See It as an Excuse to Push His Own Agenda." PBS, July 28, 2020.

OANN. "The Daily Ledger." April 7, 2020.

Office of the President. "Buy American and Hire American." Executive Order 13788, Federal Register, April 18, 2017. https://www.federalregister.gov/documents /2017/04/21/2017-08311/buy-american-and-hire-american.

Oliver, J. Eric, and Taeku Lee. "Public Opinion and the Politics of Obesity in America." *Journal of Health Politics, Policy and Law* 30, no. 5 (2005): 923–54.

Oster, Emily. "Parents Can't Wait around Forever." *The Atlantic*, July 2, 2020.

Oxford Analytica. "US November Election Could Produce Crisis." September 18, 2020. https://doi.org/10.1108/OXAN-DB256343.

———. "Vaccine Diplomacy Will Earn China Friends and Money." May 17, 2021. https://doi.org/10.1108/OXAN-DB261517.

Pacheco, Julianna, Jake Haselswerdt, and Jamila Michener. "The Affordable Care Act and Polarization in the United States." *RSF: The Russell Sage Foundation Journal of the Social Sciences* 6, no. 2 (2020): 114–30.

Palmer, Carl L., and Rolfe D. Peterson. "Toxic Mask-ulinity: The Link between Masculine Toughness and Affective Reactions to Mask Wearing in the COVID-19 Era." *Politics & Gender* 16, no. 4 (2020): 1044–51.

Panebianco, Angelo. *Political Parties: Organization and Power.* New York: Cambridge University Press, 1988.

Panetta, Grace. "Trump Reportedly Threatened to Fire a Top Doctor at the CDC for Sounding the Alarm about the Coronavirus in February." Business Insider, April 22, 2020.

Paradies, Yin, Mandy Truong, and Naomi Priest. "A Systematic Review of the Extent and Measurement of Healthcare Provider Racism." *Journal of General Internal Medicine* 29, no. 2 (2014): 364–87.

Parker, Ashley, and Josh Dawsey. "Seven Days: Following Trump's Coronavirus Trail." *Washington Post,* December 5, 2021.

Parker, Kim, Rachel Minkin, and Jesse Bennett. "Economic Fallout from COVID-19 Continues to Hit Lower-Income Americans the Hardest." Pew Research Center, September 25, 2020. https://www.pewresearch.org/social-trends /2020/09/24/economic-fallout-from-covid-19-continues-to-hit-lower -income-americans-the-hardest/.

Parrott, Sharon, Chad Stone, Chye-Ching Huang, Michael Leachman, Peggy Bailey, Aviva Aron-Dine, Stacy Dean, and LaDonna Pavetti. "CARES Act Includes Essential Measures to Respond to Public Health, Economic Crises, but More Will Be Needed." Center on Budget and Policy Priorities, March 27, 2020. https://www.cbpp.org/sites/default/files/atoms/files/3-27-20econ .pdf.

Pedroso, Rodrigo. "Brazil's Bolsonaro Says He Will Not Be Vaccinated against Covid-19." CNN, October 13, 2021.

Pekar, Jonathan, Michael Worobey, Niema Moshiri, Konrad Scheffler, and Joel O. Wertheim. "Timing the SARS-CoV-2 Index Case in Hubei Province." *Science* 372, no. 6540 (2021): 412–17.

Pepinsky, Thomas B. "Americans Are Already Set to Conclude That the 2020 Presidential Elections Were Rigged." October 28, 2020. https://tompepinsky .com/2020/10/28/americans-are-already-set-to-conclude-that-the-2020 -presidential-elections-were-rigged/.

———. "Political Economy and Democratic Capacity to Respond to Pandemics." Social Science Research Council, May 21, 2020. https://items.ssrc.org/covid-19 -and-the-social-sciences/democracy-and-pandemics/political-economy-and -democratic-capacity-to-respond-to-pandemics/.

———. "Why the Impeachment Fight Is Even Scarier Than You Think." Politico, October 31, 2019.

Pérez, Efrén O. "Explicit Evidence on the Import of Implicit Attitudes: The IAT and Immigration Policy Judgments." *Political Behavior* 32, no. 4 (2010): 517–45.

Pérez-Peña, Richard. "Nurse Who Contracted Ebola in the U.S. Sues Her Hospital Employer." *New York Times*, March 2, 2015.

Peritz, Aki. "The Intelligence Community Got the Pandemic Right. Then Politicians Botched It." *Washington Post*, September 11, 2020.

Peters, Jeremy W., and Michael M. Grynbaum. "How Right-Wing Pundits Are Covering Coronavirus." *New York Times*, March 11, 2020.

Petersen, Melody, and Emily Baumgaertner. "Bottlenecks in Coronavirus Testing Means Excruciating Wait Times for the Sick." *Los Angeles Times*, March 30, 2020.

Petersen, Michael Bang. "COVID Lesson: Trust the Public with Hard Truths." *Nature* 598, no. 7880 (2021): 237–37.

Petersen, Ruth, Liping Pan, and Heidi M. Blanck. "Racial and Ethnic Disparities in Adult Obesity in the United States: CDC's Tracking to Inform State and Local Action." *Preventing Chronic Disease* 16 (2019).

Petri, Alexandra. "Opinion: Big Bird Is a Communist." *Washington Post*, November 9, 2021.

Pew Research Center. "COVID-19 Discussion Increasingly Popular in Twitter Posts Sent by Members of Congress." April 2, 2020. https://www.pewresearch.org/fact-tank/2020/04/02/tweets-by-members-of-congress-tell-the-story-of-an-escalating-covid-19-crisis/ft_2020-04-02_congressionaltweets_01/.

———. "Many Black and Asian Americans Say They Have Experienced Discrimination amid the COVID-19 Outbreak." June 7, 2020. https://www.pewresearch.org/social-trends/2020/07/01/many-black-and-asian-americans-say-they-have-experienced-discrimination-amid-the-covid-19-outbreak/.

Phoenix, Davin L. *The Anger Gap: How Race Shapes Emotion in Politics.* New York: Cambridge University Press, 2019.

Piccoli, Lorenzo, Jelena Dzankic, Andreas Perret, Didier Ruedin, and Timothy Craig Jacob-Owens. "International Travel Restrictions in Response to the COVID-19 Outbreak Dataset." EUI Research Data, Robert Schuman Centre for Advanced Studies, 2020. https://hdl.handle.net/1814/68359.

Pickup, Mark, Dominik Stecula, and Clifton Van Der Linden. "Novel Coronavirus, Old Partisanship: COVID-19 Attitudes and Behaviours in the United States and Canada." *Canadian Journal of Political Science/Revue canadienne de science politique* 53, no. 2 (2020): 357–64.

Pollak, Joel B. "Democrats Pushed Impeachment While Coronavirus Spread." Breitbart, March 13, 2020.

Population Reference Bureau. "Who Votes in America?" October 1, 2000. https://www.prb.org/resources/who-votes-in-america/.

Power, Lis, and Rob Savillo. "Fox News Has Promoted Hydroxychloroquine Nearly 300 Times in a Two-Week Period." Media Matters for America, April 7, 2020.

"President Trump Calls Coronavirus 'Kung Flu.'" BBC, June 24, 2020.

Quinn, Allison. "California Gov Was Reportedly Told He'd Have to Do the White House a Favor to Get Help with Testing Swabs." Daily Beast, July 18, 2020.

Quinn, Sandra C., and Michele P. Andrasik. "Addressing Vaccine Hesitancy in BIPOC Communities—Toward Trustworthiness, Partnership, and Reciprocity." *New England Journal of Medicine* 385 (2021): 97–100.

Ray, Rashawn. "Why Are Blacks Dying at Higher Rates from COVID-19?" Brookings Institution, March 2, 2020, https://www.brookings.edu/blog/fixgov/2020/04/09/why-are-blacks-dying-at-higher-rates-from-covid-19/.

Ray, Rashawn, Jane Fran Morgan, Lydia Wildeden, Samantha Elizondo, and Destiny Wiley-Yancy. "Examining and Addressing COVID-19 Racial Disparities in Detroit." Brookings Institution, March 2, 2021. https://www.brookings.edu/research/examining-and-addressing-covid-19-racial-disparities-in-detroit/.

Reichert, Corinne. "Amazon Plans to Prosecute Sellers for Price Gouging during Coronavirus Outbreak." CNET, March 6, 2020.

Reinecke, Carmen. "How the Pandemic and a Rise in Targeted Hate Crimes Has Shifted Spending for Asian Americans." NBC News, June 2, 2021.

ReliefWeb. "Public Health Experts Urge U.S. Officials to Withdraw Order Enabling Mass Expulsion of Asylum Seekers." ReliefWeb, May 19, 2020. https://reliefweb.int/report/united-states-america/public-health-experts-urge-us-officials-withdraw-order-enabling-mass.

Relman, Eliza. "Just 45% of House Republicans Say They've Been Vaccinated While 100% of Congressional Democrats Say They've Gotten the Shot." Business Insider, May 14, 2021.

Rentsch, Christopher T., Farah Kidwai-Khan, Janet P. Tate, Lesley S. Park, Joseph T. King Jr., Melissa Skanderson, Ronald G. Hauser, et al. "Patterns of COVID-19 Testing and Mortality by Race and Ethnicity among United States Veterans: A Nationwide Cohort study." *PLOS Medicine* 17, no. 9 (2020): e1003379.

Reny, Tyler T. "Masculine Norms and Infectious Disease: The Case of Covid-19." *Politics & Gender* 16, no. 4 (2020): 1028–35.

Reny, Tyler T., and Matt A. Barreto. "Xenophobia in the Time of Pandemic: Othering, Anti-Asian Attitudes, and COVID-19." *Politics, Groups, and Identities* (2020): 1–24.

Restuccia, Andrew, and Rebecca Ballhaus. "Trump Shuns Use of Law Allowing Control over Manufacturers." *Wall Street Journal*, March 22, 2020.

Reuben, Rebekah, Devon Aitken, Jonathan L. Freedman, and Gillian Einstein. "Mistrust of the Medical Profession and Higher Disgust Sensitivity Predict Parental Vaccine Hesitancy." *PLOS One* 15, no. 9 (2020): e0237755.

Reuters. "Germany Treats First Italians as Coronavirus Care Crosses Borders." March 24, 2020.

———. "Only Three U.S. States Can Test for Coronavirus—Public Lab Group." February 21, 2020.

Roberto, Katherine J., Andrew F. Johnson, and Beth M. Rauhaus. "Stigmatization and Prejudice during the COVID-19 Pandemic." *Administrative Theory & Praxis* 42, no. 3 (2020): 364–78.

Robertson, Campbell, and Robert Gebeloff. "How Millions of Women Became the Most Essential Workers in America." *New York Times*, April 18, 2020.

Rogers, Tiana N., Charles R. Rogers, Elizabeth VanSant-Webb, Lily Y. Gu, Bin Yan, and Fares Qeadan. "Racial Disparities in COVID-19 Mortality among Essential Workers in the United States." *World Medical & Health Policy* 12, no. 3 (2020): 311–27.

Romano, Andrew. "Yahoo News/YouGov Coronavirus Poll: Most Americans Reject Anti-Lockdown Protests." Yahoo!News, April 20, 2020.

Romeo, Peter. "Half the Nation's Chinese Restaurants Have Closed, Study Finds." *Restaurant Business*, April 13, 2020.

Roose, Kevin. "What Is QAnon, the Viral Pro-Trump Conspiracy Theory?" *New York Times*, September 3, 2021.

Roseman, Ira, Martin Spindel, and Paul Jose. "Appraisals of Emotion-Eliciting Events: Testing a Theory of Discrete Emotions." *Journal of Personality and Social Psychology* 59, no. 5 (1990): 899–915.

Rothstein, Bo, and Jan Teorell. "What Is Quality of Government? A Theory of Impartial Government Institutions." *Governance* 21, no. 2 (2008): 165–90.

Rudolph, Thomas J. "Who's Responsible for the Economy? The Formation and Consequences of Responsibility Attributions." *American Journal of Political Science* 47, no. 4 (2003): 698–713.

Ruiz, Neil, Khadijah Edwards, and Mark Hugo Lopez. "One-third of Asian Americans Fear Threats, Physical Attacks and Most Say Violence against Them Is Rising." Pew Research Center, April 21, 2021.

Rummler, Orion. "Hogan Says National Guard Is Protecting Coronavirus Tests Sent from South Korea." Axios, April 23, 2020.

Sadeque, Samira. "Nearly All Fox Staffers Vaccinated for Covid Even as Hosts Cast Doubt on Vaccine." *The Guardian*, September 15, 2021.

Salama, Vivian. "Not a 'Good Look': White House Fight over Masks Signaled Covid-19 Plans Running Awry." CNN, October 2, 2020.

Samuels, Brett, and Jessie Hellman. "Trump Says Testing May Be 'Frankly Overrated.'" The Hill, May 14, 2020.

Santich, Kate. "DeSantis Suspends Work Requirements for Food Stamps until Sept. 1." *Orlando Sentinel*, July 28, 2020.

Satow, Julie. "Turning a Second Home into a Primary Home." *New York Times*, July 24, 2020.

Schedler, Andreas. "The Menu of Manipulation." *Journal of Democracy* 13, no. 2 (2002): 36–50.

"Scientist Tapped to Lead CDC Does Not Inspire Confidence." *Star Tribune*, March 22, 2020.

Schneider, Saundra. "Who's to Blame? (Mis)perceptions of the Intergovernmental Response to Disasters." *Publius: Journal of Federalism* 38, no. 4 (2008): 715–38.

Schneiker, Andrea. "Populist Leadership: The Superhero Donald Trump as Savior in Times of Crisis." *Political Studies* 68, no. 4 (2020): 857–74.

Schoeni, Robert F., Emily E. Wiemers, Judith A. Seltzer, and Kenneth M. Langa. "Association between Risk Factors for Complications from COVID-19,

Perceived Chances of Infection and Complications, and Protective Behavior in the US." *JAMA Network Open* 4, no. 3 (2021): e213984.

Seligman, Benjamin, Maddalena Ferranna, and David E. Bloom. "Social Determinants of Mortality from COVID-19: A Simulation Study Using NHANES." *PLOS Medicine* 18, no. 1 (2021): e1003490.

Segarra, Marielle. "How Did We End Up in a Ventilator Bidding War?" Marketplace, April 1, 2020.

Serdan, Tamires D. A., Laureane N. Masi, Renata Gorjao, Tania C. Pithon-Curi, Rui Curi, and Sandro M. Hirabara. "COVID-19 in Brazil: Historical Cases, Disease Milestones, and Estimated Outbreak Peak." *Travel Medicine and Infectious Disease* 38 (2020): 101733.

Shamsian, Jacob, and Sonam Sheth. "Trump and His Allies Filed More Than 40 Lawsuits Challenging the 2020 Election Results. All of Them Failed." Business Insider, February 22, 2021.

Shear, Michael D., Abby Goodnough, Sheila Kaplan, Sheri Fink, Katie Thomas, and Noah Weiland. "The Lost Month: How a Failure to Test Blinded the U.S. to Covid-19." *New York Times*, March 28, 2020.

Siegler, Kirk. "Across America, Frustrated Protesters Rally to Reopen the Economy." National Public Radio, April 18, 2020.

Singer, Merrill. "A Dose of Drugs, a Touch of Violence, a Case of AIDS: Conceptualizing the SAVA Syndemic." *Free Inquiry in Creative Sociology* 28, no. 1 (2000): 13–24.

Sirin, Cigdem V., Nicholas A. Valentino, and Jose D. Villalobos. *Seeing Us in Them: Social Divisions and the Politics of Group Empathy.* Cambridge: Cambridge University Press, 2021.

———. "The Social Causes and Political Consequences of Group Empathy." *Political Psychology* 38, no. 3 (2017): 427–48.

Sloan, Chris, Robin Duddy-Tenbrunsel, Samantha Ferguson, and Angel Valladares. "COVID-19 Projected to Worsen Racial Disparities in Health Coverage." Avalere, September 16, 2020. https://avalere.com/press-releases/covid-19-projected-to-worsen-racial-disparities-in-health-coverage.

Smialek, Jeanna, and Jack Ewing "Coronavirus Tests Limits of Central Bank Firepower." *New York Times*, February 29, 2020.

Smith, Allan. "Trump Booed at Alabama Rally after Telling Supporters to Get Vaccinated." NBC News, August 22, 2021.

Smith, Craig A., and Phoebe C. Ellsworth. "Patterns of Cognitive Appraisal in Emotion." *Journal of Personality and Social Psychology* 48, no. 4 (1985): 813–38.

@smotus. "Correlation of Biden Vote Share and Adult Covid Vaccination Rate Is Now at .847. (CDC Data)." Twitter, June 4, 2021. https://twitter.com/smotus/status/1404483957647831046?s=20.

Sniderman, Paul M., Michael Bang Petersen, Rune Slothuus, Rune Stubager, and Philip Petrov. "Reactions to Terror Attacks: A Heuristic Model." *Political Psychology* 40, no. S1 (2019): 245–58.

Sobolewska, Maria, and Robert Ford. *Brexitland: Identity, Diversity and the Reshaping of British Politics.* Cambridge: Cambridge University Press, 2020.

Soergel, Andrew. "States Competing in 'Global Jungle' for PPE." *US News and World Report*, April 7, 2020.

Sonmez, Felicia. "Texas Lt. Gov. Dan Patrick Comes under Fire for Saying Seniors Should 'Take A Chance' on Their Own Lives for Sake of Grandchildren during Coronavirus Crisis." *Washington Post*, March 24, 2020.

Sorman, Guy. "Black Lives Matter in Paris: An American Movement in France." *France-Amerique*, September 10, 2020.

Soucheray, Stephanie. "Coroner: First US COVID-19 Death Occurred in Early February." Center for Infectious Disease Research and Policy, April 22, 2020. https://www.cidrap.umn.edu/news-perspective/2020/04/coroner-first-us -covid-19-death-occurred-early-february.

Spencer, Ben. "'Racist' Oxygen Device May Explain Why Covid Hit Minorities So Hard." *Sunday Times*, November 21, 2021.

Stafford, Ned. "Covid-19: Why Germany's Case Fatality Rate Seems So Low." *BMJ* 369 (2020).

Stein, Jeff. "Top Republicans Denounced Trump's Muslim Ban on the Trail. Now They Support His Executive Order." Vox, January 28, 2017.

Stevenson, Alexandra. "Senator Tom Cotton Repeats Fringe Theory of Coronavirus Origins." *New York Times*, February 17, 2020.

Stewart, Emily. "Anti-Maskers Explain Themselves." Vox, August 7, 2020.

Stiglitz, Joseph. "Lessons from COVID-19 and Trump for Theory and Policy (Paper)." *Journal of Policy Modeling* 43, no. 4 (2021): 749–60.

Stockman, Farah. "Sick People across the U.S. Say They Are Being Denied the Coronavirus Test." *New York Times*, March 12, 2020.

Stop AAPI Hate. "New Data on Anti-Asian Hate Incidents against Elderly and Total National Incidents in 2020." News release, February 9, 2022. https:// stopaapihate.org/wp-content/uploads/2021/04/Stop-AAPI-Hate-Press -Statement-Bay-Area-Elderly-Incidents-210209.pdf.

Straus, Daniel, and Oliver Laughland. "Trump Calls Coronavirus Criticism Democrats' 'New Hoax' and Links It to Immigration." *The Guardian*, February 28, 2020.

Street, Francesca. "Dread at 30,000 Feet: Inside the Increasingly Violent World of US Flight Attendants." CNN, September 6, 2021.

Subramanian, Sabu V., and Ichiro Kawachi. "The Association between State Income Inequality and Worse Health Is Not Confounded by Race." *International Journal of Epidemiology* 32, no. 6 (2003): 1022–28.

Suliman, Adela, and Paulina Villegas. "Conservative Radio Host and Vaccine Critic Dies of Covid-19 Complications." *Washington Post*, August 12, 2021.

Sun, Lena, and Joel Achenbach. "Unvaccinated People Were 11 Times More Likely to Die of Covid-19, CDC Report Finds." *Washington Post*, September 10, 2021.

Tajfel, Henri. *The Social Psychology of Minorities,*. Vol. 38. London: Minority Rights Group, 1978.

Tajfel, Henri, and John C. Turner. "The Social Identity Theory of Intergroup Behavior." In *Political Psychology: Key Readings*, ed. J. T. Jost and J. Sidanius, 276–93: New York: Psychology Press, 2004.

Tan, Annabel X., Jessica A. Hinman, Hoda S. Abdel Magid, Lorene M. Nelson, and Michelle C. Odden. "Association between Income Inequality and County-Level COVID-19 Cases and Deaths in the US." *JAMA Network Open* 4, no. 5 (2021): e218799.

Tankersly, Jim, Maggie Haberman, and Roni Caryn Rabin. "Trump Considers Reopening Economy, over Health Experts' Objections." *New York Times*, March 23, 2020.

Taylor, Donald M., and Janet R. Doria. "Self-Serving and Group-Serving Bias in Attribution." *Journal of Social Psychology* 113, no. 2 (1981): 201–11.

Taylor, Marisa. "Exclusive: U.S. Axed CDC Expert Job in China Months before Virus Outbreak." Reuters, March 22, 2020.

Teorell, Jan, Aksel Sundström, Sören Holmberg, Bo Rothstein, Natalia Alvarado Pachon, and Cem Mert Dalli. "The Quality of Government Standard Dataset, Version Jan21." University of Gothenburg, The Quality of Government Institute, 2021. http://www.qog.pol.gu.se doi:10.18157/qogstdjan21.

Terrizzi, John A., Natalie J. Shook, and Michael A. McDaniel. "The Behavioral Immune System and Social Conservatism: A Meta-analysis." *Evolution and Human Behavior* 34, no. 2 (2013): 99–108.

Tesler, Michael. *Post-Racial or Most-Racial? Race and Politics in the Obama Era.* Chicago: University of Chicago Press, 2016.

———. "The Spillover of Racialization into Health Care: How President Obama Polarized Public Opinion by Racial Attitudes and Race." *American Journal of Political Science* 56, no. 3 (2012): 690–704.

———. "Trump Voters Think African Americans Are Much Less Deserving Than 'Average Americans.'" Huffington Post, December 19, 2016.

Tessum, Christopher W., David A. Paolella, Sarah E. Chambliss, Joshua S. Apte, Jason D. Hill, and Julian D. Marshall. "PM2.5 Polluters Disproportionately and Systemically Affect People of Color in the United States." *Science Advances* 7, no. 18 (2021): eabf4491.

Timberg, Craig, and Drew Harwell. "Government Efforts to Track Virus through Phone Location Data Complicated by Privacy Concerns." *Washington Post*, March 19, 2020.

Treisman, Rachel. "Fox Anchor Neil Cavuto Urged Viewers to Get Vaccinated. Then Came the Death Threats." National Public Radio, October 27, 2021.

Trofimov, Yaroslav, and Summer Said. "Bahrain, Facing a Covid Surge, Starts Giving Pfizer Boosters to Recipients of Chinese Vaccine." *Wall Street Journal*, June 2, 2021

Trump, Donald J. "Donald Trump's Speech at the Republican Convention, as Prepared for Delivery." CNN, July 16, 2016. https://www.cnn.com/2016/07/22/politics/donald-trump-rnc-speech-text/index.html.

Turow, Joseph, Michael Hennessy, Nora Draper, Ope Akanbi, and Diami Virgilio. *Divided We Feel: Partisan Politics Drive Americans' Emotions Regarding Surveillance of Low-Income Populations.* A Report from the Annenberg School for Communication University of Pennsylvania, 2018.

"22 Days of Dither and Delay on Coronavirus That Cost Thousands of British Lives." *The Times*, May 23, 2020.

Tworek, Heidi. "Lessons Learned from Taiwan and South Korea's Tech-Enabled COVID-19 Communications." Brookings Institution, October 6, 2020.

United States Elections Project. "National General Election VEP Turnout Rates, 1789–Present." http://www.electproject.org/national-1789-present.

Ura, Alex. "Dallas Hospital Apologizes for 'Mistakes' in Ebola Care." *Texas Tribune*, October 16, 2014.

U.S. Census Bureau. "County Population by Characteristics: 2010–2019." https://www.census.gov/data/tables/time-series/demo/popest/2010s-counties-detail.html.

———. "Population Estimates, July 1 2021, (V2021)." https://www.census.gov/quickfacts/fact/table/US/PST045219.

———. "Quarterly Residential Vacancies and Homeownership, Third Quarter 2021." November 2, 2021. https://www.census.gov/housing/hvs/files/currenthvspress.pdf.

———. "Real Median Household Income by Race and Hispanic Origin: 1967 to 2017." https://www.census.gov/content/dam/Census/library/visualizations/2018/demo/p60-263/figure1.pdf.

U.S. Department of State. "Important Announcement on H2 Visas." March 26, 2020. https://travel.state.gov/content/travel/en/News/visas-news/important-announcement-on-h2-visas.html.

———. "The United States Announces Assistance to Combat the Novel Coronavirus." February 7, 2020. https://www.usaid.gov/coronavirus/updates/state/mar-20-2020-united-states-announces-assistance-combat-novel-coronavirus.

Valentino, Nicholas A., Ted Brader, and Ashley E. Jardina. "Immigration Opposition among US Whites: General Ethnocentrism or Media Priming of Attitudes about Latinos?" *Political Psychology* 34, no. 2 (2013): 149–66.

Vasilopoulos, Pavlos. "Terrorist Events, Emotional Reactions, and Political Participation: The 2015 Paris Attacks." *West European Politics* 41, no. 1 (2018): 102–27.

Vergano, Dan. "The Government Asked Us Not to Release Records from the CDC's First Failed COVID Test. Here They Are." Buzzfeed News, December 8, 2021.

Villegas, Paulina. "Birx Says Trump's Idea to Inject Disinfectant Haunts Her: 'I Still Think about It Every Day.'" *Washington Post*, March 16, 2021. https://www.washingtonpost.com/health/2021/03/16/deborah-birx-disinfectant-injection-moment-interview/.

Visontay, Elias. "NSW, Victoria Border Open for Fully Vaccinated at Midnight." *The Age*, November 4, 2021.

Voteview: Congressional Roll-Call Votes Database. https://voteview.com/.

Wagner, John, and Felicia Sonmez. "Election Highlights: Ohio Judge Rejects Governor's Efforts to Postpone Tuesday's Vote; Biden Wins Washington Primary." *Washington Post*, March 17, 2020.

Wallace-Wells, Benjamin. "What Happened to Joe Biden's 'Summer of Freedom' from the Pandemic?" *New Yorker*, August 12, 2021.

Watson, Katy. "Coronavirus: Brazil's Bolsonaro in Denial and Out on a Limb." BBC, March 29, 2020.

Weaver, Vesla M., and Amy E. Lerman. "Political Consequences of the Carceral State." *American Political Science Review* (2010): 817–33.

Weber, Max. *Economy and Society: An Outline of Interpretive Sociology*, Vol. 1. Berkeley: University of California Press, 1978.

Webster, Steven W. *American Rage: How Anger Shapes Our Politics.* Cambridge: Cambridge University Press, 2020.

Werner, Erica, and Jeff Stein. "Biden Unveils $1.9 Trillion Economic and Health-Care Relief Package." *Washington Post*, January 14, 2021.

"What We Know about Delays in Coronavirus Testing." *Washington Post*, March 16, 2020.

White House. "Executive Order on Advancing Equity, Justice, and Opportunity for Asian Americans, Native Hawaiians, and Pacific Islanders." May 28, 2021. https://www.whitehouse.gov/briefing-room/presidential-actions/2021/05/28/executive-order-on-advancing-equity-justice-and-opportunity-for-asian-americans-native-hawaiians-and-pacific-islanders/.

———. "White House Coronavirus Task Force Briefing." April 3, 2020.

White, Jeremy B. "Trump Claims 'Total Authority' over State Decisions." Politico, April 13, 2020.

Whoriskey, Peter, and Neena Satija. "How U.S. Coronavirus Testing Stalled: Flawed Tests, Red Tape and Resistance to Using the Millions of Tests Produced by the WHO." *Washington Post*, March 16, 2020.

Wieler, Lothar H., Ute Rexroth, and René Gottschalk. "Emerging COVID-19 Success Story: Germany's Push to Maintain Progress." Our World in Data, March 20, 2021. https://ourworldindata.org/covid-exemplar-germany.

Wikipedia. "List of Ethnic Groups in the United States by Household Income." https://bit.ly/3cq6qUS.

Wilson, Colleen. "Murphy 'Would Love' to Turn People away at NJ Borders, but Not Ready to Enforce Quarantine." NorthJersey.com, July 15, 2020.

Wise, Alana. "Trump Defends Testing Capacity Despite Experts' Warnings." National Public Radio, April 17, 2020.

World Health Organization. "Diagnostic Detection of 2019-nCoV by Real-Time RT-PCR." January 17, 2020. https://www.who.int/docs/default-source/coronaviruse/protocol-v2-1.pdf?sfvrsn=a9ef618c_2.

Yaffe-Bellany, David. "'The Big Guys Get Bailed Out': Restaurants Vie for Relief Funds." *New York Times*, April 20, 2020.

Yelp. "Local Economic Impact Report." September 2020. https://www.yelpeconomicaverage.com/business-closures-update-sep-2020.

Yen, Hope. "AP FACT CHECK: Trump's Inaccurate Boasts on China Travel Ban." Associated Press, March 26, 2020.

Yogeeswaran, Kumar, and Nilanjana Dasgupta. "Will the 'Real' American Please Stand Up? The Effect of Implicit National Prototypes on Discriminatory Behavior and Judgments." *Personality and Social Psychology Bulletin* 36, no. 10 (2010): 1332–45.

YouGov. "Do You Think the Coronavirus Outbreak Has Brought the UK Together, or Pulled It Further Apart?" March 30, 2020. https://yougov.co.uk/topics/politics/survey-results/daily/2020/03/30/e959b/2.

———. "Do You Think People Do, or Do Not, Have a Civic Duty to Self-Isolate for 14 Days If They Have Been in Contact with Somebody Who Has Been Diagnosed with Coronavirus?" June 12, 2020. https://yougov.co.uk/topics/politics/survey-results/daily/2020/06/12/81a5a/1.

Younis, Mohamed. "Americans Want More, Not Less, Immigration for First Time." Gallup, July 1, 2020. https://news.gallup.com/poll/313106/americans-not-less-immigration-first-time.aspx.

Yu, Qinggang, Cristina E. Salvador, Irene Melani, Martha K. Berg, Enrique W. Neblett, and Shinobu Kitayama. "Racial Residential Segregation and Economic Disparity Jointly Exacerbate COVID-19 Fatality in Large American Cities." *Annals of the New York Academy of Sciences* 1494 (2021): 18–30.

Zaller, John. "Information, Values, and Opinion." *American Political Science Review* 85, no. 4 (1991): 1215–37.

———. *The Nature and Origin of Public Opinion.* New York: Cambridge University Press, 1992.

Zeleny, Jeff. "Why These 8 Republican Governors Are Holding Out on Statewide Stay-at-Home Orders." CNN, April 4, 2020.

Zhang, Baobao, Sarah Kreps, Nina McMurry, and R. Miles McCain. "Americans' Perceptions of Privacy and Surveillance in the COVID-19 Pandemic." *PLOS One* 15, no. 12 (2020): e0242652.

Ziegler, Brett. "Health Care Rankings: Measuring How Well States Are Meeting Citizens' Health Care Needs." *US News and World Report.* https://www.usnews.com/news/best-states/rankings/health-care.

Zimmer, Ben. "Hard-to-Define 'Antifa' Becomes Election-Year Wedge Issue." *The Atlanta Journal-Constitution*, October 9, 2020.

———. "Why Trump Is So Obsessed with Antifa." *The Atlantic*, June 4, 2020.

INDEX

A NOTE ON THE TYPE

This book has been composed in Adobe Text and Gotham.
Adobe Text, designed by Robert Slimbach for Adobe,
bridges the gap between fifteenth- and sixteenth-century
calligraphic and eighteenth-century Modern styles.
Gotham, inspired by New York street signs, was designed
by Tobias Frere-Jones for Hoefler & Co.